Practical Guide to Dermatology

Henry W. Lim · Laurie L. Kohen ·
Samantha L. Schneider · Danielle Yeager
Editors

Practical Guide to Dermatology

The Henry Ford Manual

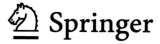 Springer

Editors
Henry W. Lim
Department of Dermatology
Henry Ford Health System
Detroit, MI, USA

Laurie L. Kohen
Department of Dermatology
Henry Ford Health System
Detroit, MI, USA

Samantha L. Schneider
Department of Dermatology
Henry Ford Health System
Detroit, MI, USA

Danielle Yeager
Department of Dermatology
Henry Ford Health System
Detroit, MI, USA

ISBN 978-3-030-18014-0   ISBN 978-3-030-18015-7   (eBook)
https://doi.org/10.1007/978-3-030-18015-7

This Springer imprint is published by the registered company Springer Nature Switzerland AG
The registered company address is: Gewerbestrasse 11, 6330 Cham, Switzerland

Preface

At the Henry Ford Department of Dermatology, there has been a long-standing guidebook, initially developed by one of the editors (LK), that provides a practical clinical reference for our residents and junior faculty. Over the years, the book has expanded and evolved to become a highly valued text among our entire department. The *Practical Guide* is an expansion of this effort. Members of Henry Ford Dermatology Department, alumni, and residents contributed to this *Practical Guide*.

We strive to be evidence-based in many of the recommendations. However, as all of us recognize, many medications used in dermatology are "off-label," and others, while widely used, may not have undergone appropriate clinical trials. Since these treatments are commonly used in clinical practice, we have included many in our algorithms. Treatment ladders presented (including the dosing of medication) are based on our experience at Henry Ford. Therefore, appropriate clinical judgement regarding the individual patient's condition must be exercised.

This *Practical Guide* is meant to complement, but not replace, an ACGME-accredited dermatology residency training program. It is our hope that it would enhance the excellent level of care that you and your team deliver to your patients.

We would like to thank all the authors for their contribution; without their time and expertise, this effort would not have come to fruition. Finally, we do sincerely hope that you will find this *Practical Guide* useful in your daily patient care.

Detroit, MI, USA
February 2019

Samantha L. Schneider, MD
Danielle Yeager, MD
Laurie L. Kohen, MD
Henry W. Lim, MD

Contents

Immune-mediated Disorders

Jennifer B. Mancuso and Pranita V. Rambhatla

Bullous Pemphigoid

What Not To Miss

- Drug induced
  - PEARL: PF ChaNGs—Penicillamine, PCN derivatives, PUVA, furosemide, captopril, NSAIDs, gold, sulfasalazine
- Early Disease
  - Urticarial plaques or pruritus alone can be early manifestation, especially in the elderly

Key DDx

- Diabetic bullae
- Bullous impetigo
- Bullous insect bite reaction
- Epidermolysis Bullosa Acquisita
- Pemphigus Vulgaris
- Cicatricial pemphigoid
- Allergic contact dermatitis
- Bullous drug eruption
- Porphyria cutanea tarda or pseudoporphyria

J. B. Mancuso
Department of Dermatology, University of Michigan, Ann Arbor, MI, USA

P. V. Rambhatla (✉)
Department of Dermatology, Henry Ford Health System, 3031 West Grand Blvd, Suite 800, Detroit, MI 48202, USA
e-mail: prambha1@hfhs.org

© Springer Nature Switzerland AG 2020
H. W. Lim et al. (eds.), *Practical Guide to Dermatology*,
https://doi.org/10.1007/978-3-030-18015-7_1

Work Up Pearls

- Do two biopsies
  - One for H&E (lesional—edge of a blister)
  - Second for immunofluorescence (perilesional)
    - Ideally, a lesion less than 72 h old
    - PEARL: If only urticarial lesions, DIF should be lesional
- Serum tests used if biopsy is inconclusive
  - Some areas, such as scalp, that may have extensive excoriation, may show nonspecific biopsy and negative DIF so IIF can be diagnostic in these cases
  - IIF for circulating anti-BMZ IgG
  - ELISA to detect Ab to BP180 and BP230
    - ELISA can also be used to monitor disease activity

Treatment Ladder

- Mild-moderate disease
  - High potency topical steroids (Class I)
    - Can be used as monotherapy in severe disease [1]
  - Minocycline or doxycycline 100 mg twice daily [2] with or without niacinamide 0.5–2.0 g three times daily
- Moderate-severe disease
  - Prednisone taper (slow), consider starting steroid sparing agent at or shortly after starting oral prednisone [3]
    - 0.5–1.0 mg/kg daily controls disease over 1–3 weeks, slowly taper once disease is controlled over 3 months
  - Methotrexate 10–25 mg weekly
    - Need lower doses in elderly and CKD patients [4]
  - Mycophenolate mofetil 1–3 g per day, divided twice daily [5]
  - Dapsone for mucosal-predominant or neutrophil/eosinophil-rich BP [6]: 50–200 mg daily
  - Azathioprine [5] titrate up to dose of 2.5 mg/kg daily
- Severe or refractory disease
  - IVIG [7] 1–2 g/kg per cycle divided into 3–5 consecutive days per month for 3–6 months
  - Pulse solumedrol 2 gm IV total, divided over 3–5 days
  - Rituximab 1000 mg once and repeated in 2 weeks is 1 cycle [8, 9]
    - Patients often need more than 1 cycle
    - May need to continue second immunosuppressive until rituximab starts to work
    - Consider ordering CD20 lab after infusion to assess effect of medication
  - Omalizumab 150–300 mg every 4 weeks [10]

Dermatomyositis

What Not To Miss

- Drug induced
  - Hydroxyurea (MC), statins, D-penicillamine, cyclophosphamide, BCG vaccine, TNF-α inhibitors
- Occult malignancy
  - Up to 40% of adults may have an occult malignancy
  - Strong association with ovarian cancer in women
- Amyopathic DM
  - Must do pulmonary and malignancy work up
- DM associated with anti-MDA5 antibody
  - Can be fatal
  - Painful palmar papules, ulcerations in oral mucosa and overlying Gottron's papules on elbows/knees
  - Rapidly progressive interstitial lung disease, panniculitis, arthritis, less muscle involvement [11]
    - ILD diagnosed with PFTs with DLCO (diffusing capacity of the lungs for carbon monoxide) and high resolution chest CT if needed
- Children with DM can present with calcinosis cutis

Key DDx

- Systemic lupus erythematosus
- Mixed connective tissue disease
- Phototoxic/photoallergic drug eruption
- PMLE
- Contact dermatitis
- CTCL

Work Up Pearls [12–14]

- Clinical findings
  - Cutaneous findings: heliotrope rash, Gottron's papules overlying joints of hands, photosensitivity, poikiloderma, shawl and V sign, holster sign, calcinosis cutis, mechanic's hands, dilated capillary loops of nail folds, jagged cuticles, scalp erythema and scaling

- o Muscle disease: progressive symmetric proximal muscle weakness +/− esophageal muscles (dysphagia), cardiac disease (mostly subclinical EKG findings)
- o Other: pulmonary (15–65% with interstitial lung disease), arthralgia/arthritis
- o Remember DM can cause panniculitis and vasculitis in addition to the more common cutaneous manifestations
- o Also consider dermatomyositis in the differential of intractable scalp pruritus/dysesthesia

- Labs
  - o +ANA in 40%, CK, aldolase, CBC, CMP, TSH, UA
  - o Antibodies to consider
    - Anti-Mi-2, anti-Jo-1, anti-SRP, anti-NXP-2, anti-PM-Scl, anti-Ku, anti-MDA5, anti-TIF-1-γ, anti-U1RNP

- Diagnostics
  - o PFTs with diffusing capacity of the lungs for carbon monoxide (DLCO), EMG, MRI or muscle biopsy, ECG, barium swallow (if esophageal symptoms).
  - o Cancer screenings (age appropriate): CT chest/abdomen/pelvis, transvaginal/testicular ultrasound, colonoscopy, pap smear and mammogram.

- Biopsy
  - o PEARL: Can be identical to lupus erythematosus

Treatment Ladder

- Skin-limited disease
  - o 1st line (will not treat muscle disease): photoprotection, topical CS/CNI +/− hydroxychloroquine 5 mg/kg daily up to 200 mg twice daily; Caution: 30% of patients will get cutaneous drug eruption
  - o 2nd line: systemic steroids, methotrexate, mycophenolate mofetil, IVIG

- Skin + muscle disease
  - 1st line:
    - systemic steroids [15] (slow taper) 0.5–1.0 mg/kg daily controls disease over 1–3 weeks, slowly taper once disease is controlled over 3 months
    - Methotrexate [16] 10–25 mg weekly
    - Mycophenolate mofetil 1.0–3.0 g daily, divided into twice daily dosing [15]
    - Azathioprine [17] titrate up to dose of 2.5 mg/kg daily
  - o 2nd line: IVIG [18] 1–2 g/kg per cycle divided into 3–5 consecutive days per month for 3–6 months

- Other: rituximab, cyclophosphamide, cyclosporine, leflunomide, chlorambucil, tacrolimus
  - If interstitial lung disease: steroids, rituximab, cyclophosphamide
- Monitoring
  - Malignancy screens [13]
    - Most important within first 2 years, risk decreases 5 years after dx
  - Review of systems

Outside the Box Treatment Options

- Tofacitinib for refractory patients
- PEARL: TNF inhibitors are contraindicated as they can worsen myositis

Lupus Erythematosus

What Not To Miss

- Active systemic involvement
  - Malar rash can be a sign so need at least CBC, CMP and UA

- PEARL: Malar rash is persistent (vs. rosacea which waxes and wanes) and spares the nasolabial folds (vs. dermatomyositis and seborrhea, which involve NLF)
- Drug induced
  - Procainamide, hydralazine, isoniazid, d-penicillamine, minocycline, TNF-α inhibitors

- Rowell Syndrome [19]
  - EM-like lesions in a lupus patient
  - +ANA, Anti-Ro, RF

Work Up Pearls

2012 SLICC criteria: need 4, at least 1 clinical and 1 immunologic OR biopsy proven lupus nephritis and +ANA or dsDNA [20]	
Dermatologic	ACLE, CCLE, non-scarring alopecia, oral/nasal ulcers
Systemic	Synovitis, serositis, renal, neurologic
Hematologic	Hemolytic anemia, leukopenia/lymphopenia, thrombocytopenia
Immunologic	ANA, anti-dsDNA, anti-Sm, antiphospholipid, low complement (C3, C4 or CH50), direct Coombs' test

- Labs including CBC with diff, CMP, UA with microscopy, ANA, dsDNA, Ro/La, Sm, RNP, anti-phospholipid Abs (anticardiolipin, b2-glycoprotein, lupus anticoagulant), C3/C4, CH50, ESR, CRP, +/− anti-histone (drug-induced), anti-U1RNP
  - Anti-dsDNA—nephritis, CNS
  - Anti-Smith—most specific for SLE
  - Ro and La—photosensitivity, Rowell's, SCLE
  - Ro—counsel females of child bearing potential risk of neonatal lupus
    - If positive, refer to maternal-fetal-medicine or high-risk OB

- Skin biopsy
- Multidisciplinary evaluation based on lab abnormalities
  - Particularly rheumatology and nephrology
  - Cardiology and pulmonary as needed based on review of symptoms

Treatment Pearls [21]

- Preventive interventions: smoking cessation, photoprotection
- Mild disease
  - Hydroxychloroquine 5 mg/kg daily actual body weight (max 400 mg daily)
  - Chloroquine <2.3 mg/kg daily
  - Quinacrine 100 mg once daily
  - NSAIDs
  - Prednisone 5–15 mg daily for mild-moderate disease

- Moderate-severe
  - Prednisone 1–2 mg/kg daily, can do IV pulse methylprednisolone 0.5–1.0 g daily for 3 days in acutely ill patients
  - Methotrexate 10–15 mg weekly
  - Azathioprine titrate up to dose of 2.5 mg/kg daily

- Severe disease with major organ involvement
  - High dose prednisone + cyclophosphamide
  - Mycophenolate mofetil 1–3 g per day, divided into twice daily dosing
  - Azathioprine titrate up to dose of 2.5 mg/kg daily

- Other
  - Thalidomide
    - PEARL: Thalidomide requires Thalomid REMS program
  - Lenalidomide
  - Dapsone

Out of the Box Treatment Options

- Recalcitrant disease
  - Rituximab or belimumab
  - Abatacept

- ○ anti-IL-6 Ab
- ○ anti-IL-10 Ab
- ○ Ustekinumab
- ○ JAK inhibitors such as tofacitinib 5 mg twice daily
- ○ IVIG 1–2 g/kg per cycle divided into 3–5 consecutive days per month for 3–6 months
- ○ Clinical trials

Discoid Lupus Erythematosus

What Not To Miss

- Progression to SLE
  - ○ Widespread (above and below the neck) and childhood DLE have higher rates of progression [22]
- Squamous cell carcinomas
  - ○ May form in chronic DLE scars

Key DDx

- Scalp: tinea capitis, CCCA, lichen planopilaris
- Face/body: seborrheic dermatitis, sarcoidosis, PMLE, granuloma faciale, Jessner's, burn scar, syphilis

Diagnostic Pearls

- Review of systems
- Rare to see DLE below the neck if there is not involvement above the neck
- ANA+ in 5–25%

Treatment Ladder [23, 24]

- Treat aggressively if active disease given risk for scarring
- Camouflage cosmetics
- Strict photoprotection
- Topical
  - ○ Topical or intralesional steroids
- Systemic
  - ○ Hydroxychloroquine 5 mg/kg daily up to 200 mg twice daily
  - ○ Chloroquine <2.3 mg/kg daily
  - ○ +/− quinacrine 100 mg daily

- Refractory disease
  - Methotrexate 10–20 mg weekly
  - Retinoids: acitretin 10–50 mg daily, isotretinoin 0.5–1.0 mg/kg daily
  - Systemic steroids (not recommended long term): 20–40 mg daily
  - Mycophenolate mofetil 1–3 g per day, divided into twice daily dosing
  - Dapsone 25–2'00 mg daily

Out Of The Box Treatment Options

- Severe refractory disease: thalidomide, lenalidomide, IVIG

Subacute Cutaneous Lupus

What Not To Miss

- Progression to SLE
  - Up to 30–50% can progress
  - Often is mild disease
- Drug induced in up to 1/3 of cases [25]
  - Hydrochlorothiazide, terbinafine, griseofulvin, statins, NSAIDS, CCBs, antihistamines, PPIs, docetaxel, ACE-I, TNF-alpha inhibitors, many others

Key DDx

- Erythema annulare centrifugum
- Erythema multiforme
- Annular psoriasis
- Secondary syphilis
- Tinea corporis
- PMLE

Diagnostic Pearls [26]

- Anti-Ro/SS-A (75–90%), Anti-La (30–40%), ANA (60–80%, usually speckled)
  - More common in Caucasians (vs. DLE)

Treatment Ladder [23, 24]

- 1st line localized disease
  - Diligent photoprotection
  - Topical corticosteroid
  - Hydroxychloroquine 5 mg/kg daily up to 200 mg twice daily

- 1st line severe disease
  - Topical corticosteroid
  - Hydroxychloroquine 5 mg/kg daily up to 200 mg twice daily + systemic corticosteroids

- 2nd line—add
  - Quinacrine 100 mg daily
  - Methotrexate 10–25 mg weekly
  - Retinoids: acitretin 10–50 mg daily, isotretinoin 0.5–1.0 mg/kg daily
  - Dapsone 25–200 mg daily
  - Mycophenolate mofetil 1–3 g per day, divided twice daily

Out Of The Box Treatment Options

- Thalidomide for severe disease

Pemphigus Vulgaris

What Not To Miss [27]

- Drug induced
  - Thiol/sulfa containing drugs, penicillamine, captopril, cephalosporins, gold, rifampin, indocin, penicillin, piroxicam, pyritinol, pyrazolone derivatives, enalapril, aspirin

- Mucosal involvement
  - Ask about and examine ALL mucosal surface areas
  - Consider consultation with ophthalmology, dentistry/ENT, gynecology/urology

Key DDx

- Paraneoplastic pemphigus
- Pemphigus foliaceus
- Bullous pemphigoid
- Cicatricial pemphigoid
- Erythema multiforme
- Stevens-Johnson syndrome
- Mycoplasma-induced rash and mucositis
  - PEARL: More common in young males

Diagnostic Pearls

- Nikolsky sign and Asboe-Hansen sign
- Biopsy

o Lesional H&E
o Perilesional DIF

o Serum to support diagnosis and monitor disease activity
   o ELISA (Dsg 1 and 3)
   o IIF (monkey esophagus)

Treatment Ladder [28, 29]

- First line
  o Systemic steroids + steroid sparing agent
  o Glucocorticoids 1.0–1.5 mg/kg daily
     • When no new lesions form, taper very slowly over months
  o Rituximab 1000 mg once and repeated in 2 weeks is 1 cycle, repeat cycles every 6 months may be necessary
     • Emerging data supports this as first line with systemic steroids
  o Azathioprine titrate up to dose of 2.5 mg/kg daily
  o Mycophenolate mofetil 2–3 g daily

- Refractory disease
  o Methotrexate 10–25 mg weekly
  o Dapsone 50–200 mg daily
  o Cyclophosphamide 1–3 mg/kg daily
  o Cyclosporine 2.5–5.0 mg/kg daily
  o IVIG (may be combined with rituximab): 1–2 g/kg per cycle divided into 3–5 consecutive days per month for 3–6 months

Out Of The Box Treatment Options

- Plasmapheresis or plasma exchange
- Immunoadsorption

Psoriasis, Cutaneous

What Not To Miss

- HIV infection
  o Can precipitate or worsen existing psoriasis

- Associated disorders
  o Cardiovascular disease
  o Metabolic syndrome
  o NASH
  o Lymphoma
  o Mood disorders
  o May need multidisciplinary care

- Erythrodermic or pustular psoriasis
  - Make sure to ask about any systemic steroids from PCP or Urgent Care
- Psoriatic arthritis
  - Affects up to 30% of patients
  - Associated with morning stiffness, nail changes, tendon/ligament involvement
- Concurrent or antecedent perianal or body fold cutaneous group A strep infection, especially in a child presenting with sudden onset guttate psoriasis

Key DDx

- Atopic dermatitis
- Contact dermatitis
- Nummular dermatitis
- Seborrheic dermatitis
- Pityriasis rubra pilaris
- Lichen planus
- Subacute cutaneous lupus erythematosus
- Mycosis fungoides
- Tinea corporis
- Crusted scabies
- Secondary syphilis
- Bowen's—if few, smaller lesions

Work Up Pearls

- Atypical appearing psoriasis can be psoriasiform drug eruption
  - Think of lithium, IFNs, B-blockers, ACE inhibitors, antimalarials, terbinafine, NSAIDs
- Biopsy
- Consider imaging for psoriatic arthritis
  - May need rheumatology consultation to help evaluate

Treatment Ladder: Cutaneous [30, 31]

- Topicals: for mild (as monotherapy) to severe disease
  - Topical corticosteroids
  - Calcipotriene
  - Coal tar
  - Anthralin
  - Calcineurin inhibitors
  - Calcitriol

- o Tazarotene or salicylic acid for hyperkeratotic lesions
- o Intralesional triamcinolone for treatment resistant plaques

- Phototherapy [32]
  - o NBUVB two to three times weekly
  - o Excimer laser (localized lesions)
  - o PUVA is 2nd line

- Systemic
  - o Methotrexate 10–25 mg weekly
  - o Acitretin (erythrodermic, pustular) 25 mg every other day to 50 mg daily
  - o Cyclosporine 3–5 mg/kg daily
  - o Apremilast 30 mg twice daily (after starter pack)

- Biologics[33]: all given subcutaneously except infliximab which is given intravenously*
  - o TNF-a inhibitors:
    - PEARL: Avoid in patients with CHF or multiple sclerosis
    - Adalimumab: 80 mg initial dose, followed by 40 mg one week later then every other week
    - Etanercept: 50 mg twice weekly for the initial 3 months, then 50 mg weekly
    - Infliximab: 5 mg/kg given at weeks 0, 2, 6, then every 8 weeks thereafter *
    - Certolizumab: 400 mg at weeks 0, 2 and 4, followed by 200 mg every other week
  - o IL-12/23 inhibitor:
    - Ustekinumab: 45 mg at weeks 0, 4, and every 12 weeks thereafter; 90 mg for patients >100 kg (dosing is good for compliance concerns)
  - o IL-23 inhibitors:
    - Guselkumab: 100 mg at weeks 0, 4, and then every 8 weeks
    - Tildrakizumab: 100 mg at weeks 0, 4, and then every 12 weeks
  - o IL-17 inhibitors:
    - PEARL: Avoid in patients with IBD. Look for mucocutaneous candidiasis
    - Secukinumab: 300 mg at weeks 0, 1, 2, 3, and 4 then every 4 weeks
    - Ixekizumab: 160 mg at week 0, followed by 80 mg at weeks 2, 4, 6, 8, 10, 12 and then every 4 weeks
    - Brodalumab: 210 mg at weeks 0, 1, 2 and then every 2 weeks
    - PEARL: requires participation in a Risk Evaluation and Mitigation Strategy program due to concerns for suicidality.
- Other
  - o Consider "day hospital" (steroid wraps and phototherapy) for severe disease—can be done in a clinic setting or with wraps alone at home

Treatment Ladder: Scalp [34]

- Topicals
  - 3 or 5% salicylic acid compounded with fluocinonide cream or ointment
  - Clobetasol or betamethasone dipropionate-calcipotriene foam/solution
  - Tar or salicylic based shampoos
  - Intralesional triamcinolone for localized thick plaques
- Excimer laser
  - PEARL: NB-UVB will not reach the scalp through hair
- Systemics as in cutaneous psoriasis section
  - Particularly apremilast and biologics

Treatment ladder, Nails [35]

- Gentle hand/foot care
  - Avoid trauma (manicures)
  - Apply emollients regularly
  - Keep nails trimmed
- High potency topical steroid under occlusion +/− vitamin D ointment to nail plate, hyponychium, proximal/lateral nail folds
- 2nd line: tazarotene or topical calcineurin inhibitors
- 1% 5FU solution or 5% 5FU cream without occlusion BID for 6 months
- Intralesional triamcinolone 2.5 mg/ml into proximal nail fold/matrix
- Systemic
  - Biologics
  - Acitretin
  - Apremilast
  - Methotrexate

Out Of The Box Treatment Options

- Tofacitinib 5 mg BID
- IVIG 1–2 g/kg per cycle divided into 3–5 consecutive days per month for 3–6 months

In The Context Of...

- Erythroderma
  - Cyclosporine usually has fastest onset of action
  - If erythroderma and impaired kidney function, consider guselkumab, which may be faster acting [36]

- Co-morbid metabolic syndrome
  - o Consider metformin
- Pregnancy
  - o Topical steroids
  - o NBUVB
  - o Biologics (anti-TNFs, IL17, IL23) are mostly category B
    - Discuss if risks outweigh benefits, consider enrolling in pregnancy registry
    - Try to stop anti-TNFs at 30 weeks gestation and postpone live vaccinations in newborn babies
    - Certolizumab showed low transfer of the drug through placenta and minimal mother-to-infant transfer from breast milk in pharmacokinetic data.
  - o Cyclosporine (Category C) for severe disease
  - o PEARL: Impetigo herpetiformis is treated with systemic corticosteroids

Pyoderma Gangrenosum

What Not To Miss

- Unusual sites
  - o Rarely PG can involve the eyes, lungs, heart, liver, gastrointestinal tract, CNS and lymphatics
- Other PG variations
  - o Pustular, bullous, vegetative and suppurative panniculitis
- PEARL: Avoid unnecessary elective surgical procedures and debridement—if absolutely necessary, perform while on immunosuppressive therapy.

Key DDx

- Infection
  - o PG is a diagnosis of exclusion and infection must be ruled out with tissue culture
- Consider underlying genetic causes including PAPA, PASH and PAPASH syndromes

Work Up Pearls [37]

- Biopsy at edge of ulcer for H&E + tissue culture to rule out infection
- Work-up (search for underlying disease)—CBC, ESR, LFTs, BUN/Cr, ANA, SPEP (IgA gammopathy), UA, hepatitis panel, ANCAs, RF, anti-phospholipid antibodies; +/− CXR, colonoscopy

Treatment Ladder [38]

- Local wound care with non-adherent dressing, avoiding pathergy, pain management (important to keep it moist)
- Topical
  - Intralesional triamcinolone 10–20 mg/ml
  - Topical corticosteroids/calcineurin inhibitors to periphery of ulcer and antimicrobial (i/e metronidazole gel) to the center of the ulcer
- Antibiotics
  - Doxycycline 100 mg twice daily
  - Minocycline 100 mg twice daily
  - Dapsone 50–200 mg daily
- Systemic
  - Glucocorticoid starting dose at 1 mg/kg
  - Cyclosporine 4–5 mg/kg daily and taper as tolerated
  - Azathioprine titrate up to dose of 2.5 mg/kg daily
  - Methotrexate 10–30 mg per week
  - Mycophenolate mofetil 2–3 g per day, divided twice daily
  - IVIG 1–2 g/kg per cycle divided into 3–5 consecutive days per month for 3–6 months
- Biologics: TNF-a inhibitors

Outside the Box Treatment Options

- Thalidomide
- Sulfasalazine
- Clofazimine
- Anakinra
- Canakinumab

Morphea

What Not To Miss

- Genital lichen sclerosus et atrophicus
  - Can occur in patients with plaque-type morphea
- Limb contractures or limb-length discrepancies
  - This can result from linear morphea

- Linear morphea of the head (En coup de sabre and Parry-Romberg syndrome) can result in alopecia, ocular, neurologic and dental abnormalities
  - Both must be treated aggressively

Key DDx

- Systemic sclerosis
- Nephrogenic fibrosing dermopathy
- Eosinophilic fasciitis
- Lipodermatosclerosis
- Drug or chemical induced sclerodermoid reaction (PEARL: Think taxanes or PVC)

Work Up Pearls

- Skin biopsy is confirmatory
  - PEARL: Biopsy containing fascia and muscle is needed if eosinophilic fasciitis is on the differential
- X-rays for linear morphea
  - MRI can evaluate for deeper involvement
- Testing for auto-Abs only indicated if signs of another autoimmune disease [39]

Treatment Ladder [40]

- Circumscribed lesions
  - Topical or intralesional corticosteroids
  - Topical calcineurin inhibitor
  - Topical calcipotriene
  - Topical imiquimod
  - UVA1 or NBUVB (if UVA not available)
    - PEARL: UVA-1 preferred because it penetrates deeper
- Generalized or localized with functional/cosmetic threat (face, over joints)
  - Methotrexate 15–25 mg weekly +/− systemic prednisone 1 mg/kg daily for 2–3 months
  - Mycophenolate mofetil 2–3 g daily, divided twice daily
- Consultation with PT/OT, Orthopedics/Plastic surgery/OMSF
- Other options
  - Cyclosporine 2–5 mg/kg daily in 2 divided doses
  - Hydroxychloroquine 5 mg/kg daily up to 200 mg twice daily
  - Acitretin 12.5–50 mg daily + PUVA
  - Extracorporeal photopheresis
  - Bosentan 31.25–62.5 mg twice daily

Outside Of The Box Treatment Options

- Fillers for improved cosmesis once morphea stabilizes
- CO2 laser to decrease contractures and increase mobility over joints
- Infliximab, rituximab, imatinib, JAK inhibitors, thalidomide

Systemic Sclerosis

What Not To Miss

- PEARL: African American patients have a more severe course and increased mortality
- Extracutaneous findings
  - Pulmonary disease is the leading cause of mortality.
  - GI is the most common site of visceral disease and associated with increased morbidity but not mortality
  - Scleroderma renal crisis risk can be decreased with ACE-I
  - Scleroderma renal crisis has been associated with use of systemic corticosteroids in retrospective studies

Key DDx

- Generalized morphea
- Scleredema
- Scleromyxedema
- Eosinophilic fasciitis
- Nephrogenic systemic fibrosis
- Chronic GVHD
- Exogeneous: polyvinyl chloride (PVC) exposure, bleomycin toxicity, radiation effects

Workup Pearls

- CBC with diff, BUN, Cr, CK, U/A,
- Auto-antibodies
  - ANA (95% +), anti-Scl-70
  - anti-centromere Ab (associated with CREST)
  - anti-RNA pol III Ab (associated with rapidly progressive skin involvement, renal disease and cancer)
- At time of diagnosis and for monitoring: high resolution CT of lungs, PFTs with DLCO, ECG, ECHO (to assess pulmonary arterial HTN), GI consultation as appropriate
- Diagnosis [41]

ACR/EULAR 2013 Criteria. ≥ 9 = definite SSc.	
Cutaneous findings:	**Systemic findings:**
Skin thickening of fingers proximal to MCP joint (9)	Pulm art. HTN (2) or ILD (2)
Skin thickening of the fingers: puffy fingers (2) or sclerodactyly (4)	Raynaud's phenomenon (3)
Fingertip lesions: ulcers (2), pitting scars (3)	Ab's (ANA, anti-Scl-70, anti-RNA pol III) (3 max)
Telangiectasia (2)	
Abnormal nail fold capillaries (2)	

Treatment Ladder (cutaneous) [42]

- Multidisciplinary approach
  - Rheumatology +/− nephrology, pulmonology, gastroenterology

- 1st line
  - Oral corticosteroids
  - Methotrexate 10–25 mg weekly
  - Mycophenolate mofetil 2–3 g per day, divided twice daily
  - PUVA or UVA1
  - Rituximab 1000 mg once and repeated in 2 weeks is 1 cycle, repeat cycles may be necessary

- 2nd line
  - Azathioprine titrate up to dose of 2.5 mg/kg daily
  - Cyclophosphamide 1–3 mg/kg daily
  - IVIG 1–2 g/kg per cycle divided into 3–5 consecutive days per month for 3–6 months
  - Bosentan
  - Sildenafil

Outside Of The Box Treatment Options

- Myeloablative autologous hematopoietic stem-cell transplantation
- Low-energy extracorporeal shock-wave therapy
- Clinical trials for refractory or progressive disease

References

1. Joly P, Roujeau JC, Benichou J, et al. A comparison of oral and topical corticosteroids in patients with bullous pemphigoid. Bullous Diseases French Study Group. N Engl J Med. 2002;346(5):321.
2. Williams HC, Wojnarowska F, Kirtschig G, et al. Doxycycline versus prednisolone as an initial treatment strategy for bullous pemphigoid: a pragmatic, non-inferiority, randomised controlled trial. UK Dermatology Clinical Trials Network BLISTER Study Group. Lancet. 2017;389(10079):1630. Epub 2017 Mar 6.
3. Kirtschig G, Middleton P, Bennett C, Murrell DF, Wojnarowska F, Khumalo NP. Interventions for bullous pemphigoid. Cochrane Database Syst Rev. 2010;10.
4. Gürcan HM, Ahmed AR. Analysis of current data on the use of methotrexate in the treatment of pemphigus and pemphigoid. Br J Dermatol. 2009;161(4):723–31.
5. Beissert S, Werfel T, Frieling U, et al. A comparison of oral methylprednisolone plus azathioprine or mycophenolate mofetil for the treatment of bullous pemphigoid. Arch Dermatol. 2007;143(12):1536.
6. Gürcan HM, Ahmed AR. Efficacy of dapsone in the treatment of pemphigus and pemphigoid: analysis of current data. Am J Clin Dermatol. 2009;10(6):383.
7. Czernik A, Toosi S, Bystryn JC, Grando SA. Intravenous immunoglobulin in the treatment of autoimmune bullous dermatoses: an update. Autoimmunity. 2012;45(1):111–8. Epub 2011 Sep 19.
8. Kurihara Y, Yamagami J, Funakoshi T, et al. Rituximab therapy for refractory autoimmune bullous diseases: a multicenter, open-label, single-arm, phase ½ study on 10 Japanese patients. J Dermatol. 2018.
9. Lourari S, Herve C, Doffoel-Hantz V, et al. Bullous and mucous membrane pemphigoid show a mixed response to rituximab: experience in seven patients. J Eur Acad Dermatol Venereol. 2011;25(10):1238–40.
10. Kremer N, Snast I, Cohen ES et al. Rituximab and omalizumab for the treatment of bullous pemphigoid: a systematic review of the literature. Am J Clin Dermatol. 2018.
11. Kurtzman DJB, Vleugels RA. Anti-melanoma differentiation-associated gene 5 (MDA5) dermatomyositis: a concise review with an emphasis on distinctive clinical features. J Am Acad Dermatol. 2018;78(4):776–85.
12. Hochberg MC, Feldman D, Stevens MB. Adult onset polymyositis/dermatomyositis: an analysis of clinical and laboratory features and survival in 76 patients with a review of the literature. Semin Arthritis Rheum. 1986;15(3):168.
13. Chen YJ, Wu CY, Shen JL. Predicting factors of malignancy in dermatomyositis and polymyositis: a case-control study. Br J Dermatol. 2001;144(4):825.
14. Bottai M, Tjärnlund A, Santoni G, et al. EULAR/ACR classification criteria for adult and juvenile idiopathic inflammatory myopathies and their major subgroups: a methodology report. RMD Open. 2017;3(2).
15. Drake LA, Dinehart SM, Farmer ER, et al. Guidelines of care for dermatomyositis. J Am Acad Dermatol. 1996;34(5 Pt 1):824.
16. Newman ED, Scott DW. The use of low-dose oral methotrexate in the treatment of polymyositis and dermatomyositis. J Clin Rheumatol. 1995;1(2):99.
17. Bunch TW. Prednisone and azathioprine for polymyositis: long-term followup. Arthritis Rheum. 1981;24(1):45.

18. Marie I, Menard JF, Hatron PY, et al. Intravenous immunoglobulins for steroid-refractory esophageal involvement related to polymyositis and dermatomyositis: a series of 73 patients. Arthritis Care Res (Hoboken). 2010;62(12):1748.
19. Zeitouni NC, Funaro D, Cloutier RA et al. Redefining Rowell's syndrome. Br J Dermatol. 2000;142(2):343–6.
20. Petri M, Orbai AM, Alarcón GS, et al. Derivation and validation of the Systemic Lupus International Collaborating Clinics classification criteria for systemic lupus erythematosus. Arthritis Rheum. 2012;64:2677.
21. Gordon C, Amissah-Arthur MB, Gayed M et al. The British Society for Rheumatology guideline for the management of systemic lupus erythematosus in adults. British Society for Rheumatology Standards, Audit and Guidelines Working Group. Rheumatology (Oxford). 2018;57(1):e1.
22. Wallace DJ, Pistiner M, Nessim S, Metzger AL, Klinenberg JR. Cutaneous lupus erythematosus without systemic lupus erythematosus: clinical and laboratory features. Semin Arthritis Rheum. 1992 Feb;21(4):221–6.
23. Kuhn A, Ruland V, Bonsmann G. Cutaneous lupus erythematosus: update of therapeutic options part II. J Am Acad Dermatol. 2011;65(6):e195.
24. Ruland V, Bonsmann G. Cutaneous lupus erythematosus: update of therapeutic options part II. Kuhn A, J Am Acad Dermatol. 2011;65(6).
25. Grönhagen CM, Fored CM, Linder M, Granath F, Nyberg F. Subacute cutaneous lupus erythematosus and its association with drugs: a population-based matched case-control study of 234 patients in Sweden. Br J Dermatol. 2012;167(2):296–305.
26. Patsinakidis N, Gambichler T, Lahner N, et al. Cutaneous characteristics and association with antinuclear antibodies in 402 patients with different subtypes of lupus erythematosus. Patsinakidis J Eur Acad Dermatol Venereol. 2016;30(12):2097–2104.
27. Brenner S, Bialy-Golan A, Ruocco V. Drug-induced pemphigus. Clin Dermatol. 1998;16(3):393.
28. Joly P, Maho-Vaillant M, Prost-Squarcioni C, et al. First-line rituximab combined with short-term prednisone versus prednisone alone for the treatment of pemphigus (Ritux 3): a prospective, multicentre, parallel-group, open-label randomised trial. French study group on autoimmune bullous skin diseases. Lancet. 2017;389(10083):2031.
29. Harman KE, Albert S, Black MM, British association of dermatologists. Guidelines for the management of pemphigus vulgaris. Br J Dermatol. 2003;149(5):926–37.
30. Menter A, Korman NJ, Elmets CA, et al. Guidelines of care for the management of psoriasis and psoriatic arthritis: section 4. Guidelines of care for the management and treatment of psoriasis with traditional systemic agents. J Am Acad Dermatol. 2009;61(3):451–85.
31. Menter A, Korman NJ, Elmets CA, et al. Guidelines of care for the management of psoriasis and psoriatic arthritis. Section 3. Guidelines of care for the management and treatment of psoriasis with topical therapies. American Academy of Dermatology. J Am Acad Dermatol. 2009;60(4):643–59.
32. Menter A, Korman NJ, Elmets CA, et al. Guidelines of care for the management of psoriasis and psoriatic arthritis: section 5: guidelines of care for the treatment of psoriasis with phototherapy and photochemotherapy. J Am Acad Dermatol. 2010;62(1):114–35.
33. Menter A, Strober B, Kaplan DH, et al. Guidelines of care for the management and treatment of psoriasis with biologics. J Am Acad Dermatol. Epub 2019 Feb.
34. Chan CS, Van Voorhees AS, Lebwohl MG, Korman NJ, Young M, Bebo BF Jr, Kalb RE, Hsu S. Treatment of severe scalp psoriasis: from the Medical Board of the National Psoriasis Foundation. J Am Acad Dermatol. 2009;60(6):962.
35. Tan ES, Chong WS, Tey HL. Nail psoriasis: a review. Am J Clin Dermatol. 2012;13(6):375.

36. Sano S, Kubo H, Morishima H, et al. Guselkumab, a human interleukin-23 monoclonal antibody in Japanese patients with generalized pustular psoriasis and erythrodermic psoriasis: efficacy and safety analyses of a 52-week, phase 3, multicenter, open-label study. J Dermatol. 2018;45(5):529–39.
37. Ahronowitz I, Harp J, Shinkai K. Etiology and management of pyoderma gangrenosum: a comprehensive review. Am J Clin Dermatol. 2012;13(3):191.
38. Reichrath J, Bens G, Bonowitz A, Tilgen W. Treatment recommendations for pyoderma gangrenosum: an evidence-based review of the literature based on more than 350 patients. J Am Acad Dermatol. 2005;53(2):273–83.
39. Dharamsi JW, Victor S, Aguwa N, Ahn C, Arnett F, Mayes MD, Jacobe H. Morphea in adults and children cohort III: nested case-control study–the clinical significance of autoantibodies in morphea. JAMA Dermatol. 2013;149(10):1159.
40. Zwischenberger BA, Jacobe HT. A systematic review of morphea treatments and therapeutic algorithm. J Am Acad Dermatol. 2011;65:925.
41. van den Hoogen F, Khanna D, Fransen J, et al. 2013 classification criteria for systemic sclerosis: an American college of rheumatology/European league against rheumatism collaborative initiative. Ann Rheum Dis. 2013;72(11):1747–55.
42. Frech TM, Shanmugam VK, Shah AA, et al. Treatment of early diffuse systemic sclerosis skin disease. Clin Exp Rheumatol. 2013;31(2 Suppl 76):166–71.

Pediatrics

Allison Zarbo, Marla Jahnke and Tor Shwayder

Atopic Dermatitis (AD)

What Not To Miss

- Secondary bacterial infection
- Eczema herpeticum
  - Requires systemic antivirals and prompt recognition and treatment to decrease mortality rate
  - Okay to treat concurrently with topical steroids [1]

Key Differential Diagnosis

- Allergic contact dermatitis
- Netherton syndrome
- HTLV-1-associated "infective dermatitis"
- Seborrheic dermatitis
- Scabies
- Primary immunodeficiency
- Acrodermatitis enteropathica/other nutritional disorders
- Mycosis fungoides

A. Zarbo · M. Jahnke · T. Shwayder (✉)
Department of Dermatology, Henry Ford Health System,
3031 West Grand Blvd, Suite 800, Detroit, MI 48202, USA
e-mail: tshwayd1@hfhs.org

© Springer Nature Switzerland AG 2020
H. W. Lim et al. (eds.), *Practical Guide to Dermatology*,
https://doi.org/10.1007/978-3-030-18015-7_2

Work Up Pearls

- Allergic contact dermatitis: patch test patients who do not respond to optimized therapy
- Evaluate for immunodeficiency if patients present with atypical or frequent infections, abnormal hair growth, failure to thrive, failure to respond to optimized therapy

Treatment Ladder

- Soak and grease
  - Mainstay of AD management
  - Instructions
    - Bathe daily for 5–10 min in lukewarm water
    - Pat dry with towel (do not rub)
    - Apply topical medications to areas of AD, then moisturizer to entire body
    - Ointments > creams > lotions; inexpensive, effective and free of additives/fragrances/perfumes [2]
- Topicals (first line)
  - Topical corticosteroids (TCS)
    - Recommend aggressive management initially for acute dermatitis rather than letting it simmer [3]
    - For those with recurrent AD in the same cutaneous location, consider maintenance therapy weekly to twice weekly to decrease relapses [4–6]
    - Remember tachyphylaxis; take a break or switch within the same class [2]
    - Discuss side effects, caution that striae are permanent.
  - Topical calcineurin inhibitors (TCI)
    - FDA approved for ≥ 2 years of age; may be used off-label in younger patients [7]
    - May use with TCS; use for acute, chronic and maintenance (twice to three times weekly)
    - Recommend using instead of TCS if:
      - Patient is recalcitrant to TCS
      - Affected area includes face (especially eyelids) or anogenital area or skin folds
      - Side effects of TCS, including steroid-induced atrophy, are present
      - Suspicion of tachyphylaxis with long-term TCS use
    - Discuss side effects of burning and pruritus (refrigerate to minimize these side effects which usually resolve within 1–2 weeks)
    - We recommend discussing the black box warning [2]
      - PEARL: The black box warning was issued in 2006 based on the theoretical risk of systemic absorption from topicals and (a) the association of increased cancer risk secondary to high-dose oral calcineurin inhibitors used in organ transplantation patients, and (b) animal studies with exposure to TCI at 25–50-fold the maximum recommended human dose [8, 9]. To date, there is no evidence of increased lymphoma or

skin cancers in humans from TCIs in large retrospective reviews [8, 10–12]. For this reason, we may limit the body surface area of application but never restrict use of TCIs.

- Wet wraps for kids
  - Use for significant flares or recalcitrant disease at home or inpatient [13, 14]
  - Increase compliance with "warm" wet wraps by placing damp pajamas in dryer (see below) [15]
  - Reminder: this increases TCS potency; recommend using 3–5 days per week for maximum of 2 weeks per month
  - Instructions
    - Bathe child in warm water or bleach bath (see instructions below)
    - Pat dry with towel
    - Apply topical steroid only to affected areas
    - Apply generous layer of petrolatum-based ointment or other thick cream to all of skin
    - Take a pair of long-sleeved, long-legged white cotton pajamas and wet them in warm water (alternatively, use white cotton socks, gloves, towels or gauze to affected areas)
    - Wring out excess water and place in dryer for 5–10 min if possible
    - Place warm, damp pajamas on child
    - Cover damp pajamas with a second pair of dry pajamas (same size or one size larger) or other warm, dry layer
    - Leave on for at least 1 h, ideally overnight especially for severe flares
- Phototherapy (second line)
  - NBUVB highly preferred over PUVA due to safety profile
  - Can be used for acute, chronic and maintenance therapy
  - Supervision by knowledgeable physician is mandatory, and modality depends on:
    - Patient age (patient must be old enough/mature enough to stand in phototherapy booth)
    - Availability
    - Cost
    - Skin type
    - Skin cancer history
    - Use of photosensitizing medications [16]
  - Should be used in conjunction with TCS but caution with TCI [17, 18]
  - Home phototherapy may be an option for select patients

- Systemics (third line)
  - May also start if significant psychosocial impact of AD
  - Many systemic medications have been studied and guidelines differ in the US versus Europe
  - Start with methotrexate and/or cyclosporine, azathioprine
    - Methotrexate is most commonly used first line in the US
    - Mycophenolate mofetil may also be considered

- o Always decrease to the minimal effective dosage once controlled
- o Dupilumab
  - FDA approved for adolescent patients ages 12–17 years old with moderate-to-severe atopic dermatitis who are not adequately controlled with topical medications
  - FDA approved for asthma in ages 12 years old and above
  - Currently undergoing trials in pediatric population for children as young as 2 years old and off-label in those < 2 years old with success
  - Consider starting this agent prior to methotrexate
- o Methotrexate
  - Dosing is 0.2–0.7 mg/kg weekly, maximum dosage of 25 mg weekly
  - Onset of action is typically 10 weeks
  - Taper and/or discontinue once clearance is obtained
  - Consider discontinuation after 12–16 weeks if no response [16]
  - Please see methotrexate section for more information
- o Cyclosporine
  - Recommend starting at 1 mg/kg daily; range is 3–6 mg/kg daily [16]
  - May pursue
    - (a) Continuous long-term treatment but try to transition to other systemic by 12 months due to risk of malignancy, hepatotoxicity, nephrotoxicity
    - (b) Intermittent short-term bursts (3–6 months) [16, 19]
  - Please see cyclosporine section for more information.
- o Azathioprine
  - Dosing is 1–4 mg/kg daily, maximum of 4 mg/kg daily but TPMT activity may affect dosing
  - Onset of action is typically 12 weeks
  - TMPT enzyme activity level must be drawn prior to treatment
  - Avoid use with phototherapy [16]
  - Please see azathioprine section for more information.
- o Mycophenolate mofetil
  - Dosing is 40–50 mg/kg daily in young children, 30–50 mg/kg daily in adolescents
  - May use in patients as young as 2 [20], and up to 24 consecutive months [16]
  - Please see mycophenolate mofetil section for more information.
- o Corticosteroids
  - Dosing is 0.5–1.0 mg/kg daily with taper
  - Extreme caution, may lead to atopic flares
  - Reserve only for severe exacerbations as a bridge to steroid-sparing agents or when indicated for non-AD conditions (i.e. acute asthma flare)
  - May decrease linear growth while on oral corticosteroids
  - Refer to pediatrician for consideration of booster immunization protocols [16]

- ○ Other agents
  - ■ Less data is available for interferon gamma, omalizumab and other biologics
- Adjunctive therapies
  - ○ Oral antihistamines
    - ■ Nonsedating antihistamines are recommended only in the setting of comorbid conditions such as urticaria or rhinoconjunctivitis
      - However, cetirizine may occasionally help pruritus in AD
    - ■ Short-term, intermittent use of sedating antihistamines may help reduce sleep loss secondary to pruritus but is only an adjunctive therapy and not mainstay
    - ■ Caution in school aged children → may affect school performance [16]
  - ○ Melatonin
    - ■ Useful for improving sleep-onset latency and disease severity with minimal adverse effects [21]
    - ■ May start at a quarter milligram and increase up to 1 mg for every year of a patient's age with maximum of 5 mg given 30 min before bedtime (i.e., 1-year-old with max of 1 mg melatonin; 2–years-old with max of 2 mg melatonin)
    - ■ >5 mg may suppress endogenous melatonin production
    - ■ Use lowest effective dosage
    - ■ MC side effects include drowsiness, dizziness, nausea, headaches [22] (no difference versus placebo in trial [21])
    - ■ No addictive properties or withdrawal symptoms [22]
- Treatment of secondary bacterial infection
  - ○ Pursue bleach baths and intranasal mupirocin to decrease disease severity in patients with frequent bacterial infections with maintenance bleach baths [2, 23]
  - ○ Note: in the setting of mild skin infections, TCS usually clear superinfections without the use of topical or oral antibiotics.
  - ○ Bleach bath instructions
    - ■ Let child swim in bath for about 10 min three times a week (may increase to daily if needed), then rinse off with fresh water
    - ■ Half bathtub (12 inches of water): Add ¼ cup of Clorox bleach
    - ■ Full bathtub (at least 12 inches of water): Add ½ cup of Clorox bleach
    - ■ Baby tub: Add 1 tablespoon of Clorox bleach
  - ○ Restrictions for bleach baths
    - ■ Do not use undiluted bleach directly on the skin
    - ■ Do not use if many breaks or open areas on the skin (may cause stinging/burning)
    - ■ Do not use if known allergy to chlorine
    - ■ Caution with asthmatics: may flare
- Not recommended: topical antihistamines, systemic antibiotics in noninfected AD

Alopecia Areata

- For more information, please see corresponding general section
- Pediatric pearl
  - We do not use intralesional kenalog until child is old enough to consent, and physician deems child is mature enough to handle discomfort of injections as patients may become traumatized and later refuse at an age where injections are typically tolerated
  - Ask about newborn screen to rule out biotinidase deficiency

Infantile Hemangiomas (IH)

What Not To Miss

- Lesions that require prompt and consideration of aggressive management
  - High risk lesions on face, periorbital region, airway or any large lesions with rapid growth [24]
  - High risk of ulceration
    - Trauma-prone areas: diaper area, lips, axillae [25]
    - Large IHs
  - Nodular superficial IHs +/− pedunculation
    - High risk of residual fibrofatty tissue requiring surgical revision in the future [26]
  - Segmental lesions at risk for associated syndromes
- Ulcerated IHs
  - Most common complication of IHs [27]
  - Be aware if dusky discoloration in patients younger than 3 months old may predict future ulceration [28]
  - Higher risk in rapidly proliferating IHs and trauma prone areas [29]
  - Leads to scarring and is a nidus for infection.
- Special sites
  - Periocular IHs
    - Especially if >1 cm, deep component, or upper eyelid involvement refer to pediatric ophthalmologist due to risk of compromising vision [30]
    - Patching may be needed to preserve eyesight
  - "Beard area"
    - Have a high suspicion for airway IHs
      - PEARL: May present with hoarse cry, noisy breathing, stridor, cough, cyanosis [25, 31]
  - Large facial segmental IHs, consider PHACE syndrome
    - IHs >5 cm [32]

- **PEARL:** *P*osterior fossa brain malformations, *H*emangiomas, *A*rterial abnormalities, *C*oarctation of the aorta and cardiac defects, *E*ye abnormalities
- If severe cerebral or cervical anomalies, may develop arterial ischemic stroke [33]
- Refer to ophthalmology, cardiology and consider evaluating airway
- Refer to neurology if MRI/MRA is concerning or if developmental delay
- Monitor growth and development
- Caution with oral propranolol in some patients
  - **PEARL:** Theoretical increased risk of stroke with oral propranolol due to hypotension or reduced cerebrovascular perfusion if pre-existing cerebral vascular abnormalities [34]
  ○ Large, segmental IHs over the lumbosacral area, consider LUMBAR (aka SACRAL, aka PELVIS) syndrome [35]
    - **PEARL:** *L*ower body hemangioma and other cutaneous defects, *U*rogenital anomalies, ulceration, *M*yelopathy, *B*ony deformities, *A*norectal hemangioma malformations, arterial anomalies, *R*enal anomalies [35]
  ○ ≥5 IHs
    - Increased likelihood for visceral involvement such as liver > gastrointestinal tract > thyroid
    - If liver is involved, congestive heart failure may occur from AV shunting and hypothyroidism may occur due to iodothyronine deiodinase production in IH tissue which degrades thyroid hormone [36]

Key Differential Diagnosis

- Other vascular tumors
  ○ Congenital hemangioma (RICH, NICH, PICH)
  ○ Pyogenic granuloma
  ○ Spindle cell hemangioma
  ○ Epithelioid hemangioma
  ○ Tufted angioma
  ○ Kaposiform hemangioendothelioma
  ○ Others
- Vascular malformation

Work Up Pearls

- Recommend taking photographs at each visit to monitor
- Large, segmental IH of lumbosacral or perineal area: evaluate for spinal dysraphism [25]
  ○ Consider spinal ultrasound in ages 3–6 months and MRI and MRA in high-risk patients ≥6 months, as ultrasound can have low sensitivity [37]
- Large IHs >5 cm, especially on the face: MRI/MRA of brain, neck, chest; echocardiogram; +/− laryngoscopy if beard area involved, ophthalmology evaluation

- ≥5 IHs: palpate for hepatosplenomegaly; abdominal ultrasound to evaluate liver involvement
  - ○ If liver is involved, measure TSH, free T3 and free T4 [32] and stool guaiac
- Consider evaluation by multidisciplinary vascular anomalies team if complex infantile IH

Treatment Ladder

- Topical timolol
  - ○ Dosing is 0.5% gel forming solution 1–2 drops two to three times daily [38]
  - ○ Use for thin, superficial IHs as alternative to observation
  - ○ May use to prevent rebound growth if tapering off oral propranolol [39, 40]
- Oral propranolol
  - ○ Dosing of generic propranolol is 0.5–1 mg/kg daily divided into twice or three times daily dosing
    - ■ Twice daily dosing initiated around age 6 months
    - ■ Dose is increased by 0.5–1 mg/kg daily over 1–2 weeks up to 3 mg/kg daily, though most respond to dosage of 2 mg/kg daily
  - ○ Available as non-generic Hemangeol with different dosing
    - ■ PEARL: We typically use generic propranolol due to cost and equivalent outcomes
  - ○ Side effects include hypotension, bradycardia, wheezing, hypoglycemia, irritability, night terrors, cold hands/feet, and diarrhea
    - ■ If wheezing: hold and decrease to lower dosage and discontinue if persistent problem
    - ■ If hypoglycemia: deliver with or after meal to minimize hypoglycemia and hold dose if poor oral intake
    - ■ PEARL: If vomiting, diarrhea, poor-feeding, wheezing, hold medication and restart when child is at baseline
  - ○ Office visits
    - ■ Baseline cardiopulmonary examination
    - ■ Obtain personal and family history of congenital cardiac disease and respiratory disease and refer for cardiology evaluation if needed
    - ■ Obtain weight, blood pressure and heart rate at initiation and each follow up visit
      - • In our clinical experience and among others, we do not believe monitoring heart rate and blood pressure in clinic after the first dose or dose increases is required [41] although this is recommended by consensus guidelines [42]
    - ■ Follow every 1–3 months for weight-based dose adjustment and monitoring of therapy
  - ○ Consider admission to hospital to initiate propranolol if patient is extremely premature or <6 weeks corrected gestational age

- If PHACE workup is necessary, consider MRI/MRA and echocardiogram prior to initiation as severe aortic coarctation is a contraindication
- High-potency topical corticosteroids
  - Rarely used with the advent of topical timolol
  - May be helpful for minor but recurrent ulcerations
- Intralesional triamcinolone
  - 10–40 mg/mL, not exceeding 3 mg/kg per dose, for nodular IHs [43] or in some cases of ulceration
  - Response usually within 2–8 weeks and may repeat every 4 weeks [44]
  - Do not inject periocular IHs due to risk of retinal artery occlusion
  - Caution with HPA axis suppression due to systemic absorption
- Pulsed-dye laser or PDL
  - Used for ulcerated IHs, post-involution erythema, telangiectasias [45] and/or small, thin superficial IHs in proliferative phase [46]
  - Provide insurance codes for the laser and IH with ulceration for the parents; in our experience, we have always had insurance cover treatment of ulcerated IHs
- Ulcerated IHs
  - Wound care
    - Topical antibiotics, barrier creams, non-stick dressings [47]
    - Gentle debridement of crusting with saline soaks 2–3 times daily or appropriate dressing, some of which may be left in place for several days [48]
  - Topical agents
    - Topical timolol [40]
    - Topical metronidazole gel +/− mupirocin [49]
  - Systemics: oral propranolol (see above) [50]
  - Pain
    - Oral acetaminophen +/− codeine
    - Topical anesthetics such as lidocaine
    - *PEARL: Do not prescribe EMLA in infants < 3 months old due to prilocaine, hydrochloride which has been associated with methemoglobinemia due to low levels of methemoglobin reductase in infants [51]*
  - Pulsed-dye laser
    - See above
    - May repeat every 2–4 weeks

Molluscum Contagiosum: Pediatric Specific Pearls

What Not To Miss

- Look for molluscum in new onset eczema, especially if localized
  - Heralds resolution [52]

- Eczematous reaction [52, 53]
- Inflamed/pimple like reaction (only infected in about 1/10)
- Giannott-Crosti syndrome-like reactions
- Immunosuppressed patients
  - If lesions are atypical or extensive, take a history for other signs of immuno-deficiency
  - If patients have known immunodeficiency, lesions are often more persistent
- In skin of color, destructive methods may result in post inflammatory hyper- or hypopigmentation (PIH); preferable to perform curettage due to low risk of PIH, or treat in winter months

Key Differential Diagnosis

- Verruca
- Condyloma accuminata
- Adnexal tumors
- Basal cell carcinoma
- Juvenile xanthogranuloma
- Melanocytic nevus
- Papular granuloma annulare
- Cryptococcus (immunocompromised)
- Histoplasmosis (immunocompromised)
- Monkeypox
- Cowpox
- Orf
- Milia
- Calcinosis cutis

Work Up Pearls

- Consider examining for molluscum bodies (Henderson-Patterson bodies) in saline preparation or H&E
- Can curette and place on glass slide with KOH to view HP bodies with microscopy

Treatment Ladder

- Cantharidin [54]
  - We prefer cantharidin 0.7% for patients who want painless treatment
    - This is safe for use on the face, but use extreme caution around the eyes due to risk of corneal abrasion [55]
    - We have parents wash the cantharidin off with soap and water after 2 h of application
    - May repeat treatment every 2–4 weeks

- In our experience, it typically takes 2–4 treatments for severe cases of molluscum for clearance
    - Scarring is rare but may occur [56]
  ○ We do not typically occlude cantharidin when used for molluscum
  ○ Use with caution in intertriginous areas/areas of occlusion, genitalia, and in areas with increased density of lesions (may consider treatment in crops)
- Curettage [57]
  ○ Apply a topical numbing agent and leave on during curettage in order to decrease friction for ease of curettage
    - This is often tolerated better than expected.
    - ~70% are cured after a single treatment [58]
    - Risk of small, depressed scars
- Cryotherapy [59]
  ○ Apply with cotton-tip swab
  ○ Pain limits use

- Other options include: salicylic acid 17%, potassium hydroxide 5–10% applied three times daily to twice weekly, electrodessication, 40% silver nitrate paste, hydrogen peroxide, topical retinoid, PDL [60], cimetidine
  ○ Localized irritation and long duration to effect may minimize tolerability and compliance but are considered reasonable options, especially when awaiting natural resolution

Morphea: Pediatric Specific Pearls

What Not To Miss

- Extracutaneous manifestations including arthritis, joint contractures, seizures, headaches (especially concerning in patients with linear or generalized morphea) [61]

- A second autoimmune disease [62]

Key Differential Diagnosis

- Lichen sclerosus et atrophicus
- Vaccination-associated morphea
- Paraffin and silicone injections/implants
- Porphyria
- Radiation-induced morphea
- Lipodermatosclerosis
- Injections of vitamin K_1 (Texier disease)
- Nephrogenic systemic fibrosis
- Chronic graft versus host disease

Work Up Pearls

- Full ROS; consider referral to rheumatology if necessary
- Refer all new diagnoses to ophthalmology (non-urgent), as patients have a higher risk of uveitis
- Refer to physical/occupational therapy if joints are involved or contractures are present
- Linear, facial/scalp lesions require imaging

Treatment Ladder

- Aggressive therapy should be pursued once diagnosis is made in order to minimize atrophy of underlying structures, growth defects, contractures, deformities

- Topical treatments are generally reserved for more superficial, localized morphea lesions with no concern for functional or cosmetic impairment

- Risk of progression and relapse are high so systemic medication should always be considered before deferring to topicals alone

- First-line
  - Methotrexate 15 mg/m^2 or 0.6–1 mg/kg per dose (maximum of 25 mg weekly) once weekly for at least 24 months [63–65] in conjunction with steroids
  - For the first 2–3 months, three consecutive days monthly of PO prednisone 1 mg/kg daily (maximum dose of 50 mg daily) or IV methylprednisolone 20–30 mg/kg daily (maximum dose to 1000 mg daily)
    - Especially in patients with en coup de sabre, we prefer to admit to hospital or infusion center for IV methylprednisolone

- Second-line
  - Mycophenolate mofetil at 500–1000 mg/m^2
  - Switch to second-line if no response with first-line after 6 months or intolerant of methotrexate [66]

- Third-line
  - Data is lacking but reports of tacrolimus, cyclophosphamide, biologics [67, 68]

- Topicals: TCS, TCI, vitamin D analogues

- Adjunct
  - UVA1 phototherapy [69–72]
    - Low-dose UVA1: 20 J/cm2 for 12 weeks (Twice or three times weekly for 6 weeks) [72] or five times weekly for 8 weeks [70]
    - Alternately, 30 J/cm^2 three times weekly for 10 consecutive weeks [69]
  - NB-UVB, if UVA1 is not available
  - Fractionated CO2 laser for joint contractures or bound down lesions
  - Surgery, fillers, autologous fat grafts should be delayed until disease is in remission and child is done growing [73–75]

Psoriasis: Pediatric Specific Pearls

Please see autoimmune; pediatric specific concerns will be discussed here

What Not To Miss

- Oropharyngeal or perianal streptococcus as a trigger for guttate psoriasis [76, 77]
  - Strep pharyngitis
    - If clinical suspicion for strep pharyngitis (test if ≥ 2–3 Centor criteria: age 3–14 years, exudate/swelling of tonsils, tender/swollen anterior cervical lymph nodes, temperature >38 Celsius, no cough [78, 79]) or perianal strep, appropriate to work up with laboratory studies (ASO) and treat
    - Options include rapid antigen test for diagnosis [80]; if negative and high clinical suspicion, perform culture
    - Current treatment: amoxicillin (immediate release) 50 mg/kg daily for 10 days or 25 mg/kg twice daily for 10 days, maximum dosage of 1000 mg per day
  - Perianal strep
    - No guidelines exist; based on case reports, we recommend treating perianal strep with systemic antibiotics in order to attempt to improve guttate psoriasis [81]
- Other autoimmune diseases
- Co-morbidities as discussed in work up

Key Differential Diagnosis

- Seborrheic dermatitis
- Mycosis fungoides
- Dermatomyositis
- Lichen planus
- Atopic dermatitis
- Dyshidrotic eczema
- Pityriasis rubra pilaris
- Small plaque parapsoriasis
- Pityriasis lichenoides
- Pityriasis rosea
- Intertrigo
- Langerhans cell histiocytosis
- Acute generalized exanthematous pustulosis

Work Up Pearls

- Counseling
  - Important to counsel on weight loss, lifestyle modifications, and exercise as patients have a higher risk of hyperlipidemia, hypertension, diabetes, obesity, cardiovascular disease and arrhythmias [82] similar to adults [83, 84]

- Screening guidelines [85]
  - o No age restrictions: full ROS for psoriatic arthritis; yearly depression/anxiety screening
  - o 2 years old: start obtaining BMI yearly to screen for overweight and obesity
  - o 3 years old: yearly blood pressure screening for hypertension
  - o 10 years old or puberty: obtain fasting serum glucose every 3 years if obese/overweight or other risk factors for type II diabetes mellitus (T2DM)
  - o 9–11 years and again at 17–21 years old
    - ■ Obtain fasting lipid panel;
    - ■ May also obtain if any additional cardiovascular risk factors
      - • Patient risk factors: hypertension, tobacco use, BMI ≥95th percentile, HDL <40 mg/dL, T1DM, T2DM, renal disease, nephrotic syndrome, heart transplant, Kawasaki disease, HIV, chronic inflammatory disease
      - • Family risk factors: parent, grandparent, aunt, uncle <55 if male and <65 if female with cardiovascular disease, myocardial infarction, angina, coronary artery bypass graft/stent/angioplasty, sudden cardiac death
  - o 9–11 years old
    - ■ Obtain ALT every 2–3 years in obese/overweight children to screen for nonalcoholic fatty liver disease
    - ■ May screen earlier if severe obesity, hypopituitarism, or family history of NALD or nonalcoholic steatohepatitis
  - o 11 years old
    - ■ Yearly substance abuse screening

Treatment Ladder

- Systemic treatment
  - o Methotrexate [86–88]
    - ■ Most commonly used agent for pediatric psoriasis
    - ■ Start at 0.3 mg/kg weekly; may increase up to 0.6 mg/kg weekly for maximum of 25 mg weekly
    - ■ Expect improvement in 4–10 weeks [73]
    - ■ Wean to lowest effective dosage once improved and stable for about 6 months by 0.1 mg/kg every month
  - o NBUVB [89–91]
    - ■ Use dependent on patient age and maturity, as patient must be able to cooperate in phototherapy booth
  - o Cyclosporine [92, 93]
    - ■ Typically reserved for severe flares due to side effects
    - ■ Dosing: 4–5 mg/kg daily
    - ■ Taper as tolerated when controlled
    - ■ Use <12 months due to side effects

- ○ Acitretin [92, 94, 95]
  - Not most efficacious treatment unless pustular psoriasis [96, 97]
  - Must avoid pregnancy for 3 years in females
  - Dosing: 0.5–1.0 mg/kg daily
  - Expect 2–3 months to improve
- ○ Biologics
  - Limited data aside from those mentioned below [98]
  - First-line etanercept
    - Longest history of use with pediatric psoriasis [99, 100], but requires weekly injections
    - FDA approved for ages 4–17 years [99]
    - Dosing: 0.8 mg/kg weekly, maximum dosage of 50 mg
  - Second-line adalimumab [101]
    - Trial with children ages 4–17 [102]
    - Consider for first line; used often first line but not FDA approved for pediatric psoriasis
      - ○ PEARL: FDA approved for juvenile idiopathic arthritis ages 2 years and older and plaque psoriasis in adults [103]. In Europe, approved since 2015 for severe plaque psoriasis in children 4 years of age or older by European Medicines Agency [104].
    - Dosing: 0.8 mg/kg at weeks 0, 1, and then every other week, maximum dosage of 40 mg
  - Ustekinumab
    - FDA approved for ages ≥ 12 years [105]
    - Weight based dosing given at weeks 0, 4, then every 12 weeks
      - ○ Weight ≤ 60 kg: 0.75 mg/kg
      - ○ Weight > 60 kg to ≤ 100 kg: 45 mg
      - ○ > 100 kg: 90 mg

Outside the Box Treatment Options

- Tonsillectomy
  - ○ Further studies are needed; case reports have shown improvement and clearance in patients with guttate psoriasis (n = 10) [106–109]
  - ○ One randomized controlled trial demonstrated improvement for plaque psoriasis in patients with flares after upper respiratory tract infections [110]

Tinea Capitis

What Not to Miss

- Severe, chronic and recurrent episodes seen in chronic mucocutaneous candidiasis, common variable immunodeficiency and HIV

Key Differential Diagnosis

- Seborrheic dermatitis
- Alopecia areata
- Trichotillomania
- Psoriasis
- Pyoderma
- Folliculitis
- Lichen planus
- Discoid lupus erythematosus
- Folliculitis decalvans

Work Up Pearls

- In our experience, you do not have to check baseline or mid-therapy labs unless patient has hepatic or renal issues, diabetes, systemic illness or prolonged treatment
- Recommend culture at baseline and to confirm mycological cure after treatment
- Counseling: ask about siblings, hair care tools, headwear, shared pillowcases, head-to-head contact sports, animals/pets [111]
- Treat empirically in endemic population such as urban settings if patient has any 1 of the following: occipital lymphadenopathy, scalp pruritus, alopecia or scaling
  - ○ Possible to have false negatives on cultures with kerion due to inflammatory response [112]

Treatment Ladder

- Oral terbinafine (250 mg tablet)
  - ○ FDA approved for children ≥4 years
  - ○ <25 kg: 125 mg daily for 6 weeks*
  - ○ 25–35 kg: 187.5 mg daily for 6 weeks*
  - ○ >35 kg: 250 mg daily for 6 weeks*
    - ▪ *minimum therapy is 6 weeks
    - ▪ Recommend test for mycological cure with culture upon completion

- Oral griseofulvin (suspension and tablet available)
  - ○ 1 month–≤2 years: microsize suspension 15–25 mg/kg daily or divided into twice daily doses for 6–8 weeks or until resolution*
  - ○ >2 years—adolescents
    - ▪ Microsize 20–25 mg/kg daily or divided into twice daily dosing for 6–8 weeks*

- Maximum dosing of 1 g daily
- May require up to 18 weeks of therapy
  - Ultramicrosize: 10–15 mg/kg daily (maximum dosage of 750 mg daily) for ~6 weeks*
    - May require up to 18 weeks of therapy
  - * Recommend test for mycological cure with culture

- Antifungal shampoo (ketoconazole or selenium sulfide)
  - Shampoo at least twice weekly during therapy and use as long-term maintenance to decrease rate of reinfection [113]

- If recurrences, consider if patient had clinical cure but not mycological cure or reinfected (consider evaluating other household members and pets)

Tinea Corporis

What Not To Miss

- Recommend using tinea capitis dosing of oral terbinafine or griseofulvin for hair bearing areas; please see above

- Consider work up for immune disorder if severe, refractory course

Key Differential Diagnosis

- Nummular eczema
- Atopic dermatitis
- Petaloid seborrheic dermatitis
- Tinea versicolor
- Pityriasis rosea
- Parapsoriasis
- Erythema annulare centrifugum
- Psoriasis
- Subacute lupus erythematosus
- Granuloma annulare
- Impetigo

Work Up Pearls

- Obtain KOH
- Obtain fungal culture

Treatment Ladder

- Topicals
  - Majority of tinea corporis can be treated with topical antifungals for at least 2 weeks
  - Recommend patients treat for 2 weeks past clearance to prevent recurrence
  - Nystatin is ineffective and only targets candida

- Oral medications
  - Indicated if refractory or extensive tinea corporis, Majocchi's granuloma, or nail involvement
  - End point: clinical resolution
  - Oral terbinafine (250 mg tablet)
    - FDA approved for children ≥4 years for tinea capitis, used off-label for tinea corporis
    - 10–20 kg: 62.5 mg daily
    - 20–40 kg: 125 mg daily
    - >40 kg: 250 mg daily
    - Recommended duration for tinea pedis, manuum: 2 weeks or until clinical clearance
    - Recommended duration for tinea corporis, cruris and faciei: 1–2 weeks or until clinical clearance
  - Oral griseofulvin
    - Approved for children >2 years-adolescents
    - Microsize: 10–20 mg/kg daily
      - Maximum daily dosage: 1000 mg daily
    - Ultramicrosize: 5–15 mg/kg daily
      - Maximum daily dosage: 750 mg daily
    - Recommended duration for tinea pedis, manuum: 4–8 weeks or until clinical clearance
    - Recommended duration for tinea corporis, cruris and faciei: 2–4 weeks or until clinical clearance
  - Oral itraconazole
    - Limited data for infants, children, adolescents
    - 3–5 mg/kg daily
    - Maximum daily dosage: 200 mg daily
    - Recommended duration for tinea pedis, manuum, corporis, cruris, faciei: 1 week
  - Oral fluconazole
    - Infants, children, adolescents
    - Initial 6 mg/kg weekly
    - Maximum daily dosage: 600 mg daily
    - Recommended duration for tinea pedis, manuum: 2–6 weeks
    - Recommended duration for tinea corporis, cruris, faciei: 2–4 weeks
  - We do not recommend oral ketoconazole due to risk of severe liver injury and adrenal insufficiency

Onychomycosis

- Topical treatment with ciclopirox lacquer alone sometimes suffices but requires prolonged use (32 weeks) [114]

Scabies

- Pediatric pearl
  - Permethrin is not approved for ages <2 months, however, we have no qualms using this agent
    - Other options include topical sulfur.
  - In prepubescent children, topicals should cover the scalp down
  - Scabetic nodules may occur and may persist for months [115]
    - Low to mid potency topical steroids may be used to treat
  - Consider scabies prep on older family members with consent if non-cooperative child

Nevus Sebaceous/Sebaceus: Pediatric Specific Pearls

What Not To Miss

- Consider nevus sebaceous (NS) syndrome if CNS, ocular, skeletal abnormalities
  - Usually only present in large NS
- Consider phakomatosis pigmentokeratotica if speckled lentiginous nevus or agminated melanocytic nevi and focal cortical dysplasia are present

Key Differential Diagnosis

- Alopecia areata
- Sebaceous hyperplasia
- Basal cell carcinoma
- Epidermal nevus
- Aplasia cutis congenita
- Solitary mastocytoma
- Juvenile xanthogranuloma
- Melanoma

Work Up Pearls

- Consider biopsy of secondary growths

Treatment Ladder

- Watchful waiting
  - Monitor every 1–3 years until puberty then yearly [116]
- Excision
  - Typically consider when child can tolerate under local anesthesia (usually around puberty when lesion becomes thicker anyway)
  - Consider sooner if lesion will always be too large for excision under local anesthesia
  - Consider sooner if potentially stigmatizing location
- CO_2 laser ablation

Verruca: Pediatric Specific Pearls

What Not To Miss

- Screen for verruca as a sign of immunodeficiency if extensive lesions or other signs (failure to thrive, frequent or atypical infections, etc.)
- Screen for verruca intraorally when lesions are present on hands
- Condyloma accuminata as sign of child maltreatment
  - Consider especially when child toilet trained/wiping self exclusively, no other family members/caregivers with known warts, or other signs of maltreatment are present on full skin exam

Key Differential Diagnosis

- Molluscum contagiosum
- Acquired digital fibrokeratoma
- Squamous cell carcinoma
- Tungiasis
- Amelanotic melanoma
- Prurigo nodularis

Work Up Pearls

- Treatment may be warranted if lesions are uncomfortable or cosmetically disconcerting; many will undergo spontaneous remission within 2 years [117]

Treatment Ladder

- For children, we prefer painless measures such as
  - Cantharidin 0.7% usually under occlusion
    - May repeat in office every 3–4 weeks [117]
  - Topical salicylic acid: may be performed at home; prefer 40–50% for palmar/plantar surfaces [117]
    - Can use at home in conjunction with in-office treatments
  - Topical fluorouracil [118]
  - Topical imiquimod [118]
  - Topical cidofovir [119]

- Other (painful) options include
  - Cryotherapy [117]
  - Intralesional candida [120]
  - Intralesional bleomycin [118]—use with caution for localized areas only in children due to risk of systemic absorption [121]
  - Topical fluorouracil
  - Intralesional fluorouracil [122]
  - Topical trichloroacetic acid [123]
  - Pulsed dye laser [124]
  - Intralesional cidofovir [125, 126]
  - Surgical removal

- Oral medications
  - Cimetidine (30–40 mg/kg daily divided twice daily for 2–3 months [127]): note that RCT have not consistently found superiority over placebo [128–130]
  - Oral acitretin: one case report [131]
  - Oral zinc sulfate: zinc sulfate 10 mg/kg daily (maximum of 600 mg daily) for minimum of 3 months [132]

Outside the Box Treatment Options

- HPV vaccination: case reports of resolution of warts after vaccine [133–135]
- CO2 laser [136]
- Photodynamic therapy [137]
- Topical viable Bacillus Calmette-Guérin [138]

Neonatal Concerns [139]

Neonatal rashes		
Disorder	**Clinical course**	**Treatment**
Miliaria crystallina	Dew drop like vesicles release clear sweat. Self-limited	Unnecessary other than cool baths, loose clothing, cool environment to decrease development
Miliaria rubra	Erythematous non-folliculocentric papules. Self-limited	
Transient Neonatal Pustular Melanosis	Presents in first few days of life in darker skin types in a well-appearing infant with asymptomatic superficial sterile pustules which rupture easily, and/or hyperpigmented macules with fine collarette of scale (babies may present at birth with some or all phases)	No treatment necessary
Neonatal Cephalic Pustulosis	Pustules/acneiform pustules (not comedones like neonatal acne) on head, neck, upper trunk	No treatment necessary; may use topical antifungals or low potency topical corticosteroids. Avoid baby oils, creams, ointments
Erythema toxicum neonatorum	Onset most commonly at 3-4 days of life (range is birth-10 days of life) in well-appearing neonate. Erythematous macules-patches with white/pale yellow papulopustules centrally; relapse and remits for first 2 weeks of life. Self-limited	Gentle cleansing

Diaper rashes		
Diaper dermatitis	**Presentations**	**Treatment**
Chafing/frictional dermatitis*	Redness/scaling in friction areas: inner thighs, buttocks, abdomen, genitalia, back where diaper rubs	Keep area dry and go diaperless as much as possible, frequent diaper changes, gentle cleansing, zinc oxide or petrolatum-based barrier creams, low-potency topical corticosteroid
Irritant contact dermatitis*	Erythematous patches, papules +/− vesicles, erosions notably sparing folds. Usually worse anteriorly in boys and posteriorly in girls	See chafing/frictional dermatitis
Diaper candidiasis*	Beefy-red erythematous papules, pustules and plaques on lower abdomen, genitals, buttocks, notably involving the inguinal folds. May be malodorous	Topical antifungal (azoles > nystatin), barrier creams/ointments See chafing/frictional dermatitis

Diaper rashes

Diaper dermatitis	Presentations	Treatment
Seborrheic dermatitis	May involve diaper area, scalp, face, intertriginous areas, ankles, wrists, umbilicus +/− mild/no pruritus with erythematous patches; may resolve within 6 months → 2 years [140]	Gentle shampooing and scrubbing of scale, mild topical corticosteroid twice daily, topical antifungals Mineral oil to loosen scale on scalp
Allergic contact dermatitis	Symmetrical scaly pink papules/plaques on lateral buttocks, hips, inner thighs	Sensitive diapers, wipes, mild topical corticosteroid Consider patch testing Diaper hygiene
Jacquet's dermatitis (erosive diaper dermatitis)	Erythema, vesiculation, punched out erosions	Diaper hygiene, low-mid potency topical corticosteroids
Granuloma gluteale infantum	Purple-red papulonodules in the groin, lower abdomen, inner thighs as response to chronic irritation/candidiasis	Taper high potency fluorinated topical steroids if used; address underlying etiology
Psoriasis	Sharply demarcated erythematous plaques +/− scaling; consider if recalcitrant diaper dermatitis or classic lesions elsewhere	Please see psoriasis section
Acrodermatitis enteropathica/other nutritional or metabolic deficiencies	Diaper area, perioral, hands/feet with erythema, scaling, crusting, oozing [141]. Systemic symptoms including failure to thrive may be present. In acrodermatitis enteropathica, test plasma zinc and albumin	Treatment dependent upon etiology. For acrodermatitis enteropathica, treatment depends on whether acquired versus genetic with mutation in SLC39A4); may be seen in exclusively breastfed infants with low zinc in mothers' milk Treat with 3 mg/kg/day of elemental zinc (13.2 mg/kg/day of zinc sulfate) [142, 143]
Langerhans cell histiocytosis	Consider if recalcitrant; may resemble seborrheic dermatitis, +/− erosions, petechiae	Please see section on LCH

*MCC

References

1. Aronson PL, Shah SS, Mohamad Z, Yan AC. Topical corticosteroids and hospital length of stay in children with eczema herpeticum. Pediatr Dermatol. 2013;30(2):215–21.
2. Eichenfield LF, Tom WL, Berger TG, Krol A, Paller AS, Schwarzenberger K, et al. Guidelines of care for the management of atopic dermatitis: section 2. Management and treatment of atopic dermatitis with topical therapies. J Am Acad Dermatol. 2014;71(1):116–32.
3. Thomas KS, Armstrong S, Avery A, Po AL, O'Neill C, Young S, et al. Randomised controlled trial of short bursts of a potent topical corticosteroid versus prolonged use of a mild preparation for children with mild or moderate atopic eczema. BMJ (Clin Res ed). 2002;324(7340):768.
4. Schmitt J, von Kobyletzki L, Svensson A, Apfelbacher C. Efficacy and tolerability of proactive treatment with topical corticosteroids and calcineurin inhibitors for atopic eczema: systematic review and meta-analysis of randomized controlled trials. Br J Dermatol. 2011;164(2):415–28.
5. Hanifin J, Gupta AK, Rajagopalan R. Intermittent dosing of fluticasone propionate cream for reducing the risk of relapse in atopic dermatitis patients. Br J Dermatol. 2002;147(3):528–37.
6. Glazenburg EJ, Wolkerstorfer A, Gerretsen AL, Mulder PG, Oranje AP. Efficacy and safety of fluticasone propionate 0.005% ointment in the long-term maintenance treatment of children with atopic dermatitis: differences between boys and girls? Pediatric allergy and immunology: official publication of the European Society of Pediatric Allergy and Immunology. 2009;20(1):59–66.
7. El-Batawy MM, Bosseila MA, Mashaly HM, Hafez VS. Topical calcineurin inhibitors in atopic dermatitis: a systematic review and meta-analysis. J Dermatol Sci. 2009;54(2):76–87.
8. Tennis P, Gelfand JM, Rothman KJ. Evaluation of cancer risk related to atopic dermatitis and use of topical calcineurin inhibitors. Br J Dermatol. 2011;165(3):465–73.
9. Thaci D, Salgo R. Malignancy concerns of topical calcineurin inhibitors for atopic dermatitis: facts and controversies. Clin Dermatol. 2010;28(1):52–6.
10. Berger TG, Duvic M, Van Voorhees AS, VanBeek MJ, Frieden IJ. The use of topical calcineurin inhibitors in dermatology: safety concerns. Report of the American Academy of Dermatology Association Task Force. J Am Acad Dermatol. 2006;54(5):818–23.
11. Legendre L, Barnetche T, Mazereeuw-Hautier J, Meyer N, Murrell D, Paul C. Risk of lymphoma in patients with atopic dermatitis and the role of topical treatment: a systematic review and meta-analysis. J Am Acad Dermatol. 2015;72(6):992–1002.
12. Koo JY, Fleischer AB Jr, Abramovits W, Pariser DM, McCall CO, Horn TD, et al. Tacrolimus ointment is safe and effective in the treatment of atopic dermatitis: results in 8000 patients. J Am Acad Dermatol. 2005;53(2 Suppl 2):S195–205.
13. Devillers AC, Oranje AP. Efficacy and safety of 'wet-wrap' dressings as an intervention treatment in children with severe and/or refractory atopic dermatitis: a critical review of the literature. Br J Dermatol. 2006;154(4):579–85.
14. Dabade TS, Davis DM, Wetter DA, Hand JL, McEvoy MT, Pittelkow MR, et al. Wet dressing therapy in conjunction with topical corticosteroids is effective for rapid control of severe pediatric atopic dermatitis: experience with 218 patients over 30 years at Mayo Clinic. J Am Acad Dermatol. 2012;67(1):100–6.
15. Cooper CA, DeKlotz CMC. Warming up to the idea of wet wraps. Pediatr Dermatol. 2017;34(6):737–8.
16. Sidbury R, Davis DM, Cohen DE, Cordoro KM, Berger TG, Bergman JN, et al. Guidelines of care for the management of atopic dermatitis: section 3. Management and treatment with phototherapy and systemic agents. J Am Acad Dermatol. 2014;71(2):327–49.
17. Astellas. Medication guide (tacrolimus). http://www.protopic.com/pdf/protopic_med_guide.pdf.

18. Medicis. Prescribing information (pimecrolimus). http://elidel-us.com/files/Elidel_PI.pdf.

19. Harper JI, Ahmed I, Barclay G, Lacour M, Hoeger P, Cork MJ, et al. Cyclosporin for severe childhood atopic dermatitis: short course versus continuous therapy. Br J Dermatol. 2000;142(1):52–8.

20. Heller M, Shin HT, Orlow SJ, Schaffer JV. Mycophenolate mofetil for severe childhood atopic dermatitis: experience in 14 patients. J Dermatol. 2007;157(1):127–32.

21. Chang YS, Lin MH, Lee JH, Lee PL, Dai YS, Chu KH, et al. Melatonin supplementation for children with atopic dermatitis and sleep disturbance: a randomized clinical trial. JAMA Pediatr. 2016;170(1):35–42.

22. Buscemi N, Vandermeer B, Hooton N, Pandya R, Tjosvold L, Hartling L, et al. Efficacy and safety of exogenous melatonin for secondary sleep disorders and sleep disorders accompanying sleep restriction: meta-analysis. BMJ (Clin Res ed). 2006;332(7538):385–93.

23. Huang JT, Abrams M, Tlougan B, Rademaker A, Paller AS. Treatment of Staphylococcus aureus colonization in atopic dermatitis decreases disease severity. Pediatrics. 2009;123(5):e808–14.

24. Darrow DH, Greene AK, Mancini AJ, Nopper AJ. Diagnosis and management of infantile hemangioma. Pediatrics. 2015;136(4):e1060–104.

25. Jahnke MN. Vascular lesions. Pediatr Ann. 2016;45(8):e299–305.

26. Luu M, Frieden IJ. Haemangioma: clinical course, complications and management. Br J Dermatol. 2013;169(1):20–30.

27. Haggstrom AN, Drolet BA, Baselga E, Chamlin SL, Garzon MC, Horii KA, et al. Prospective study of infantile hemangiomas: demographic, prenatal, and perinatal characteristics. J Pediatr. 2007;150(3):291–4.

28. Maguiness SM, Hoffman WY, McCalmont TH, Frieden IJ. Early white discoloration of infantile hemangioma: a sign of impending ulceration. Arch Dermatol. 2010;146(11):1235–9.

29. Chamlin SL, Haggstrom AN, Drolet BA, Baselga E, Frieden IJ, Garzon MC, et al. Multicenter prospective study of ulcerated hemangiomas. J Pediatr. 2007;151(6):684–9, 9.e1.

30. Samuelov L, Kinori M, Rychlik K, Konanur M, Chamlin SL, Rahmani B, et al. Risk factors for ocular complications in periocular infantile hemangiomas. Pediatr Dermatol. 2018;35(4):458–62.

31. Orlow SJ, Isakoff MS, Blei F. Increased risk of symptomatic hemangiomas of the airway in association with cutaneous hemangiomas in a "beard" distribution. J Pediatr. 1997;131(4):643–6.

32. Frieden IJ, Reese V, Cohen D. PHACE syndrome. The association of posterior fossa brain malformations, hemangiomas, arterial anomalies, coarctation of the aorta and cardiac defects, and eye abnormalities. Arch Dermatol. 1996;132(3):307–11.

33. Siegel DH, Tefft KA, Kelly T, Johnson C, Metry D, Burrows P, et al. Stroke in children with posterior fossa brain malformations, hemangiomas, arterial anomalies, coarctation of the aorta and cardiac defects, and eye abnormalities (PHACE) syndrome: a systematic review of the literature. Stroke. 2012;43(6):1672–4.

34. Metry DW, Garzon MC, Drolet BA, Frommelt P, Haggstrom A, Hall J, et al. PHACE syndrome: current knowledge, future directions. Pediatr Dermatol. 2009;26(4):381–98.

35. Iacobas I, Burrows PE, Frieden IJ, Liang MG, Mulliken JB, Mancini AJ, et al. LUMBAR: association between cutaneous infantile hemangiomas of the lower body and regional congenital anomalies. J Pediatr. 2010;157(5):795–801.e1-7.

36. Huang SA, Tu HM, Harney JW, Venihaki M, Butte AJ, Kozakewich HP, et al. Severe hypothyroidism caused by type 3 iodothyronine deiodinase in infantile hemangiomas. New Engl J Med. 2000;343(3):185–9.

37. de Graaf M, Pasmans SG, van Drooge AM, Nievelstein RA, Gooskens RH, Raphael MF, et al. Associated anomalies and diagnostic approach in lumbosacral and perineal haemangiomas: case report and review of the literature. J Plast Reconstr Aesthet Surg JPRAS. 2013;66(1):e26–8.

38. Khan M, Boyce A, Prieto-Merino D, Svensson A, Wedgeworth E, Flohr C. The role of topical timolol in the treatment of infantile hemangiomas: a systematic review and meta-analysis. Acta Dermato-Venereol. 2017;97(10):1167–71.
39. Blatt J, Morrell DS, Buck S, Zdanski C, Gold S, Stavas J, et al. Beta-blockers for infantile hemangiomas: a single-institution experience. Clin Pediatr. 2011;50(8):757–63.
40. Boos MD, Castelo-Soccio L. Experience with topical timolol maleate for the treatment of ulcerated infantile hemangiomas (IH). J Am Acad Dermatol. 2016;74(3):567–70.
41. Kumar MG, Coughlin C, Bayliss SJ. Outpatient use of oral propranolol and topical timolol for infantile hemangiomas: survey results and comparison with propranolol consensus statement guidelines. Pediatr Dermatol. 2015;32(2):171–9.
42. Drolet BA, Frommelt PC, Chamlin SL, Haggstrom A, Bauman NM, Chiu YE, et al. Initiation and use of propranolol for infantile hemangioma: report of a consensus conference. Pediatrics. 2013;131(1):128–40.
43. Chen MT, Yeong EK, Horng SY. Intralesional corticosteroid therapy in proliferating head and neck hemangiomas: a review of 155 cases. J Pediatr Surg. 2000;35(3):420–3.
44. Ceisler EJ, Santos L, Blei F. Periocular hemangiomas: what every physician should know. Pediatr Dermatol. 2004;21(1):1–9.
45. Frieden IJ. Which hemangiomas to treat–and how? Arch Dermatol. 1997;133(12):1593–5.
46. Stier MF, Glick SA, Hirsch RJ. Laser treatment of pediatric vascular lesions: port wine stains and hemangiomas. J Am Acad Dermatol. 2008;58(2):261–85.
47. Morelli JG, Tan OT, Yohn JJ, Weston WL. Treatment of ulcerated hemangiomas infancy. Arch Pediatr Adolesc Med. 1994;148(10):1104–5.
48. Wang JY, Ighani A, Ayala AP, Akita S, Lara-Corrales I, Alavi A. Medical, surgical, and wound care management of Ulcerated Infantile hemangiomas: a systematic review [Formula: see text]. J Cutan Med Surg. 2018;22(5):495–504.
49. Kim HJ, Colombo M, Frieden IJ. Ulcerated hemangiomas: clinical characteristics and response to therapy. J Am Acad Dermatol. 2001;44(6):962–72.
50. Saint-Jean M, Leaute-Labreze C, Mazereeuw-Hautier J, Bodak N, Hamel-Teillac D, Kupfer-Bessaguet I, et al. Propranolol for treatment of ulcerated infantile hemangiomas. J Am Acad Dermatol. 2011;64(5):827–32.
51. Tran AN, Koo JY. Risk of systemic toxicity with topical lidocaine/prilocaine: a review. J Drugs Dermatol JDD. 2014;13(9):1118–22.
52. Berger EM, Orlow SJ, Patel RR, Schaffer JV. Experience with molluscum contagiosum and associated inflammatory reactions in a pediatric dermatology practice: the bump that rashes. Arch Dermatol. 2012;148(11):1257–64.
53. Butala N, Siegfried E, Weissler A. Molluscum BOTE sign: a predictor of imminent resolution. Pediatrics. 2013;131(5):e1650–3.
54. Coloe J, Morrell DS. Cantharidin use among pediatric dermatologists in the treatment of molluscum contagiosum. Pediatr Dermatol. 2009;26(4):405–8.
55. Jahnke MN, Hwang S, Griffith JL, Shwayder T. Cantharidin for treatment of facial molluscum contagiosum: a retrospective review. J Am Acad Dermatol. 2018;78(1):198–200.
56. Piggot C, Friedlander SF, Tom W. Poxvirus infections. In: Goldsmith LA, Katz SI, Gilchrest BA, et al. editors. Fitzpatrick's dermatology in general medicine. 2: McGraw-Hill; 2012. p. 2402.
57. Hanna D, Hatami A, Powell J, Marcoux D, Maari C, Savard P, et al. A prospective randomized trial comparing the efficacy and adverse effects of four recognized treatments of molluscum contagiosum in children. Pediatr Dermatol. 2006;23(6):574–9.
58. Harel A, Kutz AM, Hadj-Rabia S, Mashiah J. To treat molluscum contagiosum or not-curettage: an effective well-accepted treatment modality. Pediatr Dermatol. 2016;33(6):640–5.
59. Al-Mutairi N, Al-Doukhi A, Al-Farag S, Al-Haddad A. Comparative study on the efficacy, safety, and acceptability of imiquimod 5% cream versus cryotherapy for molluscum contagiosum in children. Pediatr Dermatol. 2010;27(4):388–94.

60. Isaacs SN. Molluscum contagiosum. 27 July 2017.
61. Zulian F, Vallongo C, Woo P, Russo R, Ruperto N, Harper J, et al. Localized scleroderma in childhood is not just a skin disease. Arthritis Rheum. 2005;52(9):2873–81.
62. Harrington CI, Dunsmore IR. An investigation into the incidence of auto-immune disorders in patients with localized morphoea. Br J Dermatol. 1989;120(5):645–8.
63. Li SC, Torok KS, Pope E, Dedeoglu F, Hong S, Jacobe HT, et al. Development of consensus treatment plans for juvenile localized scleroderma: a roadmap toward comparative effectiveness studies in juvenile localized scleroderma. Arthritis Care Res. 2012;64(8):1175–85.
64. Uziel Y, Feldman BM, Krafchik BR, Yeung RS, Laxer RM. Methotrexate and corticosteroid therapy for pediatric localized scleroderma. J Pediatr. 2000;136(1):91–5.
65. Torok KS, Arkachaisri T. Methotrexate and corticosteroids in the treatment of localized scleroderma: a standardized prospective longitudinal single-center study. J Rheumatol. 2012;39(2):286–94.
66. Martini G, Ramanan AV, Falcini F, Girschick H, Goldsmith DP, Zulian F. Successful treatment of severe or methotrexate-resistant juvenile localized scleroderma with mycophenolate mofetil. Rheumatology (Oxford, England). 2009;48(11):1410–3.
67. Li SC, Feldman BM, Higgins GC, Haines KA, Punaro MG, O'Neil KM. Treatment of pediatric localized scleroderma: results of a survey of North American pediatric rheumatologists. J Rheumatol. 2010;37(1):175–81.
68. Martini G, Campus S, Raffeiner B, Boscarol G, Meneghel A, Zulian F. Tocilizumab in two children with pansclerotic morphoea: a hopeful therapy for refractory cases? Clin Exp Rheumatol. 2017;35 Suppl 106(4):211–3.
69. Camacho NR, Sanchez JE, Martin RF, Gonzalez JR, Sanchez JL. Medium-dose UVA1 phototherapy in localized scleroderma and its effect in CD34-positive dendritic cells. J Am Acad Dermatol. 2001;45(5):697–9.
70. Kreuter A, Hyun J, Skrygan M, Sommer A, Bastian A, Altmeyer P, et al. Ultraviolet al-induced downregulation of human beta-defensins and interleukin-6 and interleukin-8 correlates with clinical improvement in localized scleroderma. Br J Dermatol. 2006;155(3):600–7.
71. De Rie MA, Bos JD. Photochemotherapy for systemic and localized scleroderma. J Am Acad Dermatol. 2000;43(4):725–6.
72. Kerscher M, Volkenandt M, Gruss C, Reuther T, von Kobyletzki G, Freitag M, et al. Low-dose UVA phototherapy for treatment of localized scleroderma. J Am Acad Dermatol. 1998;38(1):21–6.
73. Sengezer M, Deveci M, Selmanpakoglu N. Repair of "coup de sabre," a linear form of scleroderma. Ann Plast Surg. 1996;37(4):428–32.
74. Lapiere JC, Aasi S, Cook B, Montalvo A. Successful correction of depressed scars of the forehead secondary to trauma and morphea en coup de sabre by en bloc autologous dermal fat graft. Dermatol Surg Off Publ Am Soc Dermatol Surg. 2000;26(8):793–7.
75. Palmero ML, Uziel Y, Laxer RM, Forrest CR, Pope E. En coup de sabre scleroderma and Parry-Romberg syndrome in adolescents: surgical options and patient-related outcomes. J Rheumatol. 2010;37(10):2174–9.
76. Patrizi A, Costa AM, Fiorillo L, Neri I. Perianal streptococcal dermatitis associated with guttate psoriasis and/or balanoposthitis: a study of five cases. Pediatr Dermatol. 1994;11(2):168–71.
77. Herbst RA, Hoch O, Kapp A, Weiss J. Guttate psoriasis triggered by perianal streptococcal dermatitis in a four-year-old boy. J Am Acad Dermatol. 2000;42(5 Pt 2):885–7.
78. Centor RM, Witherspoon JM, Dalton HP, Brody CE, Link K. The diagnosis of strep throat in adults in the emergency room. Med Decis Making Int J Soc Med Decis Making. 1981;1(3):239–46.
79. McIsaac WJ, Kellner JD, Aufricht P, Vanjaka A, Low DE. Empirical validation of guidelines for the management of pharyngitis in children and adults. JAMA. 2004;291(13):1587–95.

80. Shulman ST, Bisno AL, Clegg HW, Gerber MA, Kaplan EL, Lee G, et al. Clinical practice guideline for the diagnosis and management of group a streptococcal pharyngitis: 2012 update by the Infectious Diseases Society of America. Clin Infect Dis Off Public Infect Dis Soc Am. 2012;55(10):1279–82.

81. Garritsen FM, Kraag DE, de Graaf M. Guttate psoriasis triggered by perianal streptococcal infection. Clin Exper Dermatol. 2017;42(5):536–8.

82. Kwa L, Kwa MC, Silverberg JI. Cardiovascular comorbidities of pediatric psoriasis among hospitalized children in the United States. J Am Acad Dermatol. 2017;77(6):1023–9.

83. Augustin M, Glaeske G, Radtke MA, Christophers E, Reich K, Schafer I. Epidemiology and comorbidity of psoriasis in children. Br J Dermatol. 2010;162(3):633–6.

84. Koebnick C, Black MH, Smith N, Der-Sarkissian JK, Porter AH, Jacobsen SJ, et al. The association of psoriasis and elevated blood lipids in overweight and obese children. J Pediatr. 2011;159(4):577–83.

85. Osier E, Wang AS, Tollefson MM, Cordoro KM, Daniels SR, Eichenfield A, et al. Pediatric psoriasis comorbidity screening guidelines. JAMA Dermatol. 2017;153(7):698–704.

86. van Geel MJ, Oostveen AM, Hoppenreijs EP, Hendriks JC, van de Kerkhof PC, de Jong EM, et al. Methotrexate in pediatric plaque-type psoriasis: long-term daily clinical practice results from the Child-CAPTURE registry. J Dermatol Treat. 2015;26(5):406–12.

87. Kaur I, Dogra S, De D, Kanwar AJ. Systemic methotrexate treatment in childhood psoriasis: further experience in 24 children from India. Pediatr Dermatol. 2008;25(2):184–8.

88. Collin B, Vani A, Ogboli M, Moss C. Methotrexate treatment in 13 children with severe plaque psoriasis. Clin Exper Dermatol. 2009;34(3):295–8.

89. Pavlovsky M, Baum S, Shpiro D, Pavlovsky L, Pavlotsky F. Narrow band UVB: is it effective and safe for paediatric psoriasis and atopic dermatitis? J Eur Acad Dermatol Venereol JEADV. 2011;25(6):727–9.

90. Zamberk P, Velazquez D, Campos M, Hernanz JM, Lazaro P. Paediatric psoriasis–narrowband UVB treatment. J Eur Acad Dermatol Venereol JEADV. 2010;24(4):415–9.

91. Tan E, Lim D, Rademaker M. Narrowband UVB phototherapy in children: a New Zealand experience. Australas J Dermatol. 2010;51(4):268–73.

92. van Geel MJ, Mul K, de Jager ME, van de Kerkhof PC, de Jong EM, Seyger MM. Systemic treatments in paediatric psoriasis: a systematic evidence-based update. J Eur Acad Dermatol Venereol JEADV. 2015;29(3):425–37.

93. Di Lernia V, Stingeni L, Boccaletti V, Calzavara Pinton PG, Guarneri C, Belloni Fortina A, et al. Effectiveness and safety of cyclosporine in pediatric plaque psoriasis: a multicentric retrospective analysis. J Dermatol Treat. 2016;27(5):395–8.

94. Di Lernia V, Bonamonte D, Lasagni C, Belloni Fortina A, Cambiaghi S, Corazza M, et al. Effectiveness and safety of acitretin in children with plaque psoriasis: a multicenter retrospective analysis. Pediatr Dermatol. 2016;33(5):530–5.

95. Charbit L, Mahe E, Phan A, Chiaverini C, Boralevi F, Bourrat E, et al. Systemic treatments in childhood psoriasis: a French multicentre study on 154 children. Br J Dermatol. 2016;174(5):1118–21.

96. Lebwohl M, Ali S. Treatment of psoriasis. Part 2. Systemic therapies. J Am Acad Dermatol. 2001;45(5):649–61; quiz 62-4.

97. Brecher AR, Orlow SJ. Oral retinoid therapy for dermatologic conditions in children and adolescents. J Am Acad Dermatol. 2003;49(2):171–82; quiz 83-6.

98. Garber C, Creighton-Smith M, Sorensen EP, Dumont N, Gottlieb AB. Systemic treatment of recalcitrant pediatric psoriasis: a case series and literature review. J Drugs Dermatol JDD. 2015;14(8):881–6.

99. Paller AS, Siegfried EC, Langley RG, Gottlieb AB, Pariser D, Landells I, et al. Etanercept treatment for children and adolescents with plaque psoriasis. New Engl J Med. 2008;358(3):241–51.

100. Paller AS, Siegfried EC, Eichenfield LF, Pariser D, Langley RG, Creamer K, et al. Long-term etanercept in pediatric patients with plaque psoriasis. J Am Acad Dermatol. 2010;63(5):762–8.

101. Papp K, Thaci D, Marcoux D, Weibel L, Unnebrink K, Williams D. Efficacy and safety of adalimumab versus methotrexate treatment in pediatric patients with severe chronic plaque psoriasis: Results from the 16-week randomized, double-blind period of a phase 3 study. In: 4th World Psoriasis and Psoriatic Arthritis Conference on Psoriasis 2015. J Investig Dermatol.

102. Papp K, Thaci D, Marcoux D, Weibel L, Philipp S, Ghislain PD, et al. Efficacy and safety of adalimumab every other week versus methotrexate once weekly in children and adolescents with severe chronic plaque psoriasis: a randomised, double-blind, phase 3 trial. Lancet (London, England). 2017;390(10089):40–9.

103. FDA. Full prescribing information: adalimumab. https://www.accessdata.fda.gov/drugsat-fda_docs/label/2012/125057s232lbl.pdf.

104. Kivelevitch D, Menter A. Adalimumab in paediatric psoriasis. Lancet (London, England). 2017;390(10089):5–6.

105. Johnson J. Janssen announces U.S. FDA approval of Stelara (Ustekinumab) for the treatment of adolescents with moderate to severe plaque psoriasis Horsham, PA: Johnson & Johnson; 2017. https://www.jnj.com/media-center/press-releases/janssen-announces-us-fda-approval-of-stelara-ustekinumab-for-the-treatment-of-adolescents-with-moderate-to-severe-plaque-psoriasis.

106. McMillin BD, Maddern BR, Graham WR. A role for tonsillectomy in the treatment of psoriasis? Ear Nose Throat J. 1999;78(3):155–8.

107. Saita B, Ishii Y, Ogata K, Kikuchi I, Inoue S, Naritomi K. Two sisters with guttate psoriasis responsive to tonsillectomy: case reports with HLA studies. J Dermatol. 1979;6(3):185–9.

108. Hone SW, Donnelly MJ, Powell F, Blayney AW. Clearance of recalcitrant psoriasis after tonsillectomy. Clin Otolaryngol Allied Sci. 1996;21(6):546–7.

109. Wu W, Debbaneh M, Moslehi H, Koo J, Liao W. Tonsillectomy as a treatment for psoriasis: a review. J Dermatol Treat. 2014;25(6):482–6.

110. Thorleifsdottir RH, Sigurdardottir SL, Sigurgeirsson B, Olafsson JH, Sigurdsson MI, Petersen H, et al. Improvement of psoriasis after tonsillectomy is associated with a decrease in the frequency of circulating T cells that recognize streptococcal determinants and homologous skin determinants. J Immunol (Baltimore, Md: 1950). 2012;188(10):5160–5.

111. Ely JW, Rosenfeld S, Seabury Stone M. Diagnosis and management of tinea infections. Am Fam Phys. 2014;90(10):702–10.

112. John AM, Schwartz RA, Janniger CK. The kerion: an angry tinea capitis. Int J Dermatol. 2018;57(1):3–9.

113. Bennassar A, Grimalt R. Management of tinea capitis in childhood. Clin Cosmet Investig Dermatol. 2010;3:89–98.

114. Friedlander SF, Chan YC, Chan YH, Eichenfield LF. Onychomycosis does not always require systemic treatment for cure: a trial using topical therapy. Pediatr Dermatol. 2013;30(3):316–22.

115. Hashimoto K, Fujiwara K, Punwaney J, DiGregorio F, Bostrom P, el-Hoshy K, et al. Post-scabetic nodules: a lymphohistiocytic reaction rich in indeterminate cells. J Dermatol. 2000;27(3):181–94.

116. Wali GN, Felton SJ, McPherson T. Management of naevus sebaceous: a national survey of UK dermatologists and plastic surgeons. Clin Exp Dermatol. 2018;43(5):589–91.

117. Sterling JC, Gibbs S, Haque Hussain SS, Mohd Mustapa MF, Handfield-Jones SE. British Association of Dermatologists' guidelines for the management of cutaneous warts 2014. Br J Dermatol. 2014;171(4):696–712.

118. Kwok CS, Gibbs S, Bennett C, Holland R, Abbott R. Topical treatments for cutaneous warts. The Cochrane database of systematic reviews. 2012;(9):Cd001781.

119. Field S, Irvine AD, Kirby B. The treatment of viral warts with topical cidofovir 1%: our experience of seven paediatric patients. Br J Dermatol. 2009;160(1):223–4.
120. Horn TD, Johnson SM, Helm RM, Roberson PK. Intralesional immunotherapy of warts with mumps, Candida, and Trichophyton skin test antigens: a single-blinded, randomized, and controlled trial. Arch Dermatol. 2005;141(5):589–94.
121. Herschthal J, McLeod MP, Zaiac M. Management of ungual warts. Dermatol Ther. 2012;25(6):545–50.
122. Iscimen A, Aydemir EH, Goksugur N, Engin B. Intralesional 5-fluorouracil, lidocaine and epinephrine mixture for the treatment of verrucae: a prospective placebo-controlled, single-blind randomized study. J Eur Acad Dermatol Venereol JEADV. 2004;18(4):455–8.
123. Pezeshkpoor F, Banihashemi M, Yazdanpanah MJ, Yousefzadeh H, Sharghi M, Hoseinzadeh H. Comparative study of topical 80% trichloroacetic acid with 35% trichloroacetic acid in the treatment of the common wart. J Drugs Dermatol JDD. 2012;11(11):e66–9.
124. Sparreboom EE, Luijks HG, Luiting-Welkenhuyzen HA, Willems PW, Groeneveld CP, Bovenschen HJ. Pulsed-dye laser treatment for recalcitrant viral warts: a retrospective case series of 227 patients. Br J Dermatol. 2014;171(5):1270–3.
125. Broganelli P, Chiaretta A, Fragnelli B, Bernengo MG. Intralesional cidofovir for the treatment of multiple and recalcitrant cutaneous viral warts. Dermatol Ther. 2012;25(5):468–71.
126. Blouin MM, Cloutier R, Noel R. Intralesional cidofovir in the treatment of cutaneous warts in a renal transplant patient. J Cutan Med Surg. 2012;16(6):462–4.
127. Orlow SJ, Paller A. Cimetidine therapy for multiple viral warts in children. J Am Acad Dermatol. 1993;28(5 Pt 1):794–6.
128. Yilmaz E, Alpsoy E, Basaran E. Cimetidine therapy for warts: a placebo-controlled, double-blind study. J Am Acad Dermatol. 1996;34(6):1005–7.
129. Lee SH, Rose B, Thompson CH, Cossart Y. Plantar warts of defined aetiology in adults and unresponsiveness to low dose cimetidine. Australas J Dermatol. 2001;42(3):220–1.
130. Rogers CJ, Gibney MD, Siegfried EC, Harrison BR, Glaser DA. Cimetidine therapy for recalcitrant warts in adults: is it any better than placebo? J Am Acad Dermatol. 1999;41(1):123–7.
131. Simone CD, Capizzi R, Carbone A, Fossati B, Valenzano F, Amerio P. Use of acitretin in a case of giant common warts in an HIV-infected patient. Eur J Dermatol EJD. 2008;18(3):346–7.
132. Stefani M, Bottino G, Fontenelle E, Azulay DR. Efficacy comparison between cimetidine and zinc sulphate in the treatment of multiple and recalcitrant warts. Anais Brasileiros Dermatol. 2009;84(1):23–9.
133. Daniel BS, Murrell DF. Complete resolution of chronic multiple verruca vulgaris treated with quadrivalent human papillomavirus vaccine. JAMA Dermatol. 2013;149(3):370–2.
134. Venugopal SS, Murrell DF. Recalcitrant cutaneous warts treated with recombinant quadrivalent human papillomavirus vaccine (types 6, 11, 16, and 18) in a developmentally delayed, 31-year-old white man. Arch Dermatol. 2010;146(5):475–7.
135. Abeck D, Folster-Holst R. Quadrivalent human papillomavirus vaccination: a promising treatment for recalcitrant cutaneous warts in children. Acta Dermato-Venereol. 2015;95(8):1017–9.
136. Sloan K, Haberman H, Lynde CW. Carbon dioxide laser-treatment of resistant verrucae vulgaris: retrospective analysis. J Cutan Med Surg. 1998;2(23):142–5.
137. Schroeter CA, Kaas L, Waterval JJ, Bos PM, Neumann HA. Successful treatment of periungual warts using photodynamic therapy: a pilot study. J Eur Acad Dermatol Venereol JEADV. 2007;21(9):1170–4.
138. Salem A, Nofal A, Hosny D. Treatment of common and plane warts in children with topical viable Bacillus Calmette-Guerin. Pediatr Dermatol. 2013;30(1):60–3.
139. Chadha A, Jahnke M. Common neonatal rashes. Pediatr Ann. 2019;48(1):e16–22.
140. Elish D, Silverberg NB. Infantile seborrheic dermatitis. Cutis. 2006;77(5):297–300.

141. Al Rashed A, Al Shehri M, Kaliyadan F. Acrodermatitis enteropathica in a pair of twins. J Dermatol Case Rep. 2016;10(4):65–7.
142. Maverakis E, Fung MA, Lynch PJ, Draznin M, Michael DJ, Ruben B, et al. Acrodermatitis enteropathica and an overview of zinc metabolism. J Am Acad Dermatol. 2007;56(1):116–24.
143. Neldner KH, Hambidge KM. Zinc therapy of acrodermatitis enteropathica. New Engl J Med. 1975;292(17):879–82.

Procedural Dermatology

Danielle Yeager, Mark Balle and David Ozog

Anticoagulants Prior to Surgery [1–5]

What Not To Miss

- Increased bleeding risk
  - Newer antiplatelet agents (i.e. clopidogrel) and novel oral anticoagulant agents (i.e. dabigatran, apixiban, rivaroxaban etc.) may have an increased risk of bleeding complications [1, 2]
  - Patients on dual/combination agents may also have an increased risk of bleeding complications [2]
  - Special attention should be made to achieve good hemostasis in patients taking the above agents!

Pearls

- It is recommended to *continue* all medically necessary anticoagulants in patients undergoing Mohs and cutaneous surgery [4]
  - Increased risk of thrombotic event(s) if discontinued in perioperative period

D. Yeager · M. Balle · D. Ozog (✉)
Department of Dermatology, Henry Ford Health System,
3031 West Grand Blvd, Suite 800, Detroit, MI 48202, USA
e-mail: dozog1@hfhs.org

D. Yeager
e-mail: dyeager2@hfhs.org

© Springer Nature Switzerland AG 2020
H. W. Lim et al. (eds.), *Practical Guide to Dermatology*,
https://doi.org/10.1007/978-3-030-18015-7_3

In the context of…

- Herbal supplements
  - If *not medically* necessary, they should be discontinued [5]
  - Examples of herbal supplements that increase the risk of perioperative bleeding include vitamin E, fish oil, feverfew, garlic, ginger, ginkgo biloba, glucosamine and ginseng

Antiseptics [6–9]

What Not To Miss

- Chlorhexidine use caution around the ears (ototoxicity if it enters the external auditory canal and penetrates the tympanic membrane) and the eyes (conjunctivitis or corneal toxicity; keratitis, corneal ulceration) [6]
- Alcohol is *flammable*! Be cautious around lasers and electrosurgery

Pearls

- Betadine (povidone-iodine) is inactivated by body fluids; you must wait for it to dry to be effective
- Chlorhexidine is *not* inactivated by bodily fluids and is the longest acting topical antiseptic that has residual activity of up to 6 h
- Table below shows onset and antimicrobrial coverage [6–9]

Antimicrobial agent	Onset	Residual activity	Advantages	Disadvantages
Alcohol (isopropyl and ethanol)	Immediate *(fastest)*	None	Very broad spectrum (gram +/−, mycobacteria and most viruses)	- Inactive against spores and nonenveloped viruses - Not effective for soiled hands - *Flammable!* Caution with lasers/electrosurgery
Chlorhexidine (2–4%)	Rapid	*Longest Acting, >6 h*	Broad spectrum (gram +/−,, enveloped viruses, and fungi,) *NOT* inactivated by body fluids	- Inactive against spores and biofilms - Some mycobacterium are intrinsically resistant- Ototoxicity, corneal keratitis, ulceration and conjunctivitis - use caution around the ears/eyes

Antimicrobial agent	Onset	Residual activity	Advantages	Disadvantages
Chloroxylenol (parachloro-metaxylenol)	Slow	Good	Fairly spectrum (gram + > −, viruses, and mycobacterium)	- Not as broad spectrum, fast acting or long lasting as chlorhexidine - Decreased efficacy with body fluids - Ineffective against pseudomonas (unless combined w/EDTA)
Iodine and idophors	Rapid	Minimal	Very broad spectrum (gram +/−, mycobacterium, fungi, viruses, and *bacterial spores*)	- Skin irritation and discoloration - Inactivated by body fluids - Must wait for it to dry to be effective

Infiltrative Anesthesia [7–11]

What Not To Miss

- Side effects of lidocaine overdose [7, 8]
  - Mild toxicity (1–5 mcg/ml): circumoral numbness, and "tingling" of the hands
    - First signs of lidocaine overdose, so you must observe these patients closely
  - Moderate toxicity (6–9 mcg/ml): nausea, vomiting, tinnitus, nystagmus, slurred speech, and blurred vision
  - Severe toxicity (9–12 mcg): seizures and cardiopulmonary depression
- Treatment of lidocaine toxicity
  - Stop any injections immediately and assess the patient for symptoms to determine extent of overdose
  - Basic steps include maintaining adequate oxygenation and monitoring vital signs
  - If concerns of cardiac or CNS toxicity, patient should be transported to an emergency center for higher level of care
- Keep in mind that *not all reactions* following local anesthetic injection are due to toxicity, the easiest way to distinguish is by vital signs
  - Vasovagal reaction: low heart rate and low blood pressure
    - Treatment: Trendelenburg positioning and cold compresses
  - Epinephrine reaction: high heart rate and high blood pressure
    - Treatment: reassurance (usually resolves within minutes), phentolamine and propranolol
  - Anaphylactic reaction: high heart rate and low blood pressure
    - Treatment: epinephrine injection, antihistamines, corticosteroids, oxygen and fluids

Pearls

- To reduce the pain associated with injection [8, 10]
  - Inject into follicular openings
  - Infiltrate slowly forming a visible bleb
  - Use vibration of the skin, cold air skin cooling or verbal distraction
  - Buffer with sodium bicarbonate at a ratio of 1:10 of 8.4% bicarbonate
    - Reduces the pain of injection by increasing pH
    - Increases the speed of anesthesia onset
    - PEARL: Epinephrine activity is lost in this alkaline or neutral environment
- Bupivocaine has delayed onset of action, longer duration of action and greater risk of cardiac toxicity
- For highly vascular sites (i.e. scalp), allow 15 min for onset of vasoconstrictive effect of epinephrine to take place
- Diphenhydramine (Benadryl) is safe in amide and ester allergic patients [11]
  - Dilute 1% diphenhydramine in 4:1 ratio with normal saline for 5% solution
  - Reports of local necrosis; do not use in areas of poor perfusion

In the Context Of …

- Pregnancy
  - Lidocaine is the local anesthetic of choice (category B)
    - Avoid bupivacaine and mepivacaine (category C); risk of fetal brady-cardia
- End-stage liver disease
  - There is increased risk of lidocaine toxicity since it is metabolized by the liver
- Table below shows onset, duration and maximal dosing [7, 8]

Amide anesthetics	Onset	Duration	Max Dose (mg/kg)
Lidocaine 1%, 2% *Trade name: Xylocaine*	Rapid (sec)	0.5–2 h	4.5 mg/kg *(peds: 1.2–2.0 mg/kg)*
Lidocaine 0.5% with Epinephrine 1:200,000 *Trade name: Xylocaine + epi*	Rapid (sec)	1–4 h	7.5 mg/kg *(peds: 3.0–4.5 mg/kg)*
Bupivacaine 0.5% *Trade name: Marcaine or sensorcaine*	5–8 min	2–4 h	2.5 mg/kg
Bupivacaine 0.5% with Epinephrine 1:200,000 *Trade name: Marcaine or sensor-caine + epi*	5–8 min	4–8 h	3 mg/kg

Topical Anesthesia [10, 12]

What Not To Miss

- Methemoglobinemia
  - EMLA (which is eutectic mix of lidocaine 2.5%/prilocaine 2.5%) has an increased risk of methemoglobinemia attributed to its prilocaine component.
- Caution with occlusion or large surface areas, as this may increase absorption [10]
  - Large surface areas typically are >2,000 cm^2 (i.e. entire extremity or trunk) [12]
  - Risk of toxicity is increased in children due to higher body surface to weight ratio compared to adults

Pearls

- Topical agents are recommended as first-line method for non-ablative laser treatments [10]

In the Context Of …

- Use on large body surface areas [12]
  - Exposure to high concentrations of local anesthetics may cause life threatening effects (irregular heartbeats, seizures and death)
    - 2 case reports of death following application for laser hair removal when applied to bilateral lower legs under occlusion
  - FDA warning in 2007
    - Advised against unsupervised application by patients to avoid high levels of absorption in the blood
    - Recommend applying sparingly, avoiding broken/irritated skin, and avoid applying under occlusion
- Pregnancy or nursing women
  - Topical lidocaine is considered safe but there is insufficient data on the use of other topical anesthetics
- Pediatric patients
  - Topical anesthesia is first line method for repair of dermal lacerations and minimally invasive procedures
  - When infiltrated anesthesia is needed, it is recommended to use adjunctive topical anesthesia to minimize discomfort

Tumescent Anesthesia [13]

What Not To Miss

- Maximum dosing is 55 mg/kg [13]
    - Valid for weight range studied, which included patients 43.6–81.8 kg for liposuction purposes
    - Sample calculation of max dose of lidocaine in a 70 kg patient
        - 70 kg × 55 mg/kg = 3,850 mg of lidocaine
            - When using basic formula below, patients receive only 500 mg of lidocaine
    - Basic formula has final concentrations: lidocaine 0.05%, epinephrine 1: 1,000,000
        - 50 ml 1% lidocaine (500 mg)
        - 1 ml 1:1000 epinephrine from ampule (1 mg)
        - 10 ml sodium bicarbonate (of an 8.4% $NaHCO_3$ solution)
        - 1 L of normal saline (0.9% NaCl solution)

Pearls

- Advantageous because it is associated with decreased bleeding and increased duration of anesthesia while avoiding complications of general anesthesia
- Facilitates in tissue dissection due to the volume injected
- Useful for liposuction, excision of interconnected sinus tracts in hidradenitis suppurativa patients, ambulatory phlebectomy and more

In the Context Of …

- Reducing patient discomfort
    - The use of warm anesthetic solution and slow infiltration is recommended

Surgery Site Infection [2, 7, 14]

What Not To Miss

- Contamination that occurs during the surgery is the #1 cause of surgical site infection
- Risk factors for infection
    - Studies have found that shaving with a *razor* increases the risk (may be due to microscopic cuts in the skin)

- PEARL: If hair must be removed, this should be done just before the surgical procedure in a careful manner so that the skin remains intact without cuts or scratches
  - Recommend using electric shaver or depilatory cream, NOT a razor
- ○ Host factors
  - Diabetes, obesity, smoking, chronic renal failure, skin neoplasm, *S. aureus* nasal carrier, immunosuppression, patient at high risk of endocarditis or recent total joint replacement (within 2 years)
- ○ Body site
  - Below the knee, nose, ear, groin, and genitalia
- ○ Complex surgery
  - Prolonged procedure (greater than 3 h), flap or graft repair, and longer incision

Pearls

- Most dermatologic surgeries fall into the *clean* or *clean contaminated* categories and *do not* require prophylaxis
  - ○ However, it should be considered in patients who have the above risk factors; especially in patients at high risk of infectious endocarditis and those with recent total joint replacement (within 2 years).
- The American Heart Association updated its recommendations for antibiotic prophylaxis for infective endocarditis in 2017 [14]
  - ○ Limit antibiotic prophylaxis to patients with the following conditions
    - Prosthetic valve or prosthetic material used in valve repair, including transcatheter-implanted prostheses as well as, homografts (cadaveric donor grafts)
    - Prosthetic material used for cardiac valve repair, such as annuloplasty rings or chords
    - Previous infectious endocarditis
    - Cardiac transplantation patients who developed cardiac valvulopathy
    - Certain congenital heart conditions (CHD)
      - Unrepaired cyanotic CHD
      - Completely repaired CHD with residual shunts or valvular regurgitation at the site of or adjacent to the site of prosthetic patch or prosthetic device
      - Repaired CHD with residual defects or adjacent prosthetic device

- *Staphylococcus aureus* is the most common organism in surgical site infections
  - ○ Signs and symptoms typically present 4–8 days post operatively

In the Context Of ...

- Prophylactic antibiotics
  - o Table below shows some common recommendations for prophylactic regimens based on bacterial flora in certain body locations
  - o It is important to give *1 hour prior* to surgery to ensure adequate distribution into the tissue and wound coagulum [2, 7]

Surgical site/procedure	Antibiotic
Non- oral sites (lip, ear, or nasal flap)	*No allergies:* - Keflex (cephalexin) 2 g PO
	Penicillin allergy: - Clindamycin 600 mg PO -OR- - Azithromycin 500 mg PO
Oral mucosa breached	*No allergies:* - Amoxicillin 2 g PO
	Penicillin allergy: - Clindamycin 600 mg PO -OR- - Azithromycin 500 mg PO
Lesions in the groin or on the legs	*No allergies:* - Keflex 2 g PO -OR- - TMP- SMX DS 1 tablet
	Penicillin allergy: - TMP- SMX DS 1 tablet -OR- - Levofloxacin 500 mg PO

Surgical Anatomy [7, 8, 14, 15]

MOTOR NERVE ANATOMIC DANGER ZONES

What Not To Miss

- There are several key danger zones [15]
  - o Temporal branch of facial nerve
    - Greatest risk of injury: superficial to deep temporalis fascia as it crosses the zygomatic arch
    - Runs diagonal 0.5 cm below the tragus to 1.5 cm above the lateral brow
    - Injury causes brow ptosis, flattening of forehead due to frontalis paralysis and inability to raise the eyebrow

- ○ Zygomatic branch of facial nerve
  - Greatest risk of injury: malar cheek
  - Runs fairly deep so it is less commonly injured
  - Injury causes inability to completely close eyes, possible ectropion and trouble elevating upper lip
- ○ Marginal mandibular nerve
  - Greatest risk of injury: 2–3 cm inferolateral to oral commissure as it passes over the mandible
  - Runs just anterior to the masseter muscle where it crosses over the body of mandible
  - Injury causes facial asymmetry when smiling (inability to depress lip on ipsilateral side), and inability to show the lower teeth
- ○ Spinal accessory nerve
  - Greatest risk of injury: at Erb's point where cervical plexus emerges (see figure below)
  - Runs along the posterior triangle, exiting at posterior border of sterno-cleidomastoid and then entering the anterior border of the trapezius
  - Injury causes winged scapula, inability to shrug shoulder, difficulty initiating abduction of arm and chronic shoulder pain
- ○ Ulnar nerve
  - Greatest risk of injury: medial epicondyle of humerus
  - Injury causes "claw-hand deformity", weakness in risk flexion, loss of flexion of 4th and 5th digits and loss of sensation in ulnar distribution

Pearls

- Motor nerves all run deep to the superficial musculoaponeurotic system (SMAS)
  - ○ Staying above the SMAS during facial surgery may prevent motor nerve damage
- Sensory nerves all run superficial to the SMAS
  - ○ Often transected during facial surgery causing numbness

In the Context Of ...

- Locating motor nerve danger areas
  - ○ Facial danger zones (Fig. 1)
  - ○ Spinal accessory nerve (Fig. 2)
- Sensory nerve blocks [7, 8, 14, 15]
  - ○ Aim is to inject NEAR the nerve and avoid entering nerve foramen for risk of nerve injury and needle breakage
  - ○ Most nerves can be blocked with 1–2 mLs of anesthetic

Nerve block	Area of anesthesia achieved	Technique
Supraorbital nerve	Forehead and frontal scalp above eyebrows	Injection of anesthetic infiltrated immediately superficial to periosteum at orbital rim in mid-pupillary line.
Supratrochlear	Midforehead, glabella, and frontal scalp	Injection of anesthetic immediately superficial to periosteum at superomedial orbital rim at the junction of glabella and eyebrow
Greater auricular nerve branches and auriculotemporal nerve	Frontal scalp and forehead	Injection of anesthetic into subcutaneous plane laterally from the supraorbital nerve to region immediately superior and posterior to attachment of ear pinna
Infraorbital nerve	Medial cheek, upper lip and nasal ala	1. Injection anesthetic ~1 cm inferior to orbital rim in the mid-pupillary line, superficial to maxillary bone periosteum -OR- 2. Intraoral approach: insert needle between 1st and 2nd premolars, moving cephalad parallel to periosteum until maxillary bone is reach
Infratrochlear nerve	Lateral and dorsal nose	Inject anesthetic superficial to periosteum at inferomedial orbital rim at superior end of nose-cheek concavity
Anterior ethmoidal nerve	Nasal tip	Anesthetic infiltrated along cartilage at junction of nasal cartilage and bone, slightly lateral from midline
Mental nerve	Lower lip and chin	1. Inject anesthetic at level of periosteum in mid-pupillary line halfway cephalad along mandible -OR- 2. Intraoral approach: insert needle between 1st and 2nd premolars, moving caudally along periosteum to halfway down the mandible
Digital nerve	Fingers and toes	Inject anesthetic distal to MCP/MTP until lightly tap bone. Then, withdrawal slightly, position dorsally and inject. Next, position needle ventrally and inject. Repeat on other side of the digit. (2 dorsal and 2 ventral injections per digit) *Do not use epinephrine and use small volumes (<1.5 mL on each side of digit) to avoid ischemia*

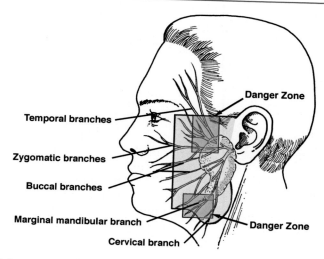

Fig. 1 Facial danger zones. Illustration by: Jay Knipstein

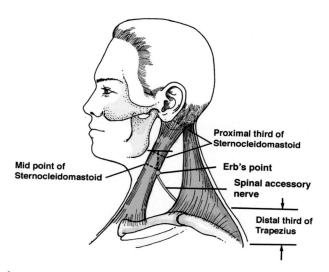

Fig. 2 Spinal accessory nerve. Illustration by: Jay Knipstein

Excisions [16]

What Not To Miss

- Fusiform ellipse
  - In most cases, an optimal scar results when you place the fusiform ellipse within major skin folds or relaxed skin tension lines
  - Hold the #15 blade perpendicular to avoid beveling when creating incisions

Pearls

- The optimal angle for fusiform ellipses is 30 degrees with the length-to-width ratio of 3:1
- Undermining
  - Reduces tension to optimize surgical outcome
  - Use blunt scissors
    - Insert scissors and then spread the tissue via blunt dissection to avoid damage to surrounding nerves or arteries
  - Undermining planes
    - Cheek: mid to deep subcutaneous fat
    - Forehead: just above frontalis muscle
    - Temple: just above the superficial fascia
    - Scalp: subgaleal space
    - Nose: just above perichondrium
    - Lip: just above orbicularis oris
    - Ear: just above perichondrium
    - Eyelid: just above orbicularis oculi
    - Neck, trunk and extremities: just above superficial fascia
  - Make sure to also undermine at apical angles to help avoid standing cones

In the Context Of …

- Epidermoid cysts
  - Dissection is facilitated by injection of a generous amount of anesthesia into surrounding tissue
  - Fusiform ellipse may be smaller than the area of the cyst; may be able to dissect the cyst out

- Lipomas
  - A linear incision can be made in the middle of the lipoma

- Dermatofibromas
  - Inform patients that the scar maybe larger and more noticeable than the original lesion

- Melanoma [16]
  - WLE must be oriented longitudinally on an extremity, regardless of lesion orientation or optimal relaxed skin tension lines
  - Consider purse string closure instead of ellipse on trunk or extremity

Wound Repair [15, 17]

What Not To Miss

- In layered closures, sub-epidermal placement of sutures is performed with absorbable sutures

Pearls

- Second intention healing can be used for shallow wounds, mucosal sites, temple area, and concave sites (such as medial canthus, conchal bowl, and alar crease)
- Primary intention
  - Buried absorbable sutures
    - Help reduce wound tension to optimize cosmetic results
    - Used for large deeper wounds
    - Reduce risk of wound dehiscence
  - Epidermal sutures
    - Simple interrupted stitches can be helpful in high-tension wounds and help fix uneven edges
      - To correct uneven edges: place the suture more superficially on higher side and deeper on the lower side (Fig. 3)

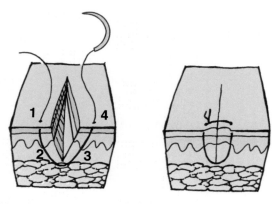

Fig. 3 Simple interrupted sutures. Illustration by: Jay Knipstein

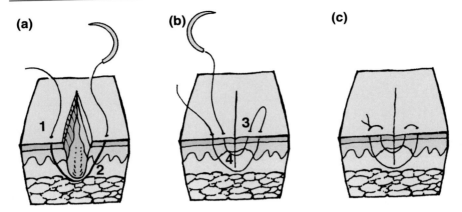

Fig. 4 Vertical mattress sutures. Illustration by: Jay Knipstein

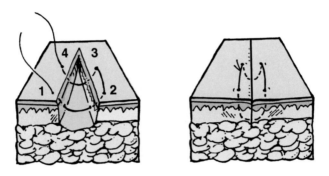

Fig. 5 Horizontal mattress sutures. Illustration by: Jay Knipstein

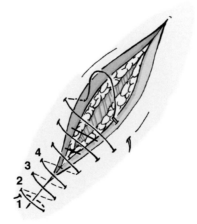

Fig. 6 Running simple sutures. Illustration by: Jay Knipstein

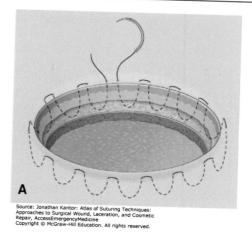

Fig. 7 Purse string sutures Suturing Technique and Other Closure Materials. In: Kantor, J. *Atlas of Suturing techniques: Approaches to Surgical Wound, Laceration, and Cosmetic Repair.* New York: McGraw-Hill; 2016, with permission from McGraw-Hill

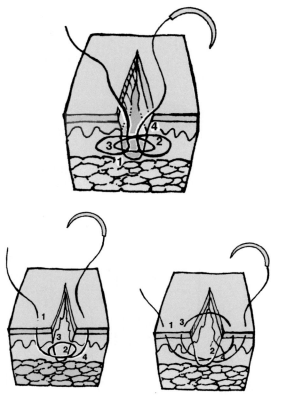

Fig. 8 Pulley sutures. Illustration by: Jay Knipstein

- Vertical mattress suture may be helpful in achieving wound eversion (Fig. 4)
  - Horizontal mattress suture may be helpful in reducing tension and achieving hemostasis (Fig. 5)
  - Running sutures can be used for quick closures for wounds under minimal tension (Fig. 6)
  - Purse string closures can be used to close round circular defects and decreases wound size and healing time (Fig. 7)
    - PEARL: Consider a purse string suture in an excisional biopsy of any pigmented lesion concerning for melanoma to minimize the overall size of the future re-excision (See above) [16]
  - Pulley stitches help close wounds under high tension
    - PEARL: Performed by stitching from far-near-near-far (Fig. 8)

In the Context Of …

- Suture removal
  - Head and neck: <7 days
  - Extremities and torso: 10–14 days

Suture Characteristics [7, 15]

What Not To Miss

- Select the smallest suture that will provide enough strength for wound closure

Pearls

- Suture spitting can result from placing deep sutures too superficially in the dermis
- Suture track marks can be prevented by avoiding tying sutures too tight and early suture removal
- Popular sutures for facial repairs
  - Deep absorbable sutures
    - 4–0 or 5–0 Polyglactin 910 (Vicryl®) or Poliglecaprone 25 (Monocryl®)
  - Epidermal sutures
    - 5–0 or 6–0 Fast-absorbing gut, Nylon, or Polypropylene (Prolene®)
- Popular sutures for high tension sites
  - Deep absorbable sutures
    - Polydioxanone (PDS®) offers prolonged tensile strength (50% at 4 weeks) [7]

In the Context Of ...

- Table below lists non-absorbable sutures [7, 15]

Suture	Configuration	Ease of handle	Knot security	Tissue reactivity	Uses
Silk	Braided	*The Best*	Good	High (*#2 to plain gut*)	Mucosal surfaces
Nylon (Ethilon, Dermalon)	Monofilament	Good to fair	Poor	Very low	Surface closure
Polypropylene (Prolene, surgilene)	Monofilament	Good to fair	Poor	Least of non-absorbables	Ideal for running sub-cuticular
Polyester (Ethibond, Dacron, Mersilene)*	Braided	Very Good	Good	Minimal	Highest strength of non-absorables; mucosal surfaces
Polybutester (novafil)*	Monofilament	Good to fair	Poor	Low	Used when significant edema since high elasticity

*Not commonly used in dermatology

- Table below lists absorbable sutures [7, 15]

Suture	Configuration	Complete absorption	Ease of handle	Knot security	Tissue reactivity	Uses
Surgical gut (plain)	Virtually monofilament	70 days	Fair	Poor	Moderate—High (#1)	Rare
Surgical gut (chromic)	Virtually monofilament	90 days	Poor	Poor	Less than plain	Grafts, mucosa
Surgical gut (fast-absorbing)	Virtually monofilament	21–42 days	Fair	Poor	Low	Grafts, epidermal closure
Polyglycolic acid (Dexon)	Braided	90 days	Good	Good	Low	Subcutaneous closure, vessel ligation
Polyglactin 910 (Vicryl, Polysorb)	Braided	56–70 days	Good	Good	Low	Subcutaneous closure, vessel ligation

Suture	Configuration	Complete absorption	Ease of handle	Knot security	Tissue reactivity	Uses
Polydioxanone (PDS II)	Monofilament	180–240 days *longest*	Poor	Moderate	Low	Subcutaneous closure for high tension sites (i.e. trunk)
Polyglyconate (Maxon)	Monofilament	180 days	Fair	Good	Low	Subcutaneous closure for high tension sites
Poliglecaprone 25 (Monocryl)	Monofilament	90–120 days	Fair	Moderate	Minimal *least inflammatory*	Subcutaneous closure (NOT high tension sites)

Flap Basics [7, 15]

What Not To Miss

- Primary movement: motion of flap required to close primary defect
- Primary tension vector: tension vector that opposes primary movement of flap
- Secondary movement: movement of surrounding tissue in reaction to flap
- Flap survival is based on the preservation of the blood supply
  - In the case of random pattern flaps, depends on subdermal plexus
  - In the case of interpolation/axial flaps, depends on named arteries or their tributaries

Pearls

- Mnemonic STARTS represents basic reconstructive options [7, 15]
  - Simple closures, Transposition flaps, Advancement flaps, Rotation flaps, Tissue importation flaps and Skin grafts

In the Context Of …

- Complications
  - Post-operative bleeding and infection are most common in immediate post-operative period
    - Highest risk of bleeding in first 48 h
    - Post-operative infections tend to occur 4–8 days following surgery
  - Evacuation is required if a hematoma develops to prevent flap necrosis
  - Smoking increases risk of flap and graft necrosis

Incision and Drainage [15]

What Not To Miss

- Be mindful of regional anatomy
- Make a small incision over the point of greatest fluctuance

Pearls

- Local anesthesia is often less effective in infected tissues because of its low pH [15]
- Shield area when you make initial incision with gauze to prevent spraying of contents

In the Context Of…

- Previously removed cysts: may be surrounded by fibrotic scar

Post-operative Complications [1–3, 15, 19]

What Not To Miss

- Bleeding is most common complication [1–3]
  - Highest risk in the first 48 h following a procedure
  - Higher risk in patients on dual antiplatelet/anticoagulant agents
  - Also higher in patients taking new antiplatelet agents (i.e. clopidogrel) and novel oral anticoagulant agents (i.e. dabigatran, apixiban, rivaroxaban etc.)
  - Hematomas can lead to the terrible tetrad [18]
    - Hematoma → infection → dehiscence → necrosis
  - A large expanding hematoma requires immediate attention and removal of sutures to release tension
    - Expanding hematomas in the neck and periorbital region are considered medical emergencies
- Infection rate is overall low in dermatologic surgeries (0.1–2.29%) [15, 19]
  - Typically occur 4–8 days following procedure
  - Higher risk in clean-contaminated wounds
  - Higher risk if host has poor blood supply to surgical site
  - Hematomas are a growth medium for bacteria and increase risk of infection (see above)

Pearls

- To prevent dehiscence
  - o Avoid crushing tissue, excessive electrocautery, ineffective hemostasis, dead space in the wound, excessive wound tension and overly tight sutures

In the Context Of …

- Allergic reaction to suture material
  - o This is very rare
  - o Hypersensitivity to chromic catgut suture is the most common
  - o Patient's should be patch tested

References

1. Koenen W, Kunte C, Hatmann D. Prospective multicenter cohort study on 9154 surgical procedures to assess the risk of postoperative bleeding- a DESSI study. J Eur Acad Dermatol Venereol. 2017;31(4):724–31.
2. Eilers RE, Goldenberg A, Cowan NL. A retrospective assessment of postoperative bleeding complications in anticoaulated patients following Mohs micrographic surgery. Dermatol Surg. 2018;44(4):504–11.
3. Cook-Norris RH, Michaels JD, Weaver AL. Complications of cutaneous surgery in patients taking clopidogrel-containing anticoagulation. J Am Acad Dermatol. 2011;65(3):584–91. Rosengren H, Heal C, Smith S. Curr Derm Rep. 2012;1:55.
4. Brown DG, Wilkerson EC, Love WE. A review of traditional and novel oral anticoagulant and antiplatelet therapy for dermatologists and dermatologic surgeons. J Am Acad Dermatol. 2015;72(3):524–34.
5. Collins SC, Dufresne RG Jr. Dietary supplements in the setting of mohs surgery. Dermatol Surg. 2002;28:447–52.
6. Steinsapir KD, Woodward JA. Chlorhexidine keratitis: safety of chlorhexidine as a facial antiseptic. Dermatol Surg. 2017;43(1):1–6.
7. Bolognia Jean, Jorizzo Joseph L, Schaffer Julie V. Dermatology. Philadelphia: Elsevier Saunders; 2012. p. 2556–69.
8. Alikhan A, Hocker TL, Chavan R. Review of dermatology. Edinburgh: Elsevier; 2017.
9. Williamson DA, Carter GP, Howden BP. Current and emerging topical antibacterials and antiseptics: agents, action, and resistance patterns. Clin Microbiol Rev. 2017;30(3):827–60.
10. Kouba DJ, LoPiccolo MC, Alam M et al. Guidelines for the use of local anesthesia in office-based dermatologic surgery. J Am Acad Dermatol. 2016;74(6):1201–19.
11. Pavlidakey PG, Brodell EE, Helms SE. Diphenhydramie as an alternative local anesthetic agent. J Clin Aesthet Dermatol. 2009;2(10):37–40.
12. Sobanko JF, Miller CJ, Alster TS. Topical anesthetics for dermatologic procedures: a review. Derm Surg. 2012;1–13.
13. Ostad A, Kageyama N, Moy RL. Tumescent anesthesia with a lidocaine dose of 55 mg/kg is safe for liposuction. Dermatol Surg. 1996;22:921–7.
14. Nishimura RA, Otto CM, Bonow RO, Carabello BA, Erwin JP, 3rd, Fleisher LA, et al. 2017 AHA/ACC focused update of the 2014 AHA/ACC guideline for the management of patients with valvular heart disease: a report of American College of Cardiology/ American Heart Association Task Force on Clinical Practice Guidelines. Circulation. 2017.

15. Robinson JK, Hanke WC, Siegal DM, et al. Surgery of the skin, 3th ed. Philadelphia: Elsevier Saunders; 2015. p. 1–285 Print.
16. Oberlin, D, Porto DA, Lopiccolo M, Kohen LL. Modified purse-string closure: a lymphatic channel and tissue sparing technique for biopsy of suspicious pigmented lesions on extremities. J Am Acad Dermatol. 2018;S0190–9622(18):30347–5.
17. Kantor J. Atlas of suturing techniques: approaches to surgical wound, laceration, and cosmetic repair. New York: McGraw-Hill; 2016.
18. Hendi A. Surgical complications: the terrible tetrad, AAD Young Physician Focus, vol 6, No. 4, Winter 2007.
19. James WD, Berger TG, Elston DM. "Dermatologic Surgery" Andrews' Diseases of the Skin. Ed. John Updike, Ed. Katrina Kenison, vol. 37. Philadelphia: Elsevier Saunders; 2016. p. 874–900 Print.

Malignancy, Staging and Surgical Management

Chelsea Luther, Jesse Veenstra, Laurie L. Kohen and Molly Powers

Actinic Keratosis [1–8]

What Not To Miss

- SCC *in situ*
- Pigmented AKs are extremely difficult to differentiate from early lentigo maligna

Key DDx

- SCC *in situ*
- If pigmented, lentigo maligna
- Benign lichenoid keratosis

Treatment Ladder

- Cryotherapy for solitary lesions
- Field therapy [1, 2]
  - 5-Fluorouracil
    - 5-Fluorouracil 5% cream BID for 2–4 weeks—warn healing may not be evident for 1 to 2 months following treatment
    - 5-Fluorouracil 5% cream mixed with 0.005% calcipotriol ointment (1:1) BID for at least 4 days [3]

C. Luther · J. Veenstra · M. Powers
Department of Dermatology, Henry Ford Health System,
3031 West Grand Blvd,Suite 800, Detroit, MI 48202, USA

L. L. Kohen (✉)
Henry Ford Health System, 3031 West Grand, Blvd, Suite 800, Detroit, MI 48202, USA
e-mail: lkohen1@hfhs.org

© Springer Nature Switzerland AG 2020
H. W. Lim et al. (eds.), *Practical Guide to Dermatology*,
https://doi.org/10.1007/978-3-030-18015-7_4

- 5-Fluorouracil 0.5% cream daily for 1–4 weeks
- 5-Fluorouracil 1% cream BID for 2–6 weeks
- Generic topical 5-FU available as 0.5 or 5% cream or 2 or 5% solution
  - Imiquimod 5% cream nightly. Leave on for ~8 h, then remove with mild soap and water twice to three times weekly for 12–16 weeks
  - Ingenol mebutate 0.015% gel daily for 3 days for face and scalp or 0.05% gel daily for 2 days for trunk and extremities
  - Diclofenac 3% gel BID for 60–90 days
  - Photodynamic therapy (PDT). 2 treatments, about 4 weeks apart (see photo-therapy section for details)

Outside the Box Treatment Options

- Medium depth chemical peels with 35–50% TCA alone or at 35% + Jessner's solution, 70% glycolic acid, or solid CO_2 [4]
- Fractional CO_2 (70 mJ, 9 W, density 4) or Erbium-YAG (2.0 J, fluence of 10 J/cm^2) [5–8]

In the Context Of ...

- Multiple lesions:
  - Consider field therapy with treatment regimens listed above
- Pigmented actinic keratoses:
  - Need to utilize dermoscopy and clinical gestalt
  - Small lesions with gritty scale favor AKs; broader lesions without scale and dermoscopic features including annular-granular pattern, rhomboids or circle-within-a-circle (targets) would be concerning for lentigo maligna

SCC in Situ [9–15]

What Not To Miss

- Invasive SCC

Key DDx

- Superficial basal cell carcinoma
- Squamous cell carcinoma
- Psoriasis
- Actinic keratosis
- Inflamed or irritated seborrheic keratosis
- Benign lichenoid keratosis

Treatment Ladder

- Mohs: based on Mohs Appropriate Use Criteria (AUC) [9]
  - Location: head, neck, hands, feet, or anterior legs
  - Size >2 cm
  - Immunocompromised
  - PEARL: for full recommendations, please refer to the Mohs AUC at the end of this chapter
- Electrodessication and curettage [10]
- 5-Fluorouracil 5% cream BID for 4–8 weeks (may require 12 weeks) +/– occlusive dressing or with topical keratolytic agent (e.g. salicylic acid, lactic acid, ammonium lactate) or retinoic acid [11]
- Imiquimod 5% cream daily for 6–16 weeks [12]
- PDT
  - PDT with aminolevulinic acid or methylaminolevulinate gel or cream 3 h prior to illumination with broadband red light (75 J/cm^2, 570–670 nm). Repeat session 7 days later. [13]
    - PEARL: Recommend red light as it penetrates more deeply [14, 15]
- Cryotherapy
  - Tumor including ≥3 mm surrounding rim of normal-appearing skin for two freeze-thaw cycles of ten seconds [16]

Outside the Box

- Chemowraps (weekly 5-fluorouracil 5% cream under Unna wraps) [17]

Basal Cell Carcinoma [16–20]

What Not To Miss

- Approximately 70% of BCCs occur on the head and neck [18]—look for pearly or lucent quality, with small telangiectasias and a rolled edge or border
- Patients may believe that lesions on the lower extremity represent scars, areas of trauma or old insect bites
  - Dermoscopy may help elucidate superficial BCC from scar

Key DDx

- Trichoepithelioma (particularly desmoplastic)
- Bowen's disease
- Fibrous papule of the nose
- Scar
- Microcystic adnexal carcinoma

Treatment Ladder

- Principles of Treatment
  - The primary goals of treatment of BCCs are the complete removal of the tumor and the maximal preservation of function and cosmesis
  - Surgical approaches often offer the most effective and efficient means for accomplishing cure, but considerations of function, cosmesis, and patient preference may lead to choosing radiation therapy as primary treatment
    - Refer to appropriate use criteria (AUC) [19]. May use Mohs AUC app to help guide clinical judgment or refer to the AUC at the end of this chapter
- High risk:
  - Refer to Mohs
- Low risk:
  - Areas include trunk and extremities, excluding the pretibial surface, hands, feet, nail units, and ankles
  - If <2 cm, superficial type, lacks perineural invasion; primary lesion (not recurrent including other failed treatment options), low risk locations may consider [11]:
    - Imiquimod 5% cream 5 times weekly for 6 weeks
    - 5-Fluorouracil 5% cream BID for 3–6 weeks (may require 10–12 weeks)
    - PDT with pulse dye laser (PDL)
      - PDT as above, followed by 585-PDL (spot size = 7 mm, fluence = 10 J/cm^2, pulse duration = 10 ms, 10% overlap, three passes, and cooling) [20]
    - ED&C (see below)
    - Surgical excision [21]

Outside the Box Treatment Options

- If metastatic, locally advanced, or not a surgical or radiation candidate, may consider:
  - Vismodegib 150 mg daily until disease progression or unacceptable toxicity [22]
  - Sonidegib 200 mg daily until disease progression or unacceptable toxicity [23]
- Use of nicotinamide may be effective in reducing the development of BCCs.

NCCN Guidelines for Basal Cell Carcinoma [24]

- Risk Factors for Local Recurrence or Metastases
  - Location/Size
    - Size ≥20 mm in area L
    - Size ≥10 mm in area M
    - Any size in area H
  - Poorly defined borders
  - Recurrent lesion
  - Immunosuppression
  - Site of prior radiation or chronic inflammatory process

- Aggressive features: infiltrative, micronodular, morpheaform, basosquamous, sclerosing, or carcinosarcomatous differentiation
- Perineural involvement

Squamous Cell Carcinoma [17, 21, 22]

What Not To Miss

- Metastatic disease
  - SCC on the oral mucosa and lip carry much greater risk of metastases
  - For a complete list of risk factors for local recurrence or metastases, please refer to NCCN Guidelines for SCCs in the Staging and Surgical Management of Dermatologic Malignancies chapter
- Atypical presentation
  - Closely monitor burn scars, radiation sites, chronic wounds such as those with hidradenitis for risk of SCC formation
- High risk features (do not consider standard excision if any of these are present!):
  - ≥1 cm on the cheeks, forehead, scalp, neck, or pretibial; ≥0.6 cm on central face, eyelids, eyebrows, periorbital skin, nose, cutaneous or vermillion lip, chin, mandible, preauricular and postauricular skin, temple, and ear, genitalia, hands, and feet; recurrent tumors; location in chronic wound, scar, or previous site of radiation; neurologic symptoms; poorly differentiated; tumor thickness >2 mm; perineural invasion

Key DDx

- Actinic keratosis
- Bowen's disease
- Basal cell carcinoma
- Verruca vulgaris

Work Up Pearls

- History with full review of systems
- Physical exam including lymph node exam
- Biopsy

Treatment Ladder

- Principles of Treatment
  - Primary goals of treatment are complete removal of the tumor and the maximal preservation of function and cosmesis

- o Surgical approaches often offer the most effective and efficient means for accomplishing cure, but considerations of function, cosmesis, and patient preference may lead to choosing radiation therapy as primary treatment
- Refer to appropriate use criteria (AUC) [19]. May use Mohs AUC app to help guide clinical judgment or refer to the AUC at the end of this chapter
  - o High risk—Early and aggressive surgical excision with 6 mm margins
  - o Low risk—(NO high risk features, see below), can excise with 4 mm margins [25]
  - o If on the trunk or extremities and the only high-risk feature is size greater than 2 cm, can consider WLE with 1 cm margin
- To prevent recurrence in patients with multiple high-risk features (especially those that exhibit extensive perineural or large-nerve (>1 mm in diameter) involvement), can consider adjuvant radiation therapy (ART) with surgery [26]
- If locally advanced or non-surgical candidate, etc., may consider chemotherapy +/− radiation

Outside the Box Treatment Options

- If metastatic, locally advanced, or not a surgical or radiation candidate, may consider (in conjunction with oncology)
  - ■ Cetuximab IV: Initial loading dose: 400 mg/m^2, followed by maintenance dose: 250 mg/m^2 weekly until disease progression [27]
  - o Nivolumab 240 mg once every 2 weeks or 480 mg once every 4 weeks until disease progression or unacceptable toxicity [28]
  - o Pembrolizumab 200 mg IV once every 3 weeks until disease progression or unacceptable toxicity [29]

In the Context Of …

- Keratoacanthoma
  - o Solidary keratoacanthoma
    - ■ Surgical excision is the preferred treatment; can perform standard excision with 4 mm margins or refer to Mohs surgery [30]
    - ■ Alternate therapies
      - • ED&C [31]
      - • Intralesional methotrexate-injection of 1 mL of methotrexate in a concentration of 12.5 or 25 mg/mL every two to three weeks for one to four treatment sessions (until resolution) [32]
      - • Intralesional 5-FU undiluted in a concentration of 50 mg/mL on a weekly basis for three to eight treatment sessions [33]
  - o Multiple or giant keratoacanthomas
    - ■ Acitretin 25–60 mg per day [34]
    - ■ Isotretinoin 1.0–1.5 mg/kg per day [35]

- Multiple NMSC
  - Consider chemoprevention with nicotinamide 500 mg BID, or low dose acitretin, 10 mg daily
- Follow up
  - Patients with local disease: every 3–6 months for two years, then every 6–12 months for three years, then annually for life
  - Patients with regional disease: every 1–3 months for one year, then every 2–4 months for one year, then every 4–6 months for three years, then every 6–12 months for life
  - Patients with high-risk tumors should be taught how to perform self-lymph node examinations and complete these weekly for life.
- PEARL: Any LINEAR nail lesion, especially those treated as verruca with no response, must be biopsied to rule out Bowens/SCC

NCCN Guidelines for Squamous Cell Carcinoma [36]

- Risk Factors for Local Recurrence or Metastases
  - Location/Size
    - Size ≥20 mm in area L
    - Size ≥10 mm in area M
    - Any size in area H
  - Poorly defined borders
  - Recurrent lesion
  - Immunosuppression
  - Site of prior radiation or chronic inflammatory process
  - Rapid growth
  - Neurologic symptoms
  - Poorly differentiated
  - Depth > 6 mm or invasion beyond subcutaneous fat
  - Perineural, lymphatic, or vascular involvement
- Identification of High-risk Patients
  - Organ transplant patients or other settings of immunosuppression
  - Genetic conditions that predispose patients to the development of SCC
  - High number of total tumors
  - High frequency of developing tumors
  - Aggressive tumors (extension beyond cutaneous structures, perineural involvement, large and poorly differentiated, having ≥3 risk factors for recurrence)
- Sentinel Lymph Node Biopsy (SLNB) for SCC
  - SLNB has been used to try to identify patients who may be candidates for complete lymph node dissection or adjuvant RT/immunotherapy.
    - Sub-clinical nodal metastases have been identified in 7–21% of patients with high-risk SCC (most studies reporting rates between 12 and 17%)
    - It remains unclear if SLNB followed by complete lymph node dissection or adjuvant RT improves survival

Clinical Staging of Cutaneous SCC [37]

Stage	T	N	M	Clinical
I	T1	N0	M0	Tumor <2 cm in diameter
II	T2	N0	M0	Tumor 2-4 cm in diameter
III	T3	N0	M0	Tumor >4 cm in diameter or minor bone erosion or perineural invasion or deep invasion*
III	T1	N1	M0	
III	T2	N1	M0	Metastasis in a single ipsilateral lymph node, ≤3 cm and ENE–
III	T3	N1	M0	
IV	T1	N2	M0	Metastasis in a single ipsilateral node >3 cm but <6 cm and ENE–; or
IV	T2	N2	M0	Metastases in multiple ipsilateral lymph nodes (none >6 cm in
IV	T3	N2	M0	greatest dimension and ENE–); or In bilateral or contralateral lymph nodes (none >6 cm in greatest dimension and ENE–)
IV	Any T	N3	M0	Metastasis in a lymph node >6 cm in greatest dimension and ENE–; or Metastasis in any node(s) and clinically overt ENE+
IV	T4	Any N	M0	Tumor with gross cortical bone/marrow, skull base invasion and/or skull base foramen invasion
IV	Any T	Any N	M1	Distant metastases

* Deep invasion is defined as invasion beyond the subcutaneous fat or >6 mm; perineural invasion is defined as tumor cells within the nerve sheath of a nerve lying deeper than the dermis or measuring 0.1 mm or larger in caliber.

ENE: extranodal extension

Used with the permission of the American College of Surgeons. Amin, M.B., Edge, S.B., Greene, F.L., et al. (Eds.) AJCC Cancer Staging Manual. 8th Ed. Springer New York, 2017

Melanoma

What Not To Miss

- Nail Lesion
    - Biopsy any new or changing dark, solitary, irregular, >3 mm lesions that are wider proximally or have periungual pigmentation (Hutchinson's sign)
    - New onset single nail melanonychia in an adult must be scrutinized
    - Ethnic pigmentation and lentigines are more gray-brown in color, whereas nevi and melanoma are more brown or black
    - Dermoscopy can easily help diagnose subungual hemorrhage
    - DO NOT let a history of "trauma" to the nail dissuade from biopsy of suspicious lesion, as 25% of nail melanomas had a coincident history of recent trauma [38]

Work Up Pearls

- History including full review of systems
- Perform thorough exam including full skin exam and lymph node palpation
    - Teach patient to perform self-lymph node examinations to be completed weekly

- Consider obtaining 31-gene expression profiling (GEP) for invasive melanomas (dermatologist or pathologist to order), although this is not currently recommended by NCCN guidelines
- Biopsy
  - Initial biopsy should be complete full-thickness excisional biopsy with 1–3 mm margin to subcutaneous fat—can do punch or deep shave if lesion is small enough, but make sure deep enough (there is no pigment after biopsy) [39]
  - BIOPSY tips by SITE and dermoscopic features [40]:
    - Facial lesions concerning for lentigo maligna:
      - Do not PUNCH. If you believe the melanoma is not yet invasive, give the pathologist the most contiguous epidermis possible. Broad thin shave is best but may also perform multiple smaller shaves from same lesion representing dermoscopically heterogeneous areas
      - Features on dermoscopy that lesion is invasive: targets (circle-within-a-circle), follicles obliterated with pigment, heavy regression, shiny white structures
        - In these cases, excisional biopsy is best
    - Extra-facial lesions concerning for non-invasive lentigo maligna:
      - Broad thin shave is best
    - Acral lesions:
      - As with lentigo maligna, diagnosing acral melanoma requires context; thus, submitting more contiguous epidermis is the goal
      - A deep shave is acceptable for flat larger pigmented lesions on the hands or feet
        - PEARL: At our institution, we have found that, for flat lesions <8 mm or smaller, scoring the lesion with a punch tool to penetrate the thicker epidermis and then using a forceps to lift the edge allows for a more accurate and deeper saucerization with the blade
      - If most or all of the lesion fits into a punch tool, that may be preferred, as the depth will be captured—depends on ability to close the wound
      - In the case of larger lesions (>1.5 or 2 cm), where the clinical diagnosis is likely melanoma, incisional (punch) biopsy into the elevated or most dermoscopically concerning areas is acceptable as an attempt to obtain the true depth
        - If the depth is > or = 2 mm (even if transected at the base), then the lesion is stage T4 and would require maximal margins versus amputation depending on full staging and other parameters
    - Spitzoid lesions:
      - Radial peripheral streaks or double tier of peripheral globules *suggest* spitzoid architecture
      - Excisional or punch biopsy is preferred, as to allow the pathologist to evaluate the presence or absence of maturation at the base of the lesion

- Regressed lesions:
  - Heavy regression present clinically or on dermoscopy (grey-black peppering of dots, shiny white lines or scar-like areas) should be excised to fat so that the pathologist can evaluate for any tumor present beneath the lymphoid infiltrate
- Blue grey veil:
  - Lesions that are palpable and have features of nodular melanoma or larger tumor aggregates should be excised to fat
- Melanoma within pre-existing nevus:
  - Lesions that demonstrate benign-appearing areas of nevus should also be excised to fat in order for any deeper perifollicular melanocytes to be visualized as distinct from the adjacent melanoma in order to assess true depth

Treatment Ladder [41]

- MIS—0.5–1 cm margins
  - WLE to subcutaneous fat
- ≤1 mm (T1)—1 cm margin [42]
  - WLE to fascia
- >1 mm (T2, T3, T4)—2 cm margin [43]
  - WLE to fascia
- For melanomas on the head, neck, hands, feet, and genitalia, consider Mohs Surgery or staged excisions for complete margin assessment
- Clinically negative LNs
  - MIS or T1a ->No SLNB
  - T1b ->discuss SLNB with patient
  - T2a or higher ->do SLNB [44]
- Sentinel Lymph Node Biopsy (SNLB) for Melanoma [45]
  - Purpose:
    - To help determine prognosis
    - To help select patients who may benefit from adjuvant therapy or clinical trials
    - SLNB has NOT been shown to improve overall survival
  - Should be considered in patients with melanoma >0.8 mm or those <0.8 mm with ulceration, very high mitotic index, or lymphovascular invasion.
    - Not indicated for patients with a melanoma <0.8 mm and no other factors placing the patient at increased risk for nodal involvement (i.e. risk of a positive SLN <5%)
    - Patient's age (<40), low level of tumor-infiltrating lymphocytes, and location of tumor on the trunk or lower extremity may negatively impact metastasis risk and could warrant discussion regarding appropriateness of SLN biopsy [46].

- For those with a positive SLNB, consider clinical observation with ultrasound surveillance versus completion lymph node dissection (CLND).
  - CLND provides additional prognostic information as well as improvement in regional control/recurrence at the expense of increased morbidity.
  - CLND has fallen out of favor due to the results of the Multicenter Selective Lymphadenectomy Trial II (MSLT II) → may still be appropriate in head and neck tumors due to questionable validity of the trial for this subset of melanomas [47].
- Chemotherapy in conjunction with medical oncology for BRAF mutated or non-mutated melanoma as follows:
  - BRAF positive lesions
    - Vemurafenib 960 mg twice daily on days 1–28 of each 28-day cycle plus cobimetinib 60 mg once per day on days 1–21 of each 28-day cycle [48]
    - Dabrafenib 150 mg twice per day plus trametinib 2 mg once per day [49]
  - BRAF negative
    - Ipilimumab 3 mg/kg IV every three weeks for four doses [50]
    - Nivolumab 240 mg once every 2 weeks or 480 mg once every 4 weeks until disease progression or unacceptable toxicity [51]
    - Pembrolizumab 200 mg IV once every 3 weeks until disease progression or unacceptable toxicity [52]

Outside the Box Treatment Options

- Adjuvant radiation therapy (ART)—for head and neck melanomas if satisfactory margins cannot be achieved [53]
- For cutaneous metastatic lesions, consider metastectomy with MMS or excisions; referral for Talimogene laherparepvec (T-Vec)

In the Context Of …

- Lentigo maligna
  - Surgical excision (first line)—wide local excision with margins of at least 6–10 mm and staged excision with rush permanent sections ("slow Mohs") [54–56]
  - Traditional Mohs is an excellent choice at centers where MART-1 staining is routinely utilized and read by experts
  - Imiquimod 5% cream for patients who are not surgical candidates [56]

Melanoma TNM Staging [37, 57]

T CLASSIFICATION	THICKNESS (mm)	ULCERATION STATUS
T1	≤1.0	a: Breslow < 0.8 mm w/o ulceration b: Breslow 0.8-1.0 mm w/o ulceration or ≤ 1.0 mm w/ ulceration.
T2	1.1-2.0	a: w/o ulceration b: w/ ulceration
T3	2.1-4.0	a: w/o ulceration b: w/ ulceration
T4	>4.0	a: w/o ulceration b: w/ ulceration

Regional Lymph Nodes (N)

NX Patients in whom the regional nodes cannot be assessed (for example previously removed for another reason)

N0 No regional metastases detected

N1-3 Regional metastases based on the number of metastatic nodes, number of palpable metastatic nodes on clinical exam, and presence or absence of MSI[2]

NOTE: N1-3 and a-c subcategories assigned as shown below:

N CLASSIFICATION	# NODES	CLINICAL DETECTABILITY/MSI STATUS
N1	0-1 node	a: clinically occult[1], no MSI[2] b: clinically detected[1], no MSI[2] c: 0 nodes, MSI present[2]
N2	1-3 nodes	a: 2-3 nodes clinically occult[1], no MSI[2] b: 2-3 nodes clinically detected[1], no MSI[2] c: 1 node clinical or occult[1], MSI present[2]
N3	>1 nodes	a: >3 nodes, all clinically occult[1], no MSI[2] b: >3 nodes, ≥1 clinically detected[1] or matted, no MSI[2] c: >1 nodes clinical or occult[1], MSI present[2]

[1] Nodes are designated as clinically detectable if they can be palpated on physical exam and are confirmed melanoma following excision/biopsy.

[2] Microsatellite instability (MSI) comprise any satellite, locally recurrent, or in transit lesions.

Figure courtesy of Dr. Mike Gormally. Used with the permission of the American College of Surgeons. Amin, M.B., Edge, S.B., Greene, F.L., et al. (Eds.) AJCC Cancer Staging Manual. 8th Ed. Springer New York, 2017

| ANATOMIC STAGE/PROGNOSTIC GROUPS | | | | | | | |
Clinical Staging[1]				Pathologic Staging[2]			
Stage 0	Tis	N0	M0	0	Tis	N0	M0
Stage IA	T1a	N0	M0	IA	T1a	N0	M0
Stage IB	T1b	..	..		T1b	..	..
	T2a	..	..	IB	T2a	..	..
Stage IIA	T2b	N0	M0	IIA	T2b	M0	M0
	T3a	..	..		T2a	..	..
Stage IIB	T3b	..	..	IIB	T3b	..	..
	T4a	..	..		T4a	..	..
Stage IIC	T4b	..	..	IIC	T4b	..	..
Stage III	Any T	≥N1	M0	IIIA	T1-2a	N1a	M0
	..	..	..		T1-2a	N2a	..
	..	..	..	IIIB	T0	N1b-c	M0
	..	..	..		T1-2a	N1b-c	..
	..	..	..		T1-2a	N2b	..
	..	..	..		T2b-3a	N1a-2b	..
	..	..	..	IIIC	T0	N2b-c	M0
	..	..	..		T0	N3b-c	..
	..	..	..		T1a-3a	N2c-3c	..
	..	..	..		T3b-4a	Any N	..
	..	..	..		T4b	N1a-2c	..
	..	..	..	IIID	T4b	N3a-c	M0
Stage IV	Any T	Any N	M1	IV	Any T	Any N	M1

[1] Clinical staging includes microstaging of the primary melanoma and clinical/radiologic evaluation for metastases. By convention, it should be used after complete excision of the primary melanoma with clinical assessment for regional and distant metastases.

[2] Pathologic staging includes microstaging of the primary melanoma and pathologic information about the regional lymph nodes after partial or complete lymphadenectomy.

Figure courtesy of Dr. Mike Gormally. Used with the permission of the American College of Surgeons. Amin, M.B., Edge, S.B., Greene, F.L., et al. (Eds.) AJCC Cancer Staging Manual. 8th Ed. Springer New York, 2017

AJCC Eighth Edition Melanoma Pathologic Stage III Subgroups

N	T Category								
Category	T0	T1a	T1b	T2a	T2b	T3a	T3b	T4a	T4b
N1a	N/A	A	A	A	B	B	C	C	C
N1b	B	B	B	B	B	B	C	C	C
N1c	B	B	B	B	B	B	C	C	C
N2a	N/A	A	A	A	B	B	C	C	C
N2b	C	B	B	B	B	B	C	C	C
N2c	C	C	C	C	C	C	C	C	C
N3a	N/A	C	C	C	C	C	C	C	D
N3b	C	C	C	C	C	C	C	C	D
N3c	C	C	C	C	C	C	C	C	D

Legend	
A	Stage IIIA
B	Stage IIIB
C	Stage IIIC
D	Stage IIID

Adapted from Gershenwald et al. CA Cancer J Clin. 2017. Used with the permission of the American College of Surgeons. Amin, M.B., Edge, S.B., Greene, F.L., et al. (Eds.) AJCC Cancer Staging Manual. 8th Ed. Springer New York, 2017

Clinical Staging of Melanoma—Key Features [37]

Stage	T	N	M	Clinical
IA	T1a	N0	M0	≤0.8 mm w/o ulceration
IB	T1b	N0	M0	0.8-1.0 mm w/o ulceration or ≤1.0 mm w/ ulceration
	T2a	N0	M0	1-2 mm w/o ulceration
IIA	T3a	N0	M0	1-2 mm w/ ulceration
	T3b	N0	M0	2-4 mm w/o ulceration
IIB	T4a	N0	M0	2-4 mm w/ ulceration
	T4b	N0	M0	>4 mm w/o ulceration
IIC	T4b	N0	M0	>4 mm w/ ulceration
III	Any	≥N1	M0	Determined by occult nodes (w/SLNB) or clinically detected nodes
IV	Any	Any	M1	Spread to distant nodes or organs

Merkel Cell Carcinoma [58]

What Not To Miss

- This aggressive carcinoma favors older adults and presents as an asymptomatic solitary nodule usually on the head or neck

Key DDx

- Melanoma
- Lymphoma
- Metastatic carcinoma
- Atypical fibroxanthoma

- Dermatofibroma
- Pseudolymphoma
- Cutaneous lymphoid hyperplasia

Work Up Pearls

- Refer to tumor board
- History including full review of systems
- Perform thorough exam including full skin exam and lymph node palpation
  - Teach patient to perform self-lymph node examinations to be completed weekly
- Can consider baseline and post-treatment antibody titers to MCV (polyomavirus) to track treatment response
  - PEARL: Not officially recommended per NCCN guidelines yet

Treatment Ladder [59, 60]

- Biopsy-confirmed MCC without palpable lymph nodes on physical exam:
  - Refer patient for sentinel lymph node biopsy [60]
  - If negative SLNB → WLE with at least 1 to 2 cm margins
    - If unable to obtain these margins (anatomic location), consider ART [61]
- Biopsy-confirmed MCC with clinically palpable node:
  - Refer to surgical subspecialty for regional lymph node dissection [59]
- Follow up cutaneous skin exams
  - Every 3 months for two years, then every 4 months for two years and then every 6 months [51]

Outside the Box Treatment Options

- If locally advanced or non-surgical candidate
  - Radiation +/− chemotherapy or adjuvant immunotherapy
    - Pembrolizumab 2 mg/kg IV once every 3 weeks for two years or until complete response or unacceptable toxicity

In the Context Of …

- NCCN Guildelines for Excision [62]
  - Obtain histological negative margins when clinically feasible
  - Surgical margins should be balanced with morbidity of surgery
    - If appropriate, avoid delay in proceeding to radiation therapy
- Surgical Approach
  - Regardless of the surgical approach, sentinel lymph node biopsy (SLNB) should be performed at the time of definitive excision. Excision options include:

- ▪ Wide excision with 1–2 cm margins down to facia or pericranium when feasible
- ▪ Mohs surgery or complete circumferential peripheral and deep margin assessment, provided they do not interfere with SLNB
- Reconstruction
  - ○ Any reconstruction involving extensive undermining or tissue movement should be delayed until negative histologic margins are verified and SLNB is performed if indicated
  - ○ If adjuvant radiation therapy is planned, extensive tissue movement should be minimized, and closure should be chosen to allow for expeditious initiation of radiation therapy

Clinical Staging of Merkel Cell Carcinoma [37, 62]

Stage	T	N	M	Clinical
I	T1	N0	M0	Tumor ≤2 cm in diameter
IIA	T2-3	N0	M0	Tumor 2-5 cm in diameter (T2) or >5 cm (T3)
IIB	T4	N0	M0	Tumor invades fascia, muscle, cartilage, or bone
III	Any	N1-3	M0	Nodal involvement
IV	Any	Any	M1	Distant metastasis

Used with the permission of the American College of Surgeons. Amin, M.B., Edge, S.B., Greene, F.L., et al. (Eds.) AJCC Cancer Staging Manual. 8th Ed. Springer New York, 2017

Mycosis Fungoides

What Not To Miss

- Often requires multiple biopsies for definitive diagnosis; if there is strong suspicion may need to repeat biopsies with adequate sampling of epidermis

Key DDx

- Atopic dermatitis
- Small and large plaque parapsoriasis
- Chronic actinic dermatitis

Work Up Pearls

- History including full review of systems
- Physical examination
  - ○ Full skin examination
  - ○ Complete lymph node exam
  - ○ Abdominal exam (look for hepatosplenomegaly)

- Biopsy
- T-Cell gene rearrangement (dermatologist/dermatopathologist to order)
- Routine MF labs (surveillance or on systemic therapy):
  - CBC w/diff
  - CMP
  - LDH
  - +/− fasting lipids
  - TSH and free T4
    - PEARL: especially important if on bexarotene because it causes central hypothyroidism [63, 64]
- Special MF labs:
  - Sezary count
  - Peripheral flow cytometry
  - Peripheral T-cell gene rearrangement

Treatment Ladder

- Treatment based on extent of disease, which is determined by stage. Please refer to staging below for details

- IA, IIA
  - Topical
    - Corticosteroids
    - Nitrogen mustard (extremely expensive)
    - Bexarotene 1% gel (start daily, slowly increase to four times daily as tolerated, hold for 1 month before follow up visit) (extremely expensive)
    - Tazorac
    - Imiquimod 5% cream daily
    - Phototherapy—NBUVB or PUVA [65–70]

- IIB
  - Phototherapy—PUVA, NBUVB
  - Oral
    - Interferon
    - PO bexarotene 150–300 mg/m^2 daily
    - Photopheresis
    - Vorinostat
    - MTX +/− IFN [71, 72]
  - Other—total skin electron beam (TSEB) [73]

- IIIB, IVB
  - Chemotherapy
  - Photopheresis +/− IFN
  - TSEB
  - Pralatrexate (folate antagonist)
  - Romidepsin (histone deacetylase inhibitor)
  - Brentuximab [71, 72, 74–76]

- PEARL: Cyclosporine is contraindicated in MF→ transformation to more aggressive disease

Outside the Box Treatment Options

- Local radiation 8 Gray single fraction—can be effective at any stage for individual lesions [77]

In the Context Of …

- Pregnancy
  - Cannot use nitrogen mustard, bexarotene, tazorac, imiquimod, PUVA, TSEB, MTX, vorinostat, romidepsin, or chemotherapy
- Erythrodermic MF
  - Photopheresis
  - Alemtuzumab
    - PEARL: Also known as Campath. It is a CD56 monoclonal antibody—only appropriate for patients with erythrodermic MF

TNMB Classification and Staging [78, 79]

T (Skin)	
T1	Limited patch / plaque (<10% of BSA)
T2	Generalized patch /plaque (>10% of BSA)
T3	Tumors (>1 cm diameter)
T4	Generalized erythroderma (>80% BSA)
N (Nodes)	
N0	No clinically abnormal peripheral lymph nodes (LN)
N1	Clinically abnormal peripheral LN; histopathology Dutch Gr 1 or NCI LN 0-2
N2	Clinically abnormal peripheral LN; histopathology Dutch Gr 2 or NCI LN 3
N3	Clinically abnormal peripheral LN; histopathology Dutch Gr 3-4 or NCI LN 4
Nx	Clinically abnormal peripheral LN; histopathology not performed
M (Viscera)	
M0	No visceral involvement
M1	Visceral involvement
Mx	Abnormal visceral site; no histologic confirmation
B (Blood)	
B0	Absence of significant blood involvement: <5% of peripheral blood lymphocytes or <250/mcL are atypical (Sezary) cells or <15% CD4/CD26 or CD4/CD7 cells of total lymphocytes
B1	Low blood tumor burden: >5% of peripheral blood lymphocytes are atypical (Sezary) cells but <1000/mcL; or ≥15% CD4/CD26 or CD4/CD7 cells of total lymphocytes but doesn't meet criteria for B3
B2	High blood tumor burden: ≥1000/mcL Sezary cells (CD4/CD26 or CD4/CD7 cells on flow cytometry) or CD4/CD8 ratio ≥10:1 or CD4CD26 ≥30% or CD4CD7 ≥40%

Clinical Staging of Mycosis Fungoides [78]

Stage	T	N	M	B	Clinical
IA	T1	N0	M0	B0-1	Localized patch / plaque <10% BSA
IB	T2	N0	M0	B0-1	Diffuse patch / plaque >10% BSA
IIA	T1-2	N1-2	M0	B0-1	Patch / plaque and lymphadenopathy
IIB	T3	N0-2	M0	B0-1	Tumor
IIIA	T4	N0-2	M0	B0	Erythroderma
IIIB	T4	N0-2	M0	B1	Erythroderma and B1 Blood
IVA1	T1-4	N0-2	M0	B2	Leukemic disease (B2 Blood)
IVA2	T1-4	N3	M0	B0-2	Nodal disease
IVB	T1-4	N0-3	M1	B0-2	Metastatic disease
*Bold red color indicates key differences between stages					

Dermatofibrosarcoma Protuberans

What Not To Miss

- Deep fungal infection
  - Consider concomitant tissue culture with biopsy

Key DDx

- Keloid
- Hypertrophic scar
- Dermatofibroma
- Dermatomyofibroma
- Deep fungal infection

Work Up Pearls

- History including full review of systems
- Physical examination including complete lymph node examination
- Biopsy
- In certain lesions (particularly large or recurrent tumors), MRI to assess depth of infiltration
- Evaluation for the t(17;22) translocation should be performed prior to initiating therapy

Treatment Ladder

- Complete resection with pathologically negative margins.
  - Mohs—either traditional or slow Mohs using CD34 immunostaining → lowest recurrence rate (about 1%) [80].
  - Wide local excision: NCCN recommends margins of 2–4 cm to the investing fascia of muscle or pericranium with clear pathologic negative margins

Outside the Box Treatment Options

- Radiation therapy—for unresectable tumors, recurrent tumors, postoperatively for positive surgical margins when further surgery is not possible or as adjuvant to prevent the rate of local recurrence [81]

In the Context Of ...

- t(17;22)-positive tumors
  - Imatinib mesylate, an oral tyrosine kinase inhibitor, for t(17;22)-positive unresectable, recurrent or metastatic lesions at 800 mg daily [82]

Quick Reference for Recommended Surgical Margins of Common Lesions

- Low-risk Basal Cell Carcinoma = 4 mm [83]
  - Mohs surgery recommended for high-risk BCC (see below)
- Low-risk Squamous Cell Carcinoma in situ (Bowen's Disease) = 4–5 mm [84]
- SCC < 2 cm in diameter and well differentiated in low-risk areas (see below) = 4–6 mm [85]
- SCC > 2 cm in diameter or high-risk lesions (see SCC risk factors) = Mohs or 6 mm with complete margin assessment [85]
- Melanoma [45, 55]
  - In situ = 0.6–1.0 cm
  - ≤1.0 mm = 1 cm
  - 1.01–2.0 mm = 1–2 cm
  - >2 mm = 2 cm

- Moderate to severely atypical nevi = clear margins
  - For severely atypical nevi that are clinically concerning or in a high-risk patient → 5 mm margin re-excision would be appropriate
- Atypical Spitz tumor = 0.5–1 cm [86]

AAD 2012 Mohs Appropriate Use Criteria [87]

	Appropriate	Uncertain	Inappropriate
Area H - mask areas of the face, ears, genitalia, nipples, hands, feet, and ankles			
BCC	Primary or recurrent: - Any type		
SCC	Primary or recurrent: - Any type except AK with focal SCCis		Primary or recurrent: - AK with focal SCCis
MIS and LM	Any		
Area M - cheeks, forehead, scalp, neck, jawline, and pretibial surface			
BCC	Primary or recurrent: - Aggressive - Nodular - Superficial (IC) Primary: - Superficial $\geq$0.6 cm	Primary: - Superficial $\leq$0.5 cm	
SCC	Primary or recurrent: - Any type except AK with focal SCCis		Primary or recurrent: - AK with focal SCCis
MIS and LM	Any		
Area L - trunk and extremities (excluding nipples, hands, feet, pretibial surfaces, and ankles)			
BCC	Recurrent: - Aggressive - Nodular Primary: - Aggressive $\geq$0.6 cm - Nodular >2 cm - Nodular $\geq$1.1 cm (IC)	Primary: - Aggressive $\leq$0.5 cm - Nodular 1.1-2 cm - Nodular 0.6-1 cm (IC) - Superficial $\geq$1.1 cm (IC)	Recurrent: - Superficial Primary: - Nodular $\leq$1 cm - Nodular $\leq$0.5 cm (IC) - Superficial - Superficial $\leq$1 cm (IC)
SCC	Primary or recurrent: - Aggressive Recurrent: - KA type SCC - Nonaggressive Primary >2 cm: - Nonaggressive - SCCis Primary $\geq$1.1 cm: - Nonaggressive or SCCis (IC) - KA type SCC KA type SCC $\geq$0.6 cm (IC)	Recurrent: - SCCis Primary 1.1-2 cm: - Nonaggressive - SCCis Primary $\leq$1 cm: - Nonaggressive (IC) Primary 0.6-1 cm: - Nonaggressive (IC) Primary $\leq$0.5 cm: - KA type SCC (IC)	Primary or recurrent: - AK with focal SCCis Primary $\leq$1 cm: - Nonaggressive - KA type SCC - SCCis Primary $\leq$0.5 cm: - SCCis (IC)
MIS and LM	Recurrent	Primary	

Listed indications are for both healthy and immunocompromised (IC) patients, and tumors of any size unless otherwise specified.

AK, Actinic keratosis; KA, keratoacanthoma; LM, lentigo maligna; MIS, melanoma in situ; SCCis, squamous cell carcinoma in situ.

Adapted from the American Academy of Dermatology 2012 appropriate use criteria for Mohs micrographic surgery.

Mohs Appropriate Use Criteria Treatment Areas

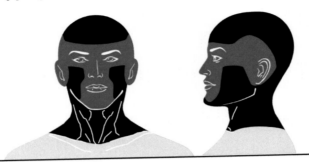

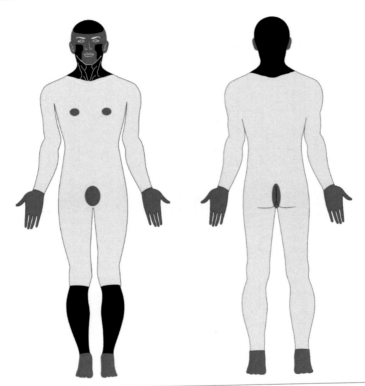

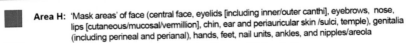

Area H: 'Mask areas' of face (central face, eyelids [including inner/outer canthi], eyebrows, nose, lips [cutaneous/mucosal/vermillion], chin, ear and periauricular skin /sulci, temple), genitalia (including perineal and perianal), hands, feet, nail units, ankles, and nipples/areola

Area M: Cheeks, forehead, scalp, neck, jawline, pre-tibial surface

Area L: Trunk and extremities (excluding pre-tibial surface, hands, feet, nail units and ankles)

Aggressive features for BCC [87]

- Morpheaform/fibrosing/sclerosing
- Infiltrating
- Perineural
- Metatypical/keratotic
- Micronodular

Aggressive features for SCC [87]

- Sclerosing
- Basosquamous (excluding keratotic BCC)
- Small cell
- Poorly or undifferentiated (characterized by a high degree of nuclear polymorphism, high mitotic rate, or low degree of keratinization)
- Perineural/perivascular
- Spindle cell
- Pagetoid
- Infiltrating
- Keratoacanthoma (KA) type: central facial
- Clear cell
- Lymphoepithelial
- Sarcomatoid
- Breslow depth 2 mm or greater
- Clark level IV or greater

Other high-risk considerations [87]

- Prior radiated skin
- Traumatic scar
- Area of osteomyelitis
- Area of chronic inflammation/ulceration
- Patients with genetic syndromes
- Immunocompromised patients
  - Organ or bone marrow transplant recipients
  - HIV
  - Select malignancies (lymphoma, leukemia), use of chemotherapy
  - Congenital or acquired immunodeficiencies
  - Use of TNFα inhibitors

Appropriate Use Criteria for Other Cutaneous Malignancies [12]

Cancer type	Area H	Area M	Area L
Adenocystic carcinoma	A (9)	A (8)	A (7)
Adnexal carcinoma	A (9)	A (8)	A (7)
Apocrine/eccrine carcinoma	A (8)	A (8)	A (8)
Angiosarcoma	U (5)	U (5)	U (5)
Atypical fibroxanthoma A	(9)	A (8)	A (7)
Bowenoid papulosis	I (3)	NA	NA
Dermatofibrosarcoma protuberans	A (9)	A (9)	A (9)
Desmoplastic trichoepithelioma	U (6)	U (5)	I (3)
Extramammary Paget disease	A (8)	A (8)	A (7)
Leiomyosarcoma	A (8)	A (8)	A (7)
Undifferentiated pleomorphic sarcoma	A (8)	A (8)	A (7)
Merkel cell carcinoma	A (8)	A (7)	U (5)
Microcystic adnexal carcinoma	A (9)	A (9)	A (8)
Mucinous carcinoma	A (8)	A (8)	A (7)
Sebaceous carcinoma	A (9)	A (8)	A (7)

Appropriate indications (A; scores 7-9) are colored green; Uncertain indications (U; scores 4-6) are colored yellow; Inappropriate indications (I; scores 1-3) are colored red. All lesions primary or recurrent in healthy or immunocompromised patients.
Adapted from the American Academy of Dermatology 2012 appropriate use criteria for Mohs micrographic surgery.

References

1. Gupta AK, et al. Interventions for actinic keratoses. Cochrane Database Syst Rev. 2012;12:CD004415.
2. Ceilley RI, Jorizzo JL. Current issues in the management of actinic keratosis. J Am Acad Dermatol. 2013;68(1 Suppl 1):S28–38.
3. Cunningham TJ, et al. Randomized trial of calcipotriol combined with 5-fluorouracil for skin cancer precursor immunotherapy. J Clin Invest. 2017;127(1):106–16.
4. Monheit GD. Medium-depth chemical peels. Dermatol Clin. 2001;19(3):413–25. vii.
5. Hantash BM, et al. Facial resurfacing for nonmelanoma skin cancer prophylaxis. Arch Dermatol. 2006;142(8):976–82.
6. Ostertag JU, et al. A clinical comparison and long-term follow-up of topical 5-fluorouracil versus laser resurfacing in the treatment of widespread actinic keratoses. Lasers Surg Med. 2006;38(8):731–9.
7. Jiang SB, et al. Er:YAG laser for the treatment of actinic keratoses. Dermatol Surg. 2000;26(5):437–40.
8. Gan SD, et al. Ablative fractional laser therapy for the treatment of actinic keratosis: a split-face study. J Am Acad Dermatol. 2016;74(2):387–9.
9. Ad Hoc Task F, et al. AAD/ACMS/ASDSA/ASMS 2012 appropriate use criteria for Mohs micrographic surgery: a report of the American Academy of Dermatology, American College of Mohs Surgery, American Society for Dermatologic Surgery Association, and the American Society for Mohs Surgery. J Am Acad Dermatol. 2012;67(4):531–50.
10. Lansbury L, et al. Interventions for non-metastatic squamous cell carcinoma of the skin: systematic review and pooled analysis of observational studies. BMJ. 2013;347:f6153.
11. Love WE, Bernhard JD, Bordeaux JS. Topical imiquimod or fluorouracil therapy for basal and squamous cell carcinoma: a systematic review. Arch Dermatol. 2009;145(12):1431–8.

12. Mackenzie-Wood A, et al. Imiquimod 5% cream in the treatment of Bowen's disease. J Am Acad Dermatol. 2001;44(3):462–70.

13. Morton C, et al. Comparison of topical methyl aminolevulinate photodynamic therapy with cryotherapy or Fluorouracil for treatment of squamous cell carcinoma in situ: results of a multicenter randomized trial. Arch Dermatol. 2006;142(6):729–35.

14. Morton CA, et al. European guidelines for topical photodynamic therapy part 1: treatment delivery and current indications-actinic keratoses, Bowen's disease, basal cell carcinoma. J Eur Acad Dermatol Venereol. 2013;27(5):536–44.

15. Zaar O, et al. Effectiveness of photodynamic therapy in Bowen's disease: a retrospective observational study in 423 lesions. J Eur Acad Dermatol Venereol. 2017;31(8):1289–94.

16. Holt PJ. Cryotherapy for skin cancer: results over a 5-year period using liquid nitrogen spray cryosurgery. Br J Dermatol. 1988;119(2):231–40.

17. Mann M, Berk DR, Petersen J. Chemowraps as an adjuvant to surgery for patients with diffuse squamous cell carcinoma of the extremities. J Drugs Dermatol. 2008;7(7):685–8.

18. Chew YK, et al. The use of paramedian forehead flap reconstruction after wide excision of basal cell carcinoma of the nose. Med J Malaysia. 2008;63(4):339–40.

19. Stuart SE, et al. Tumor recurrence of keratinocyte carcinomas judged appropriate for Mohs micrographic surgery using Appropriate Use Criteria. J Am Acad Dermatol. 2017;76(6):1131–1138.e1.

20. Carija A, et al. Single treatment of low-risk basal cell carcinomas with pulsed dye laser-mediated photodynamic therapy (PDL-PDT) compared with photodynamic therapy (PDT): a controlled, investigator-blinded, intra-individual prospective study. Photodiagnosis Photodyn Ther. 2016;16:60–5.

21. Miller SJ, et al. Basal cell and squamous cell skin cancers. J Natl Compr Canc Netw. 2010;8(8):836–64.

22. Basset-Seguin N, et al. Vismodegib in patients with advanced basal cell carcinoma: primary analysis of STEVIE, an international, open-label trial. Eur J Cancer. 2017;86:334–48.

23. Dummer R, et al. The 12-month analysis from Basal Cell Carcinoma Outcomes with LDE225 Treatment (BOLT): a phase II, randomized, double-blind study of sonidegib in patients with advanced basal cell carcinoma. J Am Acad Dermatol. 2016;75(1):113–25. e5.

24. NCCN Guidelines Basal Cell Skin Cancer. National comprehensive cancer network. Version 1; 2019.

25. Brodland DG, Zitelli JA. Surgical margins for excision of primary cutaneous squamous cell carcinoma. J Am Acad Dermatol. 1992;27(2 Pt 1):241–8.

26. Veness MJ, et al. Cutaneous head and neck squamous cell carcinoma metastatic to parotid and cervical lymph nodes. Head Neck. 2007;29(7):621–31.

27. Reigneau M, et al. Efficacy of neoadjuvant cetuximab alone or with platinum salt for the treatment of unresectable advanced nonmetastatic cutaneous squamous cell carcinomas. Br J Dermatol. 2015;173(2):527–34.

28. Ferris RL, et al. Nivolumab for recurrent squamous-cell carcinoma of the head and neck. N Engl J Med. 2016;375(19):1856–67.

29. Mehra R, et al. Efficacy and safety of pembrolizumab in recurrent/metastatic head and neck squamous cell carcinoma: pooled analyses after long-term follow-up in KEYNOTE-012. Br J Cancer. 2018;119(2):153–9.

30. Garcia-Zuazaga J, Ke M, Lee P. Giant keratoacanthoma of the upper extremity treated with mohs micrographic surgery: a case report and review of current treatment modalities. J Clin Aesthet Dermatol. 2009;2(8):22–5.

31. Kingman J, Callen JP. Keratoacanthoma. A clinical study. Arch Dermatol. 1984;120(6):736–40.

32. Annest NM, et al. Intralesional methotrexate treatment for keratoacanthoma tumors: a retrospective study and review of the literature. J Am Acad Dermatol. 2007;56(6):989–93.

33. Goette DK, Odom RB. Successful treatment of keratoacanthoma with intralesional fluorouracil. J Am Acad Dermatol. 1980;2(3):212–6.

34. Robertson SJ, et al. Severe exacerbation of multiple self-healing squamous epithelioma (Ferguson-Smith disease) with radiotherapy, which was successfully treated with acitretin. Clin Exp Dermatol. 2010;35(4):e100–2.
35. Vandergriff T, Nakamura K, High WA. Generalized eruptive keratoacanthomas of Grzybowski treated with isotretinoin. J Drugs Dermatol. 2008;7(11):1069–71.
36. NCCN Guidelines Squamous Cell Skin Cancer. National comprehensive cancer network. Version 2; 2019.
37. Amin MB, American Joint Committee on Cancer., American Cancer Society. AJCC cancer staging manual. Eight edition/editor-in-chief, Mahul B. Amin, MD, FCAP; editors, Stephen B. Edge, MD, FACS and 16 others; Donna M. Gress, RHIT, CTR-Technical editor; Laura R. Meyer, CAPM-Managing editor. ed. Chicago IL: American Joint Committee on Cancer, Springer; 2017. p. 1024. xvii.
38. Dunphy L, et al. Missed opportunity to diagnose subungual melanoma: potential pitfalls! BMJ Case Rep. 2017;2017.
39. Sober AJ, et al. Guidelines of care for primary cutaneous melanoma. J Am Acad Dermatol. 2001;45(4):579–86.
40. Elston DM. Management of atypical pigmented lesions. J Am Acad Dermatol. 2014;70(1):142–5.
41. Amin MB, et al. The eighth edition AJCC cancer staging manual: continuing to build a bridge from a population-based to a more "personalized" approach to cancer staging. CA Cancer J Clin. 2017;67(2):93–9.
42. Veronesi U, Cascinelli N. Narrow excision (1-cm margin). A safe procedure for thin cutaneous melanoma. Arch Surg. 1991;126(4):438–41.
43. Gillgren P, et al. 2-cm versus 4-cm surgical excision margins for primary cutaneous melanoma thicker than 2 mm: a randomised, multicentre trial. Lancet. 2011;378(9803):1635–42.
44. Morton DL, et al. Final trial report of sentinel-node biopsy versus nodal observation in melanoma. N Engl J Med. 2014;370(7):599–609.
45. NCCN Guidelines Melanoma. National comprehensive cancer network. 2018; Version 1; 2019.
46. Aloia TA, Gershenwald JE, Andtbacka RH, Johnson MM, Schacherer CW, Ng CS, et al. Utility of computed tomography and magnetic resonance imaging staging before completion lymphadenectomy in patients with sentinel lymph node-positive melanoma. J Clin Oncol. 2006;24(18):2858–65.
47. Faries MB, Thompson JF, Cochran AJ, Andtbacka RH, Mozzillo N, Zager JS, et al. Completion dissection or observation for sentinel-node metastasis in melanoma. N Engl J Med. 2017;376(23):2211–22.
48. Ascierto PA, et al. Cobimetinib combined with vemurafenib in advanced BRAF(V600)-mutant melanoma (coBRIM): updated efficacy results from a randomised, double-blind, phase 3 trial. Lancet Oncol. 2016;17(9):1248–60.
49. Long GV, et al. Dabrafenib and trametinib versus dabrafenib and placebo for Val600 BRAF-mutant melanoma: a multicentre, double-blind, phase 3 randomised controlled trial. Lancet. 2015;386(9992):444–51.
50. Hodi FS, et al. Improved survival with ipilimumab in patients with metastatic melanoma. N Engl J Med. 2010;363(8):711–23.
51. Robert C, et al. Nivolumab in previously untreated melanoma without BRAF mutation. N Engl J Med. 2015;372(4):320–30.
52. Eggermont AMM, et al. Adjuvant Pembrolizumab versus Placebo in Resected Stage III Melanoma. N Engl J Med. 2018;378(19):1789–801.
53. Bonnen MD, et al. Elective radiotherapy provides regional control for patients with cutaneous melanoma of the head and neck. Cancer. 2004;100(2):383–9.
54. Huilgol SC, et al. Surgical margins for lentigo maligna and lentigo maligna melanoma: the technique of mapped serial excision. Arch Dermatol. 2004;140(9):1087–92.
55. Kunishige JH, Brodland DG, Zitelli JA. Surgical margins for melanoma in situ. J Am Acad Dermatol. 2012;66(3):438–44.

56. Hazan C, et al. Staged excision for lentigo maligna and lentigo maligna melanoma: a retrospective analysis of 117 cases. J Am Acad Dermatol. 2008;58(1):142–8.
57. Gershenwald JE, Scolyer RA, Hess KR, Sondak VK, Long GV, Ross MI, et al. Melanoma staging: evidence-based changes in the American Joint Committee on Cancer eighth edition cancer staging manual. CA Cancer J Clin. 2017;67(6):472–92.
58. Harms KL, et al. Analysis of prognostic factors from 9387 merkel cell carcinoma cases forms the basis for the new 8th edition AJCC staging system. Ann Surg Oncol. 2016;23(11):3564–71.
59. Fang LC, et al. Radiation monotherapy as regional treatment for lymph node-positive Merkel cell carcinoma. Cancer. 2010;116(7):1783–90.
60. Howle JR, et al. Merkel cell carcinoma: an Australian perspective and the importance of addressing the regional lymph nodes in clinically node-negative patients. J Am Acad Dermatol. 2012;67(1):33–40.
61. Harrington C, Kwan W. Outcomes of Merkel cell carcinoma treated with radiotherapy without radical surgical excision. Ann Surg Oncol. 2014;21(11):3401–5.
62. NCCN Guidelines Merkel Cell Carcinoma. National comprehensive cancer network. Version 1; 2019.
63. Abbott RA, et al. Bexarotene therapy for mycosis fungoides and Sezary syndrome. Br J Dermatol. 2009;160(6):1299–307.
64. Scarisbrick JJ, et al. U.K. consensus statement on safe clinical prescribing of bexarotene for patients with cutaneous T-cell lymphoma. Br J Dermatol. 2013;168(1):192–200.
65. Zackheim HS. Treatment of patch-stage mycosis fungoides with topical corticosteroids. Dermatol Ther. 2003;16(4):283–7.
66. Kim YH, et al. Topical nitrogen mustard in the management of mycosis fungoides: update of the Stanford experience. Arch Dermatol. 2003;139(2):165–73.
67. Ramsay DL, Meller JA, Zackheim HS. Topical treatment of early cutaneous T-cell lymphoma. Hematol Oncol Clin North Am. 1995;9(5):1031–56.
68. Heald P, et al. Topical bexarotene therapy for patients with refractory or persistent early-stage cutaneous T-cell lymphoma: results of the phase III clinical trial. J Am Acad Dermatol. 2003;49(5):801–15.
69. Apisarnthanarax N, et al. Tazarotene 0.1% gel for refractory mycosis fungoides lesions: an open-label pilot study. J Am Acad Dermatol. 2004;50(4):600–7.
70. Deeths MJ, et al. Treatment of patch and plaque stage mycosis fungoides with imiquimod 5% cream. J Am Acad Dermatol. 2005;52(2):275–80.
71. Wilcox RA. Cutaneous T-cell lymphoma: 2016 update on diagnosis, risk-stratification, and management. Am J Hematol. 2016;91(1):151–65.
72. Jawed SI, et al. Primary cutaneous T-cell lymphoma (mycosis fungoides and Sezary syndrome): part II. Prognosis, management, and future directions. J Am Acad Dermatol. 2014;70(2):223. e1–17; quiz 240–2.
73. Jones GW, et al. Total skin electron radiation in the management of mycosis fungoides: consensus of the European Organization for Research and Treatment of Cancer (EORTC) Cutaneous Lymphoma Project Group. J Am Acad Dermatol. 2002;47(3):364–70.
74. Olsen EA, et al. Guidelines for phototherapy of mycosis fungoides and Sezary syndrome: a consensus statement of the United States Cutaneous Lymphoma Consortium. J Am Acad Dermatol. 2016;74(1):27–58.
75. Horwitz SM, et al. Identification of an active, well-tolerated dose of pralatrexate in patients with relapsed or refractory cutaneous T-cell lymphoma. Blood. 2012;119(18):4115–22.
76. Watanabe R, et al. Alemtuzumab therapy for leukemic cutaneous T-cell lymphoma: diffuse erythema as a positive predictor of complete remission. JAMA Dermatol. 2014;150(7):776–9.
77. Thomas TO, et al. Outcome of patients treated with a single-fraction dose of palliative radiation for cutaneous T-cell lymphoma. Int J Radiat Oncol Biol Phys. 2013;85(3):747–53.
78. Galper SL, Smith BD, Wilson LD. Diagnosis and management of mycosis fungoides. Oncology (Williston Park). 2010;24(6):491–501.

79. NCCN Guidelines Mycosis Fungoides/Sezary Syndrome. National comprehensive cancer network. Version 5; 2018.
80. Foroozan M, et al. Efficacy of Mohs micrographic surgery for the treatment of dermatofibrosarcoma protuberans: systematic review. Arch Dermatol. 2012;148(9):1055–63.
81. Dagan R, et al. Radiotherapy in the treatment of dermatofibrosarcoma protuberans. Am J Clin Oncol. 2005;28(6):537–9.
82. McArthur GA, et al. Molecular and clinical analysis of locally advanced dermatofibrosarcoma protuberans treated with imatinib: Imatinib Target Exploration Consortium Study B2225. J Clin Oncol. 2005;23(4):866–73.
83. Work G, Invited R, Kim JYS, Kozlow JH, Mittal B, Moyer J, et al. Guidelines of care for the management of basal cell carcinoma. J Am Acad Dermatol. 2018;78(3):540–59.
84. Westers-Attema A, van den Heijkant F, Lohman BG, Nelemans PJ, Winnepenninckx V, Kelleners-Smeets NW, et al. Bowen's disease: a six-year retrospective study of treatment with emphasis on resection margins. Acta Derm Venereol. 2014;94(4):431–5.
85. Work G, Invited R, Kim JYS, Kozlow JH, Mittal B, Moyer J, et al. Guidelines of care for the management of cutaneous squamous cell carcinoma. J Am Acad Dermatol. 2018;78(3):560–78.
86. Murphy ME, Boyer JD, Stashower ME, Zitelli JA. The surgical management of Spitz nevi. Dermatol Surg. 2002;28(11):1065–9. discussion 9.
87. American Academy of D, American College of Mohs S, American Society for Dermatologic Surgery A, American Society for Mohs S, Ad Hoc Task F, Connolly SM, et al. AAD/ACMS/ASDSA/ASMS 2012 appropriate use criteria for Mohs micrographic surgery: a report of the American Academy of Dermatology, American College of Mohs Surgery, American Society for Dermatologic Surgery Association, and the American Society for Mohs Surgery. Dermatol Surg. 2012;38(10):1582–603.

Cosmetics and Lasers

Caitlin Farmer, Matteo Lopiccolo and Alison T. Boucher

Neuromodulators

- FDA-approved for temporary improvement in the appearance of glabellar lines and lateral canthi lines [1]
- FDA-approved for axillary hyperhidrosis [1]
- Effect typically lasts about 3 months, and may take up to 1 week to demonstrate full effect, but duration of effect can vary based on patient and location of injection [1]
- *Available brands and conversion ratios*
  - 1 Botox unit = 1 Xeomin unit = approximately 2.5–3 Dysport units
- *Reconstitution strategies*
  - Botox/Xeomin 100 U vial + 2.5 ml bacteriostatic 0.9% saline = 4 U/0.1 cc
    - For axillary hyperhidrosis, dilute 100U in 4 mL instead, then inject 2 mL per axilla
  - Dysport 300 units + 3 ml bacteriostatic saline = 10U/0.1 cc = approximately 4 units of Botox/0.1 cc

---

The original version of this chapter was revised: The first author's name has been corrected. The correction to this chapter is available at https:// doi.org/10.1007/978-3-030-18015-7_15

C. Farmer · M. Lopiccolo · A. T. Boucher (✉)
Department of Dermatology, Henry Ford Health System,
3031 West Grand Blvd, Suite 800, Detroit, MI 48202, USA
e-mail: atisack1@hfhs.org

© Springer Nature Switzerland AG 2020
H. W. Lim et al. (eds.), *Practical Guide to Dermatology*,
https://doi.org/10.1007/978-3-030-18015-7_5

Botox or Xeomin 100 U vial		Botox or Xeomin 50 U vial		Dysport 300 U vial	
Diluent added	Units/1 mL	Diluent added	Units/1 mL	Diluent added	Units/1 mL
2 mL	5 units	1 mL	5 units	2.5 mL	12 units
2.5 mL	4 units	1.25 mL	4 units	3 mL	10 units
4 mL	2.5 units	2 mL	2.5 units		
5 mL	2 units				

- *Injection technique*
  - Use 31 gauge BD insulin syringes (0.3 cc) or 1 cc syringes
  - Injecting through follicular ostia may decrease pain
  - Always remember that rhytides are perpendicular to muscle fibers
  - Injections should be placed intramuscularly or in the superficial dermis depending on the thickness of the targeted muscle [1]
- *Injection dosing/site/technique based on anatomic location and desired effect:*

Upper Face

	Number of injection points	Units per point starting dose		Anatomic Landmarks
		Botox	Dysport	
Glabellar lines [1, 2]	3–5	12–30 units	30–50 units	0.5–1 cm from the upper orbital rim and internal to the mid-pupillary lines
Horizontal forehead lines [1, 2]	4–8	4–20 units	10–60 units	Under the hairline, V-shape in women and straight in men, if applicable
Crow's feet [1, 2]	1–5 per side	12–30 units	20–60 units	External part of the orbicularis oculi, 1–2 cm from the external orbital rim
Lateral eyebrow lift [1, 2]	2 per side	12–16 units	20–40 units	One point at each eyebrow tail, and the other at the external part of the frontalis

Lower Face

	Number of injection points	Units per point starting dose		Anatomic Landmarks
		Botox	Dysport	
Bunny lines [1, 2]	1 per side	1–2 units	5–10 units	1 cm above the upper lateral nostril
Perioral rhytides [1, 2]	1–2 per upper lip side and 1 per lower lip side	1–2 units	1–2 units	Vermillion border (<5 mm superiorly), philtrum (>1 mm laterally), mouth corners (>1.5 cm medially)

	Number of injection points	Units per point starting dose		Anatomic Landmarks
		Botox	Dysport	
Downturned smile [1, 2]	1 per side	2–5 units	5–10 units	1 cm lateral to oral commissure at level of angle of the mandible
Gingival smile [1, 2]	1 per side	2.5 units	2.5–5 units	Lateral nasal ala
Mental crease [3]	1–3	3–5 units per mentalis band	7–10 units	Mentalis muscle at the bony mentum
Peau D'Orange Chin [3]	1 centrally	5–10 units	10–20 units	Mentalis muscle at the prominence of the chin
Platysmal bands [1, 2]	Maximum of 10 points per side	0.5–2.5 units	5–10 units (maximum dose 100 total)	Jaw line for the superior-most injection. Continue inferiorly to the mid-band
Masseter hypertrophy [1, 2]	1–3 per side	5–10 units	10–20 units	Have patient clench jaw. 3 injection points: 1st at maximum bulge of muscle, 2nd at 1 cm lateral to anterior border of masseter muscle just superior to mandibular margin, 3rd at 1 cm medial to the lateral border of the masseter muscle just superior to mandibular margin
Hyper-hidrosis [1, 2]	1 per cm^2 (30–40 total injection points per area)	1.5–2 units/cm^2 (50–100 per axilla, 50–150 per palm, 50–200 per sole)	150–300 per axilla	Minor's starch iodine test delineates affected area

Fillers

- *General guidelines*
  - Many patients tolerate without anesthesia. Can consider topical 30% lidocaine 1 h before treatment. May consider nerve blocks for lip injections (Fig. 1)
  - High patient satisfaction due to immediate result. Last 6 months to 2 years depending on filler

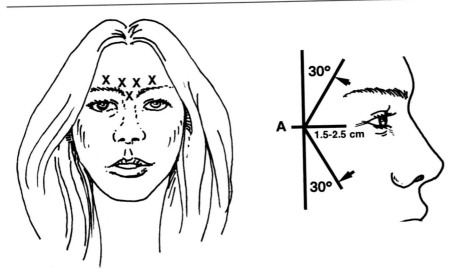

Fig. 1 Upper face botulinum toxin injection points. Illustrations by Jay Knipstein

o   Cost depends on volume injected

	Name of Filler	Source	Best for which location?	Anesthetic in the product?	How long does it last?
Hyaluronic Acid Fillers					
Thin	Belotero Balance [4–6]	Bacteria-Derived	Vertical lip lines	No	Up to 6 months
Thinner	Juvederm Volbella XC [5–7]	Bacteria-Derived	Plump and contour lips	Yes (if XC)	Up to 1 year
	Juvederm Ultra Plus XC [5–7]	Bacteria-Derived	Plump and contour lips	Yes (if XC)	Up to 1 year
	Juvederm Ultra XC [5–7]	Bacteria-Derived	Plump lips	Yes (if XC)	Up to 1 year
	Juvederm XC [5–7]	Bacteria-Derived	Lifting cheeks, plump lips, marionette lines	Yes (if XC)	Up to 1 year
Thicker	Juvederm Voluma XC [5–7]	Bacteria-Derived	Plump cheeks and mid-face	Yes (if XC)	Up to 2 years

	Name of Filler	Source	Best for which location?	Anesthetic in the product?	How long does it last?
Thinner	Restylane Silk [5, 6, 8]	Bacteria-Derived	Plump lips and marionette lines, tear troughs	Yes	Up to 6 months
	Restylane [5, 6, 9]	Bacteria-Derived	Fine face wrinkles, marionette lines, tear troughs, plump lips (but more swelling than Juvederm products)	Varies (if it has an–L it has lidocaine)	Up to 1 year
	Restylane Refyne [5, 6, 10]	Bacteria-Derived	Mild to moderate marionette or laugh lines	Yes	Up to 1 year
	Restylane Defyne [5, 6, 11]	Bacteria-Derived	Nasolabial folds and moderate to severe marionette lines	Yes	Up to 1 year
	Restylane Lyft (formerly Perlane) [5, 6, 12]	Bacteria-Derived	Cheek volume	Yes	Up to 18 months
Thicker					
Calcium Hydroxylapatite					
	Radiesse [5, 6, 13]	Synthetic	Nasolabial folds and cheeks; DO NOT use in lips	No (must be added)	>12 months
Poly-L-Lactic Acid					
	Sculptra [5, 6, 14]	Synthetic	Plump cheeks, nasolabial folds	No (must be added)	18–24 months

Chemical Peels

- *General Techniques/Guidelines*
  - Pre-peel precautions [15]:
    - Priming skin with depigmenting agents such as hydroquinone (especially for darker skin types prone to post-inflammatory hyperpigmentation) or retinoic acid daily for 2–4 weeks prior to peel, stopping 3–5 days before the procedure and use of sunscreens up until and after the chemical peel

- Discontinue topical retinoids 3–7 days before the peel
- Instruct patient not to bleach, wax, scrub, massage or use depilatories 1 week prior to peel
- Use prophylaxis in patients with active herpes simplex or history of herpes simplex with an antiviral such as acyclovir 200 mg 5 times a day, or valaciclovir 1 g 3 times a day—start 2 days prior to the peel and continue for 10–14 days after peeling

  o Intra-peel precautions [15]:
  - Degrease skin with alcohol followed by a mild acetone scrub
  - After cleaning, apply solution to the face using a sable brush, cotton tipped applicators, cotton balls, or 2 × 2 gauze sponges
  - Sensitive areas like the inner canthus of the eye and nasolabial folds should be protected with petroleum jelly.
  - The neutralizing agent should be available (if applicable) prior to beginning the peel in case early termination of the peel is necessary
  - Keep normal saline readily available in case a peel makes contact with the eyes and the eyes need to be flushed
  - Feather the edges of medium and deep peels with a lower concentration peel especially in dark-skinned patients to prevent demarcation lines

  o Post-peel precautions [15]:
  - Cold water compresses and gentle moisturizers or petroleum jelly can be used in the immediate post-peel period to help minimize discomfort
  - A mild soap for cleansing can be started the same day following the peel
  - For any crusting, an antibacterial ointment should be used to prevent infection
  - Strict photoprotection should be recommended
  - Avoid glycolic acid or retinoid products until desquamation has subsided
  - Counsel patients on recognizing and reporting complications such as pustules, blisters, persistent redness, crusting or oozing so that appropriate action can be taken

- *Glycolic acid peels* [16–18]
  o Uses: fine wrinkles, melasma, dyspigmentation
  o Ranges from very superficial to superficial peel depending on concentration (30–70%)
  o Consider test spot in very dark skin.
  o Start at 30% for 4–6 min depending on patient response.
  o Must be neutralized with sodium bicarbonate. Neutralize early if pain, erythema, vesiculation.
  o May see fine frosting if deeper peel
  o Repeat monthly. Increase concentration as tolerated to 70% max

- *Salicylic acid peel* [16–18]
  o Uses: acne, fine wrinkles, photoaging

- ○ 30% for acne
- ○ No neutralization required
- ○ May notice pseudofrosting, representing crystallization
- ○ Leave on 5–7 min and no neutralization required (wash face afterwards)
- ○ Safer for darker phototypes
- *Trichloracetic acid peels (TCA)* [16–18]
  - ○ Most commonly use 15–35%. Higher concentrations OK for face, but use caution for neck and chest where concentrations of 15–20% are best.
  - ○ Superficial peel = 10–25%; Use: fine wrinkles, dyspigmentation, melasma
  - ○ Medium peel = 25–50%; Use: fine to medium wrinkles, AKs, SKs, dyspigmentation
  - ○ Deep peel = > 50%; Use: fine to deep wrinkles, verruca
  - ○ Frost levels:
    - ■ <25%: Minimal frosting—just erythema (level I)
    - ■ 25–35%: Patchy frosting (level II)
    - ■ >35%: Compact, porcelain-like frost (level III)
  - ○ No neutralization required
  - ○ Place patients supine or slight Trendelenberg position to reduce risk of ocular contact when applying
  - ○ Prepare patient with petroleum jelly as barrier to medial/lateral canthi, nasolabial folds and corners of the mouth prior to beginning the peel Immediately blot any tears to avoid retrograde "wicking" of TCA into eyes
  - ○ Medium/deep TCA peels arestrong peels with significant erythema, tenderness and desquamation after treatments—recommend 1 week off work for peeling
- *Jessner's: Combination of salicylic acid, lactic acid, and resorcinol ethanol* [16–18]
  - ○ Used for acne, melasma, post-inflammatory hyperpigmentation, lentigines, freckles, and photodamage, AKs (if combined with TCA-35%)
  - ○ Cautions: Pregnancy category C, active inflammation, dermatitis, or infection of the area to be treated; isotretinoin therapy within 6 months of peeling; and delayed or abnormal wound healing, type V & VI skin
  - ○ For superficial peeling, two coats are usually applied. Additional coats increase the depth of peeling
  - ○ No neutralization required (wash face afterwards)
  - ○ No frosting
- *Baker-Gordon-Peel (Deep Phenol Peel): combination of 3 mL USP liquid phenol, 2 mL tap water, 8 drops of Septisol liquid soap, 3 drops of croton oil* [16–18]
  - ○ Full face peels must be done in a facility where IV access and sedation is available, cardiac status can be monitored and immediate emergency intervention is available
  - ○ High risk for depigmentation and significant medical risks:

- Poor candidates = Fitzpatrick skin type V and VI, freckled patients, long history of sun exposure, Asian patients, male patients with thicker and oilier skin. Phenol is absorbed through the skin, detoxified in the liver, and excreted by the kidneys and can cause cardiac arrhythmias, so avoid in patients with significant kidney, liver or heart disease
- Ideal patients = Non-freckled Fitzpatrick types I and II

Microneedling

- Multiple devices available with and without radiofrequency
  - Most come in electrical pen forms which can be stamped or applied in circular or cross-hatched patterns to affected areas [18].
    - Depth of needling ranges from 0 to 3 mm. Reduce depth in areas of thin skin and over bony prominences [18].
  - Resurfacing treatment great for improving texture, reducing pore size, acne scarring, wrinkles (especially perioral), some pigmentation [18].
  - Great for darker skin phototypes, as it has decreased risk of hyperpigmentation compared with laser [18].
  - Endpoint is erythema or pin-point bleeding [18].
  - Improved outcomes may be seen with the addition of topical application or dermal injection of platelet-rich plasma [19].
  - Can also be used to enhance topical drug delivery—however caution is needed as these products introduced dermally can cause unforeseen skin reactions [18].

Plasma-Rich Platelet Injections

- Platelet-rich plasma injections [20, 21]
  - Promising treatment for androgenetic alopecia with some early studies in cicatricial alopecias where it may have some benefit
    - Can increase hair diameter, hair density and decrease hair loss
  - Also used for facial rejuvenation via intradermal injection technique or with microneedling
  - Multiple systems available for blood draw and extraction of platelet-rich plasma via centrifugation
  - Use in scalp alopecia [20, 21]
    - Administered via injections or introduced following scalp microneedling
      - Injections
        - Recommended utilizing 3 cc syringes with 27–30 gauge needles
        - Injections placed just above periosteum with aliquots of 0.5–1 cc, spaced about 1 inch apart

  - ○ Usually pain is minimal and no pain relieving strategies other than distraction used
  - ○ Can consider cold air chiller for epidermal numbing if needed
- Microneedling
  - ○ Topical numbing likely needed
    - ▪ Treatment schedule: monthly injections for 3–5 months then for maintenance every 6–12 months
- ○ Use in facial rejuvenation
    - ▪ Recommend topical numbing with 30% lidocaine for 30–60 min prior to treatment
    - ▪ Start with intradermal injections then remainder can be microneedled into skin
    - ▪ Post-procedure apply petrolatum or other post-procedure cream
    - ▪ No make-up or application of any other lotions/fragrances/skin care products for 48 h
    - ▪ Treatment schedule: treatments every 4–6 weeks initially or every 4–6 months for maintenance

Sclerotherapy

- Hypertonic saline (11.7–23.4%) for telangiectasias (<1 mm), venulectasias (1–2 mm) [22, 23]
  - ○ Clean with alcohol before injecting
  - ○ Targets are the 1 mm venules
  - ○ When finished with each injection, immediately bandage injection site with cotton balls and tape
  - ○ Patient instructions: 2 weeks of compression stockings 24 h a day except while bathing, first 48 h keep compression stockings on at all times
  - ○ Potential side effects: necrosis, hyperpigmentation, pain/cramping
  - ○ Dose limitation: 10 mL
- Sodium tetradecyl sulfate: telangiectasias (<1 mm, 0.1–0.25%), venulectasias (1–2 mm, 0.25–0.5%), reticular veins (2–4 mm, 0.25–0.5% foam), non-saphenous varicose veins (3–8 mm, 0.5–1.0% foam), saphenous varicose trunks (>5 mm, 1.0–3.0% foam) [22, 23]
  - ○ This comes as 1 and 3% solution and can be injected in these concentrations or diluted with bacteriostatic saline to 0.1% or 0.3% solution and foamed with a 3-way stopcock
  - ○ Technique and patient instructions as above
  - ○ Potential side effects: pain, necrosis, HYPERPIGMENTATION
  - ○ Dose limitation: 10 mL of 3%

- Glycerin: for telangiectasias (<1 mm), venulectasias (1–2 mm), telangiectatic matting [22, 23]
  - o Potential side effects: pain/cramping, low risk of hyperpigmentation, hematuria w/injections >10 mL
  - o Dose limitation: 10 mL

Body Contouring

- **Deoxycholic acid (Kybella)** [22]
  - o *Dosage* [24]
    - A single treatment consists of up to a maximum of 50 injections, 0.2 mL each (up to a total of 10 mL), spaced 1 cm apart
    - Up to 6 single treatments may be administered at intervals no less than 1 month apart
  - o *Precautions* [24]
    - Screen patients for other potential causes of submental convexity/fullness (e.g., thyromegaly and cervical lymphadenopathy)
    - Give careful consideration to the use of Kybella in patients with excessive skin laxity, prominent platysmal bands or other conditions for which reduction of submental fat may result in an aesthetically undesirable outcome
  - o *Injection Technique* [24]
    - To avoid injury to the marginal mandibular nerve:
      - Do not inject above the inferior border of the mandible
      - Do not inject within a region defined by a 1–1.5 cm line below the inferior border (from the angle of the mandible to the mentum)
      - Inject only within the target submental fat treatment area (see Figs. 2, 3 and 4)
    - Avoid injection into the platysma:
      - Prior to each treatment session, palpate the submental area to ensure sufficient submental fat and to identify subcutaneous fat between the dermis and platysma (pre-platysmal fat) within the target treatment area (Fig. 3)
    - The number of injections and the number of treatments should be tailored to the individual patient's submental fat distribution and treatment goals
    - Outline the planned treatment area with a surgical pen and apply injection grid to mark the injection sites (Fig. 4)
    - Using a large bore needle, draw 1 mL of Kybella into a sterile 1 mL syringe and expel any air bubbles in the syringe barrel
    - Have the patient tense the platysma. Pinch the submental fat and, using a 30 gauge (or smaller) 0.5 inch needle, inject 0.2 mL of Kybella into the pre-platysmal fat (see Fig. 3) next to each of the marked injection sites by advancing the needle perpendicular to the skin
    - Avoid injecting into post-platysmal fat and withdraw needle if any resistance is met
  - o Counsel patients on post-procedure pain, numbness, swelling and bruising [24]

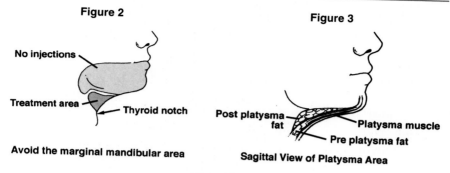

Figure 2

No injections

Treatment area

Thyroid notch

Avoid the marginal mandibular area

Figure 3

Post platysma fat

Platysma muscle

Pre platysma fat

Sagittal View of Platysma Area

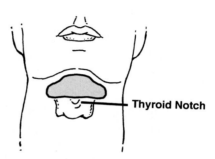

Figure 4

Thyroid Notch

Treatment Area and Injection Pattern

Fig. 2–4 Danger Zones and Injection Patterns for Kybella. Illustrations by Jay Knipstein

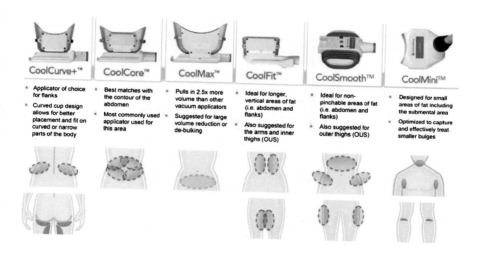

CoolCurve+™

- Applicator of choice for flanks
- Curved cup design allows for better placement and fit on curved or narrow parts of the body

CoolCore™

- Best matches with the contour of the abdomen
- Most commonly used applicator used for this area

CoolMax™

- Pulls in 2.5x more volume than other vacuum applicators
- Suggested for large volume reduction or de-bulking

CoolFit™

- Ideal for longer, vertical areas of fat (i.e. abdomen and flanks)
- Also suggested for the arms and inner thighs (OUS)

CoolSmooth™

- Ideal for non-pinchable areas of fat (i.e. abdomen and flanks)
- Also suggested for outer thighs (OUS)

CoolMini™

- Designed for small areas of fat including the submental area
- Optimized to capture and effectively treat smaller bulges

- **Cryolipolysis (CoolSculpt)** [25, 26]
  - ○ FDA and off-label treatment sites shown in figure below
  - ○ Patient must have subcutaneous fat that can be pinched for applicator to be applied; treatment not effective on visceral fat
  - ○ After application of cold stimulus, the treatment area is massaged, which can be the most painful part
  - ○ Common complications = erythema, bruising, swelling, sensitivity, and pain

Lasers

- Intense pulsed light (IPL) [27]
  - ○ Wavelength and target varies based on filter used (500–1200 nm)
  - ○ Most common uses: chronic photodamage (lentigines, telangiectasias) or hair removal in Fitzpatrick skin types I–III
    - ■ Endpoint for lentigines = darkening
    - ■ Endpoint for telangiectasias = disappearance or blue discoloration
  - ○ Not ideal for skin types IV–VI
    - ■ If you are going to treat these skin types, use longer wavelength filters or lower fluences + longer pulse widths
- Pulse dye laser (595 nm) [27]
  - ○ Targets oxyhemoglobin, best for red, pink or purple vascular lesions
  - ○ Works better for small caliber, more superficial vessels
  - ○ Facial telangiectasia, rosacea, port-wine stain (PWS), spider veins, poikiloderma of civatte, cherry angiomas (if small size)
    - ■ Longer pulse duration is effective for most facial telangiectasia while also being nonpurpuric. May need longer pulse duration for some large caliber facial telangiectasia.
    - ■ Shorter pulse durations will cause purpura but more effective for treatment of PWS or cherry angiomas
  - ○ Can also treat scars or basal cell carcinomas—short pulse durations
    - ■ Scars: usually start 10 mm spot size, 1.5 ms pulse duration, 7 J/cm2 fluence (settings for V-beam 595 nm pulse dye laser)
    - ■ Basal cell carcinomas: 10 mm spot size, 1.5 ms pulse duration, 7–9 J/cm2 fluence; cryo OFF, 3–4 passes to purpuric grey look. Include 3–4 mm margin around visible tumor (settings for V-beam 595 nm pulse dye laser)
- Potassium titanyl phosphate (KTP) laser (Frequency-doubled Nd:YAG laser) (532 nm) [27]
  - ○ Wavelength is close to an absorption peak of hemoglobin (542 nm) so useful for some vascular lesions, like telangiectasias
  - ○ Rarely causes purpura
  - ○ Also useful for lentigines
  - ○ Best for Fitzpatrick skin types I–III, but can be used in darker skin for certain situations (e.g. dermatosis papulosis nigra)

- Alexandrite (755 nm) [27]
  - Best for laser hair removal in skin types I–III
- Diode (810 nm; 940 nm) [27]
  - Best for laser hair removal in skin types I–III
- Nd:Yag laser (1064 nm) [27]
  - One of the safest lasers for dark skin because absorption of melanin is limited
  - Can treat deep vascular lesions and spider veins up to 3 mm in size, but requires high fluences and long pulse widths for efficacy so can be painful
  - Cooling = critical for pain control and to reduce the risk of burns and scarring
  - Hair removal

Settings for Hidradenitis suppurativa/hair removal [28]:

Location	Fitzpatrick Skin Type	Fluence (J/cm2)	Pulse Duration (msec)
Face	I–III	40–60	10–20
	IV	35–50	15–30
	V	30–45	20–35
	VI	20–40	35
Body	I–III	45–60	10–20
	IV	40–55	15–30
	V	40–50	20–35
	VI	35–50	35

Note: When treating with **fluences above 50 J/cm2** in darker skinned patients, recommend using a PD of 35 ms or greater [28]

- **Treatment Technique**
  - APPLY thin layer of clear gel (such as ultrasound gel, except for lentigines (no gel)) for increased epidermal protection and easy gliding of the handpiece.
  - PRE-COOL the skin (full contact with skin) to prevent epidermal damage. Larger, darker vessels require longer pre-cooling.
  - START with "test pulse": Longer pulse durations (PD) and lower fluences are safer. Gradually decrease PD or increase fluence to reach desired endpoint. Do NOT stack pulses. Potential adverse reactions may take 24–48 h to appear.
  - POST-COOL by placing copper tip of handpiece back onto the treated areas and can ice afterwards.
  - AVOID: heat/sun exposure for at least 24 h
  - Recommended time interval between treatments: at least 4–6 weeks
  - Larger reticular veins may take months to resolve and should not be treated before then.

- o **Possible reactions** [27]
  - Erythema and bruising are common and resolve with time
  - Urticarial (hive-like) reaction may occur with smaller vessels
  - If blister occurs, treat like a wound
  - Hemosiderin staining (iron leaking from tissue from blood breakdown) may occur and usually resolves with time
  - Dark coagulum in larger vessels can be removed 1–2 weeks post-treatment by nicking vessel with needle and applying pressure to force out coagulum
- o **Pearls**
  - Endpoints will vary based on type, size, color, volume, pressure or location of vein.
  - Always observe epidermis during treatment, watching for signs of damage (blanching or gray coloration). If this occurs, quickly apply cooling (NOT ice)
  - If "popping" and extravasation occur (vessel rupture), reduce the fluence, lengthen PD, or cool/compress area
  - For leg veins: use gel, first treat larger/feeder veins, treat distal to proximal; palpate post-treatment to see if re-fills (can re-treat the area if refills); patients can cool the area after treatment, DO NOT wear compression stockings after treatment
- Q-switched (QS) lasers [27]
  - o Best for pigmented lesions, tattoos
  - o Examples:
    - QS Ruby
    - QS Alexandrite
    - QS Nd:Yag
- Fractional resurfacing lasers [27]
  - o Nonablative
    - Nonablative lasers work via subtle thermal effects on dermis → stimulates a wound healing response
  - o Ablative
    - Depending on settings these lasers can be used to fully ablate epidermal lesions or in deeper fractional capacity to break up scars/wrinkles and build collagen
    - No isotretinion for 1 year and no topical retinoids for 2 weeks
    - Pre/post-treatment medications
      - Valium 5 mg and Vicodin 5/500 30 min–1 h before procedure
      - HSV prophylaxis—Valtrex 500 mg BID or acyclovir 200 mg 5x/day for 5 days starting 1 day before procedure
      - Can give prednisone 20 mg/day for 3–5 days to decrease swelling
    - Examples:
      - Carbon dioxide (CO_2) laser (10600 nm)
      - Erbium: Yag laser (2940 nm)

References

1. Carruthers A, Carruthers J. Botulinum toxin. In: Bolognia JL, Jorizzo JL, Schaffer JV editors. Dermatology, 3rd ed. Elsevier Limited; 2012. p. 2561–2570.
2. Dayan SH, Bassichis BA. Appropriate products and techniques. Aesthet Surg J. 2008;28(3): 335–347.
3. Carruthers A, Carruthers J. Aesthetic botulinum A toxin in the mid and lower face and neck. Dermatol Surg. 2003;29(5):468–76.
4. Belotero Balance [Instructions for Use]. North America: Merz, Inc.; 2016.
5. Wesley N, Dover J. The filler revolution: a six year retrospective. Drugs Dermatol. 2009;8(10):903–07.
6. Alikhan A, Hocker TLH. Review of dermatology. Elsevier Limited; 2017. p. 460–64.
7. Juvederm [Injectable Gel Fillers Indications and Important Safety Information]. Irvine, California: Allergan; 2018.
8. Restylane Silk [Product & Safety Information]. Fort Worth, Texas: Galderma Laboratories, L.P.; 2017.
9. Restylane [Product & Safety Information]. Fort Worth, Texas: Galderma Laboratories, L.P.; 2016.
10. Restylane Refyne [Product & Safety Information]. Fort Worth, Texas: Galderma Laboratories, L.P.; 2016.
11. Restylane Defyne [Product & Safety Information]. Fort Worth, Texas: Galderma Laboratories, L.P.; 2016.
12. Restylane Lyft [Product & Safety Information]. Fort Worth, Texas: Galderma Laboratories, L.P.; 2018.
13. Radiesse [Instructions for Use]. Franksville, WI: Merz North America, Inc.; 2016.
14. Sculptra Aesthetic [Instructions for Use]. Fort Worth, Texas: Galderma Laboratories, L.P.; 2016.
15. Anitha B. Prevention of complications in chemical peeling. J Cutan Aesthet Surg. 2010;3(3):186–8.
16. Siegel M, Bassichis B. Advanced surgical facial rejuvenation: art and clinical practice. Berlin: Springer; 2016 Chapter 17.
17. Tosti A, Grimes PE, Pia DPM, editors. Color atlas of chemical peels. Berlin: Springer; 2006. p. 23–7.
18. Ramaut L, Hoeksema H, Pirayesh A, Stillaert F, Monstrey S. Microneedling: Where do we stand now? A systematic review of the literature. J Plast Reconstr Aesthet Surg. 2018;71(1):1–14.
19. Ibrahim ZA, El-Ashmawy AA, Shora OA. Therapeutic effect of microneedling and autologous platelet-rich atrophic scars: A randomized study. J Cosmet Dermatol. 2017;16(3):388–99.
20. Gkini MA, Kouskoukis AE, Tripsianis G, Rigopoulos D, Kouskoukis K. Study of platelet-rich plasma injections in the treatment of androgenetic alopecia through an one-year period. J Cutan Aesthet Surg. 2014;7(4):213–19.
21. Ferrando J, Garcia-Garcia, SC, Gonzalez-de-Cossio AC, Bou L, Navarra E. A proposal of an effective platelet-rich plasma protocol for the treatment of androgenetic alopecia. Int J Trichology. 2017;9(4):165–70.
22. Alikhan A, Hocker TLH. Review of dermatology. Elsevier Limited; 2017. p. 464–67.
23. Goldman MP, Weiss RA. Phlebology and Treatment of Leg Veins. In: Bolognia JL, Jorizzo JL, Schaffer JV, editors. Dermatology, 3rd ed. Elsevier Limited; 2012. p. 2509–22.
24. Kybella [Highlights of Prescribing Information]. Irvine, California: Allergan; 2018.

25. Ingargiola MJ, Motakef S, Chung MT, Vasconez HC, Sasaki GH. Cryolipolysis for Fat Reduction and Body Contouring. Plastic Reconstr Surg. 2015;135(6):1581–90.
26. Sadick N, Luebberding S, Mai SV, Krueger N. Cryolipolysis for noninvasive body contouring: clinical efacy and patient satisfaction. Clin Cosmet Investig Dermatol. 2014;7:201–5.
27. Zachary CB, Rofagha R. Laser therapy. In: Bolognia JL, Jorizzo JL, Schaffer JV, editors. Dermatology, 3rd ed. Elsevier Limited; 2012. p. 2261–79.
28. Hamzavi IH, Griffith JL, Riyaz F, Hessam S, Bechara FG. Laser and light-based treatment options for hidradenitis suppurativa. J Am Acad Dermatol. 2015;73(5 Suppl 1):S78–81.

Dermatopathology Pearls

Danielle Yeager, Samantha L. Schneider, Marsha Chaffins and Ben J. Friedman

Biopsy Technique [1, 2]

In the Context Of …

- Alopecia
  - Best to biopsy an established area of hair loss
    - Avoid the advancing border [2]
  - If the clinical differential diagnosis includes both scarring and non-scarring processes, best to perform two 4-mm punch biopsies, with one being sectioned horizontally and the other vertically
  - If the clinical differential diagnosis includes only scarring processes, a single 4-mm punch biopsy specimen sent for vertical sectioning is usually sufficient
  - If clinical differential diagnosis includes only non-scarring processes, a single 4-mm biopsy specimen sent for horizontal sectioning is usually sufficient
  - Trichoscopy can help target highest yield areas where pathology is present

D. Yeager · S. L. Schneider
Department of Dermatology, Henry Ford Health System,
3031 West Grand Blvd, Sutie 800, Detroit, MI 48202, USA
e-mail: dyeager2@hfhs.org

S. L. Schneider
e-mail: samantha.schneider@gmail.com

M. Chaffins
Department of Dermatology, Department of Pathology and Laboratory Medicine,
Henry Ford Health System, 3031 West Grand Blvd, Suite 800, Detroit, MI 48202, USA

B. J. Friedman (✉)
Department of Dermatology and Department of Pathology and Laboratory Medicine,
Henry Ford Health System, 3031 West Grand Blvd, Suite 800, Detroit, MI 48202, USA
e-mail: bfriedm1@hfhs.org

© Springer Nature Switzerland AG 2020
H. W. Lim et al. (eds.), *Practical Guide to Dermatology*,
https://doi.org/10.1007/978-3-030-18015-7_6

- Bullous disorders
  - o Ideal biopsy captures both portions of the blister and intact skin so that the level of the split and the nature of the accompanying inflammatory infiltrate can be characterized.
  - o Saucerization removal of an entire intact small bullae or vesicle is optimal
  - o Alternative: Saucerization or punch at the very edge of a large bullae
  - o Avoid old bullae (>12 h), as these are more likely to develop secondary epidermal necrosis and introduce diagnostic difficulty with SJS/TEN
  - o For DIF: see: immunodermatology methods below

- Inflammatory disorders (NOS)
  - o >/= 4-mm punch (standard) from clinically inflamed-appearing skin
  - o AVOID areas of suspected secondary change/trauma
  - o Saucerization through upper reticular dermis is usually adequate for processes suspected to be epidermal (e.g. psoriasis versus spongiotic dermatitides)
  - o Sometimes two 4-mm punch biopsies at different sites can be helpful, especially if there is some morphologic variation by anatomic location

- Melanocytic lesions
  - o The biopsy should contain the entire lesion whenever possible, as complete architectural evaluation by the pathologist is critical for making an accurate diagnosis
  - o Excisional biopsy down to subcutis with 1-to-2 mm margins of normal skin is considered the gold standard (can take the form of a punch biopsy for small lesions)
  - o Saucerization removal with 1-to-2 mm margins of normal skin is adequate in the majority of macular lesions
  - o Acral lesions:
    - ▪ Score the biopsy specimen perpendicular to the dermatoglyphs and inform the lab to section parallel to the nicked edge to prevent the artifactual appearance of melanocyte confluence and the overdiagnosis of melanoma
    - ▪ PEARL: Can score around acral lesions with a #15 blade to better guide saucerization and minimize the likelihood of too superficial a sample and a positive margin
  - o Facial lesions:
    - ▪ When lentigo maligna is a clinical possibility, a broad thin saucerization or multiple thin saucerizations from within the lesion are an acceptable alternative to a deep excisional biopsy
    - ▪ Choose representative areas based on dermoscopy within a heterogeneous lesion
  - o Partial sampling of large lesions via a punch biopsy can lead to an incorrect diagnosis, and therefore should be avoided whenever possible [3]

- Livedo reticularis/ livedo racemosa
  - Incisional (wedge) biopsy from center of the lesion down to deep subcutis with a #15 blade
  - Alternative is the telescoping punch technique (e.g. 6-mm punch down to adipose, followed by 4-mm punch to obtain deeper subcutis)
- Lymphoma
  - Patches or thin plaques suspicious for mycosis fungoides/CTCL
    - Broad thin saucerization taken to the upper reticular dermis is often superior to small punch biopsies
    - Provides more surface area for morphologic examination (especially epidermotropism) and increases the potential yield for TCR gene rearrangement studies
  - Nodules suspected to be lymphoproliferative disorders
    - Large incisional or (>/= 6-mm) punch biopsies including subcutis to allow for thorough architectural evaluation and adequate tissue for the performance of immunostains and molecular analysis
- Panniculitis
  - A incisional/wedge biopsy down to deep subcutis or fascia is best
  - Telescoping punch technique is alternative (see above)
- Pigmentary anomalies and connective tissue nevi/hamartomas
  - Perform two >/= 4-mm punch biopsies (normal and abnormal skin) to allow for histopathologic comparison
- Retiform purpura
  - Incisional/wedge or telescoping punch technique from both center and edge of painful lesion [4]
  - Avoid frankly necrotic or ulcerated foci
- Ulcers (NOS)
  - If the setting of a broad clinical differential diagnosis, a perilesional wedge or telescoping punch biopsy of the edge is best
  - Avoid ulcer bed in most cases (will show non-specific vascular damage)
- Vasculitis
  - For H&E: >/= 4-mm punch biopsy of an established purpuric lesion (>/= 72 h) [5]
  - For DIF: see: immunodermatopathology methods below

Immunodermatopathology

- Direct immunofluorescence study (DIF)
  - Media
    - Transport media such as Michel's (most commonly used) or Zeus'
    - Alternatives include normal saline (saline soaked gauze) or liquid nitrogen (cannot be allowed to thaw)
  - Where to take biopsy:
    - Immunobullous disorders [6]
      - >/= 4-mm punch specimen taken from non-bullous lesional skin or perilesional skin within 1 cm of bullae
      - DIF is the gold standard for diagnosis => slightly more sensitive than indirect immunofluorescence and ELISA studies when performed correctly [7]
    - Vasculitis
      - >/= 4-mm punch specimen taken from lesional skin <24 h old [8]
- Salt-split skin
  - Technique that induces separation at the lamina lucida
  - Can be performed as adjunct to DIF or IIF study to help localize the site of antibody binding (above or below the lamina lucida) and narrow the differential diagnosis particularly for bullous diseases
  - For DIF:
    - Upon request can be performed on specimens initially placed in Michel's media, which are then transferred to 1 M sodium chloride (NaCl) or ethylenediaminetetraacetic acid (EDTA) to induce split
- Indirect immunofluorescence study (IIF)
  - Often only performed in specialized testing centers (can send specimen out)
  - Specimen is blood drawn from the patient (plain red top or serum separator tube).
    Depending on the differential diagnosis, the lab will use animal substrate or human skin [not from the actual patient] incubated with progressive dilutions of the patient's serum to detect and localize pathogenic antibodies
- Enzyme-linked immunosorbent assay (ELISA)
  - This is a type of antigen specific serologic test
  - Commercially available tests available for detection of IgG antibodies directed at:
    - Dsg1 and Dsg 3 => pemphigus foliaceous and pemphigus vulgaris
    - BPAG1 and BPAG2 => bullous pemphigoid
    - Collagen VII => epidermolysis bullosa acquisita and bullous lupus erythematosus
  - Sample is blood drawn from the patient (plain red top or serum separator tube)
  - Can be useful in confirming above diagnoses with supportive histopathologic findings (when DIF inconclusive or not available)

○ False negatives do occur (some patients have antibodies to epitopes not recognized by the commercial tests or less common antigens)
○ Levels can be used to monitor disease activity/ track response to therapy

Ancillary Molecular Testing in Dermatopathology

- Histopathologically ambiguous melanocytic lesions
  - ○ Array comparative genomic hybridization (aCGH)
    - Identifies copy number variations throughout the entire genome
      - Unlike the FISH assay (see below) that measures variations at predefined genetic loci known to be commonly affected in melanoma
    - Performed on formalin fixed paraffin embedded (FFPE) tissue
    - Multiple copy number variations often involving portions of chromosomes 1, 6, 8, 9 and 11 support a molecular diagnosis of melanoma [9]
    - With rare exceptions, nevi do not demonstrate copy number alterations
    - Limitations:
      - Higher tumor tissue requirement, expense and unknown significance of isolated genetic alterations
      - Only available at specialized (usually academic) centers
  - ○ Fluorescence *in situ* hybridization (FISH) melanoma assay
    - Detects chromosomal copy number alterations using a combination of probes against pre-determined genetic loci known to be commonly affected in melanoma
    - 4–6 probes used in most labs that perform the test
    - False negatives (i.e. melanomas that were FISH negative) and false positives (i.e. nevi that were FISH positive) can both occur
      - Performed on FFPE tissue
      - Available at several academic centers and as a commercial service through NeoGenomics Laboratories.
      - ○ Gene expression profiling (GEP) (i.e. Myriad myPath® melanoma assay)
    - Aims to distinguish benign from malignant melanocytic lesions through gene expression profiling of 23 genes by qRT-PCR
    - Performed on FFPE tissue (can send unstained slides or tissue block)
    - Provides a single diagnostic score that corresponds to benign, indeterminate, or malignant
    - Sensitivity 72% and specificity 94% for (unequivocal) cases in one non-manufacture conducted study [10]
    - Available exclusively as commercial test through Myriad Genetics.
- Prognostication of Primary Cutaneous Melanoma
  - ○ Decision-Dx Melanoma (Castle Biosciences)

- Provides assessment of metastatic risk for biopsy-confirmed cutaneous melanoma through gene expression profiling of 31 genes by qRT-PCR
- Performed on FFPE (can send unstained slides/tissue block)
- May be able to identify high risk patients with negative sentinel lymph node biopsies (SNLB) or who are ineligible or decline SNLB [11]
- Tumors classified as:
  o Class 1 (low risk of metastasis)
  o Class 2 (high risk of metastasis)

- Cutaneous Infections
  o PCR for mycobacterial infections and various fungal species [12]
  - Can be performed on FFPE tissue and fresh tissue (higher yield)
  - Available at specialized testing centers

  o Broad range bacterial PCR and sequencing [13]
  - Can be performed on FFPE tissue and fresh tissue (higher yield)
  - Available at specialized testing centers

  o Leishmaniasis culture and PCR [14]
  - Available through Center for Disease Control and Prevention (CDC)-check website for detailed instructions
  - https://www.cdc.gov/parasites/leishmaniasis/health_professionals/index.html
  - Best to request culture medium ahead of time from CDC, but can also place specimen in sterile buffered media (e.g., buffered saline, RPMI, Eagle's growth, Schneider's, Tobie's) with a neutral pH (~7–7.4) and then send out

- Lymphoma
  - T-cell receptor clonality studies may be ordered by the dermatopathologist on skin biopsy specimens suspicious for CTCL.
  - Detection of a monoclonal population of T-cells can further support histopathology and immunophenotypic findings in establishing a diagnosis of CTCL.
  - Next generation sequencing technique is gradually replacing capillary electrophoresis as the preferred modality for clonality detection given its higher sensitivity [15]

- Sebaceous neoplasms [16]
  - Immunohistochemistry for mismatch repair proteins PMS2, MSH6, MLH1, MSH2 can be performed on biopsies (FFPE) demonstrating sebaceous adenomas, sebaceomas, and sebaceous carcinomas to screen for Muir Torre Syndrome.
- Soft Tissue
  o Dermatofibrosarcoma protuberans (DFSP) [17]
     FISH assay: Col1a-PDGFB t(17;22) (q22;q13.1)
  o Clear cell sarcoma/ Ewing's sarcoma [18]
- FISH assay: EWSR1-ATF1 t(12;22)(q13;q12) or EWSR1-CREB1 t(2;22) (q33;q12)
- If deemed appropriate, these tests are ordered by the dermatopathologist

What's the Differential Diagnosis If Your Patient's Biopsy Shows...

- Acantholysis
  - Darier's (plus dyskeratosis)
  - Grover's (small lesions; dyskeratosis sometimes)
  - Hailey Hailey (no dyskeratosis; full thickness)
  - Pemphigus Foliaceous (superficial only)
  - Pemphigus Vulgaris (suprabasilar, no necrosis, deep follicular extension)
  - Dowling Degos/Galli Galli (occurring within lentigo-like lesions)

- CD-30 positivity
  - Prudent to rule out scabies clinically
  - Can occur in other various reactive conditions
  - In the context of clinically suspected lymphoproliferative disorder:
    - Lymphomatoid papulosis
    - Anaplastic large cell lymphoma (ALCL)
    - Transformed mycosis fungoides

- Eosinophilic spongiosis
  - Erythema toxicum neonatorum
  - Bullous pemphigoid (prodromal)
  - Allergic contact dermatitis
  - Spongiotic drug eruptions
  - Arthropod bite reaction
  - Incontinentia pigmenti (with dyskeratosis)
  - Parasitic infestations
  - Herpes gestationis
  - Eosinophilic pustular folliculitis

- Granulomatous dermatitis
  - Narrow differential diagnosis by pattern:
    - Naked (sarcoidal)
    - Tuberculoid
    - Caseating
    - Palisading
    - Suppurative
  - AFB, Fite, PAS, GMS, Gram: can be used to exclude infection
    - Consider biopsy for tissue culture if clinical suspicion high
  - Examination under polarized light may identify/exclude certain foreign bodies

- Lichenoid interface dermatitis
  - Lichen planus
  - Lichenoid drug eruption
  - Fixed drug eruption (usually with eosinophils)
  - Lupus erythematosus (some forms; usually more vacuolar)

- o Pityriasis lichenoides
- o Mycosis fungoides (not a true dermatitis; necrotic keratinocytes should be rare to absent)
- o Pigmented purpuric dermatosis (lichenoid-variant)
- o Lichenoid graft versus host disease
- o Benign lichenoid keratosis
- Neutrophilic dermatitis
  - o Intraepidermal neutrophils:
    - Psoriasis
    - Transient neonatal pustular melanosis
    - Halogenoderma
    - Acropustulosis of infancy
    - Dermatophyte
    - Impetigo
    - Seborrheic dermatitis
    - Syphilis
  - o Dermal neutrophils:
    - Sweet syndrome
    - Pyoderma gangrenosum
    - Bechet disease
    - Leukocytoclastic vasculitis
    - Erythema elevatum diutinum
    - Linear IgA bullous dermatosis
    - Bullous lupus erythematosus
    - Dermatitis herpetiformis
- Psoriasiform dermatitis
  - o Psoriasis
  - o Chronic spongiotic dermatitis
  - o Pityriasis rubra pilaris
  - o Mycosis fungoides (often concurrently lichenoid)
- Spongiotic dermatitis
  - o Contact dermatitis
  - o Dyshidrotic eczema
  - o Nummular dermatitis
  - o Stasis dermatitis
  - o ID reaction
  - o Pityriasis rosea
  - o Seborrheic dermatitis
  - o Spongiotic form of pigmenting purpuric dermatosis

References

1. Elston D, Ferringer T. Dermatopathology, 2nd ed. Elsevier; 2014.
2. Elston DM, Stratman EJ, Miller SJ. Skin biopsy: biopsy issues in specific diseases. J Am Acad Dermatol. 2016;74(1):1–16. quiz 17-18.
3. Karimipour DJ, Schwartz JL, Wang TS, et al. Microstaging accuracy after subtotal incisional biopsy of cutaneous melanoma. J Am Acad Dermatol. 2005;52(5):798–802.
4. Wysong A, Venkatesan P. An approach to the patient with retiform purpura. Dermatol Ther. 2011;24(2):151–72.
5. Carlson JA, Cavaliere LF, Grant-Kels JM. Cutaneous vasculitis: diagnosis and management. Clin Dermatol. 2006;24(5):414–29.
6. van Beek N, Zillikens D, Schmidt E. Diagnosis of autoimmune bullous diseases. J Dtsch Dermatol Ges. 2018;16(9):1077–91.
7. Sardy M, Kostaki D, Varga R, Peris K, Ruzicka T. Comparative study of direct and indirect immunofluorescence and of bullous pemphigoid 180 and 230 enzyme-linked immunosorbent assays for diagnosis of bullous pemphigoid. J Am Acad Dermatol. 2013;69(5):748–53.
8. Kulthanan K, Pinkaew S, Jiamton S, Mahaisavariya P, Suthipinittharm P. Cutaneous leukocytoclastic vasculitis: the yield of direct immunofluorescence study. J Med Assoc Thai. 2004;87(5):531–5.
9. Lee JJ, Lian CG. Molecular testing for cutaneous melanoma: an update and review. Arch Pathol Lab Med. 2018.
10. Reimann JDR, Salim S, Velazquez EF, et al. Comparison of melanoma gene expression score with histopathology, fluorescence in situ hybridization, and SNP array for the classification of melanocytic neoplasms. Mod Pathol. 2018;31(11):1733–43.
11. Gerami P, Cook RW, Russell MC, et al. Gene expression profiling for molecular staging of cutaneous melanoma in patients undergoing sentinel lymph node biopsy. J Am Acad Dermatol. 2015;72(5):780–785 e783.
12. Chung J, Ince D, Ford BA, Wanat KA. Cutaneous infections due to nontuberculosis mycobacterium: recognition and management. Am J Clin Dermatol. 2018.
13. Akram A, Maley M, Gosbell I, Nguyen T, Chavada R. Utility of 16S rRNA PCR performed on clinical specimens in patient management. Int J Infect Dis. 2017;57:144–9.
14. Practical Guide for Specimen Collection and Reference Diagnosis of Leishmaniasis. In: CDC, ed: CDC's Division of Parasitic Diseases and Malaria; 2016.
15. Sufficool KE, Lockwood CM, Abel HJ, et al. T-cell clonality assessment by next-generation sequencing improves detection sensitivity in mycosis fungoides. J Am Acad Dermatol. 2015;73(2):228–236 e222.
16. Pollinger TH, Kieliszak CR, Logemann N, Gratrix ML. Analysis of sebaceous neoplasms for DNA mismatch repair proteins in muir-torre syndromfe. Skinmed. 2017;15(4):259–64.
17. Thway K, Noujaim J, Jones RL, Fisher C. Dermatofibrosarcoma protuberans: pathology, genetics, and potential therapeutic strategies. Ann Diagn Pathol. 2016;25:64–71.
18. Machado I, Yoshida A, Morales MGN, et al. Review with novel markers facilitates precise categorization of 41 cases of diagnostically challenging, "undifferentiated small round cell tumors". A clinicopathologic, immunophenotypic and molecular analysis. Ann Diagn Pathol. 2018;34:1–12.

Skin of Color

Jewell V. Gaulding and Diane Jackson-Richards

Acne Keloidalis Nuchae (AKN) [1]

Key Association

- Dissecting cellulitis of the scalp

Work Up Pearls

- Usually a clinical diagnosis; if biopsied (atypical presentation), must be a deep biopsy (below level of follicular bulbs and scar tissue)
- If pustules or draining, perform bacterial culture

Treatment Ladder

- Topical therapies
  - Benzoyl peroxide
  - Topical clindamycin
  - Topical retinoids: adapalene, tretinoin, tazarotene
  - Class II/III topical steroids, intralesional triamcinolone (ILK) injection, 10–40 mg/ml for keloidal nodules and 3–10 mg/ml for papulopustules. Explain the possibility of hypopigmentation with ILK injection.

J. V. Gaulding
Department of Dermatology, Allegheny General Hospital, Pittsburg, PA, USA

D. Jackson-Richards (✉)
Department of Dermatology, Henry Ford Health System,
3031 West Grand Blvd, Suite 800, Detroit, MI 48202, USA
e-mail: djackso1@hfhs.org

© Springer Nature Switzerland AG 2020
H. W. Lim et al. (eds.), *Practical Guide to Dermatology*,
https://doi.org/10.1007/978-3-030-18015-7_7

131

- Systemic therapies
  - o Oral doxycycline 50–100 mg BID or minocycline 50–100 mg BID

Outside of the Box Treatment Ideas

- Nd:YAG laser
  - o Often not covered by insurance—have patient check
- Excision
  - o Consider post-op intralesional steroid series (See Keloid "Protocol")
- Oral isotretinoin 0.25 mg/kg daily then 20 mg every 2–3 days

Alopecia

Alopecia Areata [2–4]

What Not To Miss

- Autoimmune thyroid disease i.e. Hashimoto's thyroiditis
- Vitiligo
- Inflammatory bowel disease

Key DDx

- Tinea capitis
- Trichotillomania
- Traction alopecia
- Secondary syphilis
- Loose anagen syndrome
- Temporal triangular alopecia

Work Up Pearls

- CBC with differential
- Iron studies
- TSH
- Vitamin D

Treatment Ladder

- Intralesional
  - o Triamcinolone (5 mg/ml for scalp, 2.5 mg/ml for eyebrow/beard) q 4–6 weeks, stop if no response after 6 treatments
  - o 0.1 ml injected at 0.5–1 cm intervals

- Topical therapies
  - PEARL: Give topical modalities a three-month trial
  - Class I or II topical steroid +/−5% minoxidil solution/foam BID
  - Anthralin 0.5–1.0% cream (at home)
    - Short contact: start 20 min daily, then increase by 10 min every 2 weeks until reach 1 h or time required to elicit mild dermatitis.
    - Continue this contact time qd × 3–6 months
    - Inform patient about staining of skin
  - In office contact allergens
    - Sensitize initially, two weeks later begin weekly for up to 30 weeks
    - Usually 8–12 weeks for response
    - Contraindications- pregnancy, children <10 years old
    - Examples of allergens:
      - SADBE (squaric acid dibutyl ester)
      - DPCP (diphenylcyclopropenone)
        - PEARL: DPCP is photosensitive
        - Apply 2% DPCP in office then in 1 week apply 0.001% solution nightly once a week AT HOME
        - Need to find compounding pharmacy that will make 0.001% solution for the patient's home application
          - This concentration can be increased if no response
          - Unclear if visible dermatitis is required to produce the Th2 shift
        - Gradually increase to 2–3 nights a week as tolerated
  - Topical compounded JAK inhibitor (eg, tofacitinib 2% cream in liposomal base)

- Oral
  - Oral prednisone 30–40 mg/day
  - Methotrexate starting at 2.5–5 mg/week increasing as needed to up to 25 mg/week
  - Cyclosporine 2.5–5 mg/kg/day
  - Tofacitinib 10–15 mg/day

Outside the Box Treatment options

- Narrowband phototherapy
- Psoralen + UVA
- Excimer laser
- PDT
- Dupilumab

Androgenetic Alopecia [5–7]

What Not To Miss

- Pathologic hyperandrogenism
  - Look for: irregular menses, infertility, hirsutism, severe cystic acne, virilization, galactorrhea
- Telogen effluvium "unmasking" underlying androgenetic alopecia

Work Up Pearls

- Need to be off birth control for 1 cycle and test in the morning while menstruating
  - Total and free testosterone
  - Dehydroepiandrosterone sulfate (DHEA-S)
  - 17-hydroxy-progesterone
  - Prolactin
  - Iron studies
  - +/– TSH

Treatment Ladder

- Men
  - Topical
    - Minoxidil 5% foam or solution twice daily
      - 4–6 months before any benefit
      - If discontinued, hair loss will resume in 4–6 months

  - Oral
    - Finasteride 1 mg daily
      - PEARL: Check baseline PSA if older male (>45). Patient needs to inform his physician when getting PSA testing as PSA will be suppressed.
      - May take up to 12 months to notice significant improvement
      - Treatment must be continued to maintain effect

- Women
  - Topical
    - Minoxidil 5% foam once daily OR 2% solution twice daily

  - Oral
    - Aldactone 50 mg twice a day × 3 months then 100 mg twice a day
    - Finasteride
      - If premenopausal, stop 1 month prior to conception
      - Extreme caution with pregnancy when prescribing to premenopausal women

- Avoid concomitant oral contraceptive pills that contain norgestrel and norethinodrone

Outside the Box Treatment Options

- Camouflage techniques, i.e powders for the illusion of increased density
  - Examples include: Derm Match, Toppik
- 650–900 nm wavelength laser
  - At 5 mW, can increase terminal hair density after 26 weeks
  - At home products include infrared "helmet" devices
- Platelet rich plasma (PRP)—monthly for 4–6 treatments and then periodically for maintenance
  - May wish to use in conjunction with newer hair "vitamins," such as Nutrafol or Viviscal
- Compounded formulas that combine topical preparations of minoxodil, spironolactone and finasteride are available
- Combination of tacrolimus 0.3% in Cetaphil cleanser, clobetasol foam, and minoxidil 5% foam BID. (Personal communication, Jerry Shapiro, MD, New York, NY)
- Hair transplantation surgery

Central Centrifugal Cicatricial Alopecia (CCCA) [8]

Key DDx

- Androgenetic alopecia
- Lichen planopilaris
- Folliculitis decalvans

Treatment Ladder

- Gentle hair care
  - Stop all relaxing, braiding, weaving and corn rowing
    - Limit relaxing to every 8–12 weeks, ideally every 12 weeks, leave relaxer on for 20 min or less
  - Limit hot combing/flat ironing to once a week or less
  - Avoid mineral oil, petrolatum and alcohol
  - Use shea butter, coconut oil, jojoba oil, almond oil, olive oil
  - Wash hair at least once every other week
- Topical
  - Corticosteroids daily until asymptomatic then tapered to 3 days/week for maintenance
  - Topical minoxidil

- Intralesional
  - Triamcinolone 2.5–5 mg/ml injections every month for 5–6 months
- Oral
  - Doxycycline 100 mg daily for at least 6 months
    - Once achieved response, you may consider tapering
    - When remission has been sustained for a year, discontinue
  - Antimalarials
    - Hydroxychloroquine 200 mg BID (or 5 mg/kg/d)
- Surgical
  - Hair transplantation, once inflammation has been controlled for at least 1 year

Lichen Planopilaris [9, 10]

Key DDx

- Central centrifugal cicatricial alopecia
- Keratosis follicularis spinulosa decalvans
- Frontal fibrosing alopecia

Treatment Ladder

- Limited:
  - Class I/II topical corticosteroids
  - ILK 2.5–5 mg/ml
    - Target depth of injection is 1–2 mm
- Extensive:
  - 1st line:
    - Oral prednisone 1 mg/kg day × 15 days, then tapered over 4 months to halt progression/improve symptoms in rapidly progressive/severe cases
    - Hydroxychloroquine 200 mg BID (or 5 mg/kg/d)
  - 2nd line:
    - Methotrexate 10–15 mg/week
  - Refractory disease
    - Cyclosporine 4–5 mg/kg/day × 4–6 months
    - Mycophenolate mofetil 0.5 g BID × 4 weeks then 1 g BID for at least 20 weeks

Outside the Box Treatment Options

- Pioglitazone 15 mg/day
- Can consider a short course of prednisone 1 mg/kg/day × 15 days, then tapered over 4 months to halt progression/improve symptoms in rapidly progressive/severe cases

- Topical calcineurin inhibitors, especially for areas displaying atrophy or other side effects of potent topical steroids
- Excimer laser
- PRP- every 3 weeks for at least 4 sessions

Telogen Effluvium [11]

Key DDx

- Anagen effluvium- attributed to chemotherapy or toxin exposure
- Androgenetic alopecia
- Loose anagen syndrome- consider in young children, especially females with blonde hair

Work Up Pearls

- Investigate for triggers
  - Physiological (postpartum)
  - Febrile states
  - Stressors
  - Drugs
  - Endocrine
  - Organ dysfunction
  - Hair cycle disorder
  - Hair dye application
  - Syphilis
  - Systemic Lupus
- Hair pull test is positive for telogen hairs

Treatment Ladder

- Counsel patient about natural history of condition
  - PEARL: Cosmetically significant regrowth can take 12–18 months
- Removal or treatment of underlying cause (if identifiable)
- Cosmetic measures such as hair styling techniques, wigs, and camouflage powders
- Treat concomitant hair or scalp disorders (such as seborrheic dermatitis)
- +/− topical minoxidil

Outside the Box management options

- Photography to monitor and assess for improvement
- Iron supplementation to ensure ferritin levels >30 mcg/L
  - Not well established, but may be helpful in those with iron deficiency anemia

Traction Alopecia [12]

What Not To Miss

- Important to diagnose early as it may later develop into an irreversible scarring alopecia

Key DDx

- Trichotillomania
- Frontal fibrosing alopecia

Treatment Ladder

- Educate high-risk populations about conditions and practices that may convey risk of hair loss (braids, weaves, dreadlocks, ponytails/buns, turban)
- Relief of traction on the hair shaft is mainstay of treatment
- Avoidance of chemical and thermal treatment of hair
- Topical corticosteroids, apply to margin of hair loss
- ILK (2.5–5 mg/ml) can down regulate the inflammation
  - Space injections 1 cm apart with approximately 0.1 mL injected at each site
- Oral/topical antibiotics for anti-inflammatory properties
  - Minocycline 50–100 mg twice daily
  - Doxycycline 50–100 mg twice daily
- Topical minoxidil in advanced cases, hair transplantation when scarring and follicular atrophy present

Hidradenitis Suppurativa [13–18]

What Not To Miss

- Anemia
- Secondary amyloidosis
- Fistulae
- Nephrotic syndrome
- Squamous cell carcinoma
- Metabolic syndrome
- Association between HS and inflammatory bowel disease
- Inflammatory syndromes such as:
  - PAPASH (pyogenic arthritis, pyoderma gangrenosum, acne and suppurative hidradenitis)
  - PASH (pyoderma gangrenosum, acne and suppurative hidradenitis)

Key DDx

- Staphylococcal furunculosis
- Crohn's disease
- Granuloma inguinale
- Tuberculosis
- Mycetoma

Treatment Ladder

- Empathy and chronic disease counseling
  - Patient support group if available (www.hopeforhs.org)
- Behavioral modifications
  - Smoking cessation
  - Diet, exercise, weight loss, minimize carbohydrates
  - Loose-fitting underwear/clothing
- Topical anti-inflammatory/antibiotics
  - Benzoyl peroxide (BPO) 10% wash
  - Clindamycin 1% lotion (less irritating than solution; lifelong treatments for almost all HS patients).
- Localized Hurley stage I
  - 1st line
    - Topical BPO + clindamycin 1% lotion/solution
  - 2nd line
    - Doxycycline 100 mg daily × 1–6 months
    - ILK 10 mg/ml for acute flares
  - 3rd line
    - Monthly Nd:YAG, need at least 3 sessions before determining efficacy
- Generalized Hurley Stage I
  - 1st line
    - BPO, clindamycin, ILK, doxycycline 100–150 mg daily
  - 2nd line
    - Nd:YAG
      - PEARL: Best for HS nodules. Not effective if any sinus tracts have formed.
- Hurley stage II/III
  - 1st line
    - 300 mg clindamycin BID + 300 mg rifampin BID × 8–10 weeks
    - +/− monthly Nd:YAG
  - 2nd line
    - Levofloxacin 500 mg daily + rifampin 300 mg BID + metronidazole 500 mg TID × up to 8 weeks
  - Surgical
    - Localized deroofing +/− curettage and/or CO_2 laser excision

Outside of the Box Treatment Options

- Oral prednisone
  - For significant flares, 0.5–0.7 mg/kg with taper over a few weeks
- Oral dapsone
  - Start 25 mg PO daily, can titrate up to 200 mg PO daily
- Cyclosporine 2–3.5 mg/kg per day
- Colchicine 0.5 mg daily + minocycline 100 mg daily × 3 months
- Oral zinc gluconate 90 mg/day
- Clinical trials if available

In the Context Of…

- Refractory disease
  - Medical
    - Adalimumab
      - FDA approved, more lifestyle friendly but less effective compared to infliximab
      - Week 0: 160 mg, week 2: 80 mg, 40 mg weekly starting at week 4
    - Infliximab
      - More effective. than adalimumab
      - 5 mg/kg IV week 0, 2, and 6, then every 8 weeks
        - May increase dosing to 10 mg/kg and frequency up to q 4 weeks depending on efficacy
    - Ertapenem
      - 1 g daily × 4–8 weeks
      - Typically used as a bridge to surgery
      - PEARL: Requires PICC line
  - Others:
    - Ustekinumab
  - Surgical
    - CO2 laser excision
    - Consult radiation oncology to consider external electron beam radiotherapy
    - Consult plastic surgery or reconstructive urology (for perianal/vulvar disease)
- Menstrual flares
  - Add anti-androgen therapy
    - OCP (containing ethinyl estradiol)
    - Spironolactone 50 mg QD (titrate up to 200 mg QD)

Keloids [19]

Key DDx

- Xanthoma disseminatum
- Lobomycosis
- Keloidal scleroderma
- Keloidal morphea
- Carcinoma en cuirasse
- Type IV Ehlers-Danlos Syndrome

Treatment Ladder

- Intralesional triamcinolone
  - Every 4–6 weeks
  - PEARL: You can lightly spray with cryotherapy to create some edema, then inject 40 mg/ml (retrograde injections)
- Surgery + IL steroids
  - Keloid "Protocol" (Weeks 0, 1, 2, 4, 6, 10, 14)
    - After closure—inject small amount (0.1–0.2 mL) of triamcinolone 40 mg/ml between the sutures in the center of the closure
    - Post-op week #1: inject ILK BEFORE removing sutures (otherwise, pressure may dehisce the wound—if this occurs steri strip with mastisol)
    - If evidence of recurrence after series, continue monthly ILK 40 until stable

Outside the Box Treatment Options

- Silicone gel sheeting: 24 h/d × 2 months
- Pressure garments: Zimmer splints for ears
- Surgery + imiquimod nightly × 2 months starting on evening of surgery
- Intralesional 5-Fluorouracil 50 mg/ml weekly
- PDT
- Pulsed dye laser
- Nd:YAG laser

Pseudofolliculitis Barbae [20]

What Not to Miss

- Women with this condition may exhibit picking behaviors and pluck hair or manipulate skin

Key DDx

- Acne vulgaris

Work Up Pearls

- Bacterial culture if concerned about infection

Treatment Ladder

- Stop shaving for at least 1 month
- Modification of shaving practices
  - Wash with warm water and mild cleanser
  - Use wash cloth in circular motion
  - Shave with skin relaxed in the direction of the hair growth with electric razor
- Warm compresses
- Low potency topical corticosteroids +/− topical antibiotics
- Topical retinoids
- Intralesional triamcinolone
- Oral antibiotics based on bacterial cultures
- Oral prednisone 20–40 mg × 1–2 weeks if lesions are very inflamed
- Topical eflornithine cream (Vaniqa)
- Laser hair removal- works best for fair skin patients with dark brown to black hair
  - Diode
  - Long-pulse Nd:YAG

References

1. Maranda EL, Simmons BJ, Nguyen AH, et al. Treatment of acne keloidalis nuchae: a systematic review of the literature. Dermatol Ther. 2016;6(3):363–78.
2. Hordinsky MK. Current treatments for alopecia areata. J Investig Dermatol Symp. 2015;17:44–6.
3. Wasserman D, Guzman-Sanchez DA, Scott K, et al. Alopecia areata. Int J Dermatol. 2007;46(2):121–31.
4. Penzi LR, Yasuda M, Manatis-Lornell A, et al. Hair regrowth in a patient with long-standing alopecia totalis and atopic dermatitis treated with dupilumab. JAMA Dermatol. 2018;154(11):1358–60.
5. Rossi A, Anzalone A, Fortuna MC, et al. Multi-therapies in androgenetic alopecia: review and clinical experiences. Dermatol Ther. 2016;29(6):424–32.
6. Levy LL, Emer JJ. Female pattern alopecia: current perspectives. Int J Women's Health. 2013;5:541–56.
7. Dhurat R, Sukesh MS. Principles and methods of preparation of platelet-rich plasma: a review and author's perspective. J Cutan Aesthet Surg. 2014;7(4):189–97.
8. Ogunleye TA, McMichael A, Olsen EA. Central centrifugal cicatricial alopecia. Dermatol Clin. 2014;32(2):173–81.

9. Errichetti E, Figini M, Croatto M, et al. Therapeutic management of classic lichen planopilaris: a systemic review. Clin Cosmet Investig Dermatol. 2018;11:91–102.
10. Jha AK. Platelet-rich plasma for the treatment of lichen planopilaris. JAAD. 2018;79(5):e95–6.
11. Malkud S. Telogen effluvium: a review. J Clin Diagn Res. 2015;9(9):WE01–WE03.
12. Billero V, Miteva M. Traction alopecia: the root of the problem. Clin Cosmet Investig Dermatol. 2018;11:149–59.
13. Saunte DML, Jemec GBE. Hidradenitis suppurativa advances in diagnosis and treatment. JAMA Rev. 2017;318(20):2019–32.
14. Canoui-Poitrine F, Thuaut AL, Revuz JE, et al. Identification of three hidradenitis suppurativa phenotypes: latent class analysis of a cross-sectional study. J Invest Dermatol. 2013;133(6):1506–11.
15. Smith MK, Nicholson CL, Parks-Miller A, Hamzavi IH. Hidradenitis suppurativa: an update on connecting the tracts. F1000 Research 6(F1000 Faculty Rev) 2017; 1272. https://doi.org/10.12688/f1000research.11337.1.
16. van Rappard DC, Leenarts MF, Meijerink-van't Oost L et al. Comparing treatment outcomes of infliximab and adalimumab in patients with severe hidradenitis suppurativa. J Dermatolog Treat. 2012;23(4):284–9.
17. van der Zee HH, Gulliver WP. Medical treatments of hidradenitis suppurativa. Dermatol Clin. 2016;34(1):91–6.
18. Gupta M, Mahajan VK, Mehta KS, et al. Zinc therapy in Dermatology: a review. Dermatol Res Pract. 2014;2014:709152.
19. Ud-Din S, Bayat A. New insights on keloids, hypertrophic scars, and striae. Dermatol Clin. 2014;32(2):193–209.
20. Alexis A, Heath CR, Halder RM. Folliculitis keloidalis nuchae and pseudofolliculitis barbae. Dermatol Clin. 2014;32(2):183–91.

Inpatient Diseases of Significance

Angad Chadha, Chelsea Fidai and Chauncey McHargue

Calciphylaxis (aka calcific uremic arteriolopathy) [1]

What Not To Miss

- Need to differentiate uremic from non-uremic calciphylaxis
- Risk factors: ESRD, dialysis, hyperphosphatemia, hypercoagulable states, hypoalbuminemia, liver disease, hyperparathyroidism, female gender, obesity, DM, rheumatic disease, long term steroid use
- Drugs: warfarin, systemic steroids, calcium-based binders, vitamin D analogs, exogenous Ca/Vit D supplementation

Key DDx

- Coumadin necrosis
- Vasculitis
- Pyoderma gangrenosum
- Cryoglobulinemia
- Ulcerative panniculitis (e.g. pancreatic panniculitis)
- Arterial thrombosis

A. Chadha · C. Fidai
Department of Dermatology, Henry Ford Health System,
3031 West Grand Blvd, Suite 800, Detroit, MI 48202, USA

C. McHargue (✉)
Henry Ford Health System, 3031 West Grand Blvd., Suite 800, Detroit, MI 48202, USA
e-mail: cmcharg1@hfhs.org

© Springer Nature Switzerland AG 2020
H. W. Lim et al. (eds.), *Practical Guide to Dermatology*,
https://doi.org/10.1007/978-3-030-18015-7_8

Work Up Pearls

- Biopsy tips
  - Telescoping punch biopsy (6-mm followed by 4-mm into the defect) down to deep fat as calcific changes can often be deep
  - Can consider a biopsy of uninvolved skin immediately adjacent to ulcer edge if there is significant induration there (can represent calcification)
- Check timing of coumadin initiation (if on coumadin)
- Check creatinine (sCr), Ca, Vit D, PTH levels

Treatment Ladder

- Avoid local skin trauma
- Discontinue causative drug (if drug related)
- Pain control with topical lidocaine and systemic medications, aggressive wound care, surgical debridement may improve survival in ESRD patients
- Consult nephrology (low-Ca dialysis, increased dialysis frequency/duration, treatment of Ca/Phos/PTH abnormalities)
- IV sodium thiosulfate 25 g three times weekly during last hour of dialysis or immediately afterwards
  - Side effects include nausea, vomiting, metabolic acidosis, hypotension, hypocalcemia, QTc prolongation, reduced bone density
- Others: pamidronate, low dose tPA, hyperbaric oxygen therapy

Outside the Box Treatment Options

- Intralesional sodium thiosulfate if very localized disease and if patient can tolerate it (very painful)

Cutaneous Metastases [2]

What Not To Miss

- Carcinoma erysipeloides
  - Sharply demarcated red patch due to brisk inflammatory response to carcinoma cells
  - Common in cutaneous metastasis from breast cancer
- Carcinoma en curiasse or sclerodermoid carcinoma
  - Indurated fibrous nodular scar-like plaques due to infiltration of skin by carcinoma cells
  - If on scalp, can lead to alopecia neoplastica

- Carcinoma telangiectoides
  - Red patches with numerous telangiectasias or lymphatic vessels
- Periumbilical nodules (Sister Mary Joseph nodule) can be a sign of advanced colorectal carcinoma due to spread along the urachus
- Vascular plaques resembling a hemangioma or pyogenic granuloma can be seen in cutaneous metastasis from renal cell carcinoma

Key DDx

- Leukemia cutis
- Erysipelas
- Dermatofibrosarcoma protuberans
- Adnexal tumors
- Extramammary Paget's disease
- Sarcoidosis
- Cutaneous endometriosis
- Erythema nodosum
- Pyogenic granuloma
- Kaposi sarcoma

Work Up Pearls

- Review slides with the pathologist; may be able to perform stains to identify primary tumor
- Ask patient about history of internal malignancies
  - Frequency of presentation: occurs in 1–10% of internal malignancies melanoma > breast > lung > oral/nasal mucosa > GI

Treatment Ladder

- Treat underlying malignancy (consult oncology)
- Local symptomatic control for inflammation (topical corticosteroids), pain (systemic and topical pain medications)

Drug Eruptions

What Not To Miss

- Organized approach to drug eruptions
  - What is the primary lesion? (macules, papules, vesicles/bullae, pustules, purpura, wheals)
  - What is the distribution? Where did it start and where did it spread? Is there flexural involvement or accentuation? Are the face, palms, and soles involved?

- o Are facial edema, mucosal involvement, or dusky lesions present?
- o Are there associated systemic signs or laboratory findings? (fever, pruritus, lymphadenopathy, visceral involvement [elevated Cr, elevated transaminases, diarrhea], abnormal CBC [e.g. peripheral neutrophilia or eosinophilia])
- Critical evaluation of the time-course of associated symptoms (e.g. fever and leukocytosis a few hours after starting ceftriaxone may mark the onset of AGEP; high fevers and new leukocytosis a few days before development of eruption may be signs of the prodrome that precedes the development of SJS/TEN)
- Trend "Fever" and check "Meds History" tabs in electronic medical record to get a visual overview of when different drugs were administered in the hospital
- Note: Drugs administered during surgery (e.g. IV antibiotics) may only be recorded in the anesthesia record

Exanthematous Drug Eruption [3]

What Not To Miss

- Drugs: aminopenicillins, sulfonamides, cephalosporins, aromatic anticonvulsants, allopurinol, abavacir, nevirapine

Key DDx

- Viral exanthem
- Infectious mononucleosis
- Evolving/early drug-induced hypersensitivity syndrome
- Early SJS/TEN
- Engraftment syndrome
- Toxic shock syndrome
- Staphylococcal scalded skin syndrome
- Scarlet fever
- Primary HIV infections
- Early acute GVHD
- The cutaneous eruption of juvenile rheumatoid arthritis
- Kawasaki disease
- Secondary syphilis
- Miliaria rubra
- PEARL: Exanthematous drug favored over viral exanthem if the eruption is more polymorphic or if there is peripheral eosinophilia
- Symmetric drug-related intertriginous and flexural exanthem (SDRIFE)
  - o Uncommon variant of exanthematous drug eruption that occurs hours to days after exposure to the offending drug
  - o Presents as sharply demarcated V-shaped erythema in the gluteal/perianal or inguinal/perigenital areas, often with involvement of at least one other flexural area (e.g. axillae, antecubital fossae, popliteal fossae)

○ Causative drugs: drugs listed above plus clindamycin, erythromycin, iodinated contrast, ASA, pseudoephedrine

Work Up Pearls

- Onset: 4–14 days (first exposure), <4 days (re-exposure)
- Check CBC with differential and CMP to evaluate for peripheral eosinophilia and internal organ involvement which may herald the development of Drug-Induced Hypersensitivity Syndrome (DIHS)
- Exanthematous drug eruption often has rostrocaudal onset of distribution and clearing; dependent lesions can have purpura
- Eruption may worsen for another 1–3 days after drug elimination; eruption resolves in 1–2 weeks

Treatment Ladder

- Discontinue offending drug unless it is absolutely necessary and more toxic exanthems have been ruled out
- Supportive measures for exfoliation and pruritus

Outside the Box Treatment Options

- Can treat through if drug is absolutely necessary
  ○ eruption will usually disappear but may progress to erythroderma

---

Drug Reaction with Eosinophilia and Systemic Symptoms (DRESS) and Drug-Induced Hypersensitivity Syndrome (DIHS) [4, 5]

What Not To Miss

- Drugs: aromatic anticonvulsants, lamotrigine, sulfonamides, abacavir, allopurinol, dapsone, minocycline, nevirapine, vancomycin, bupropion, fluoxetine, amlodipine, captopril, NSAIDs
- Internal organ involvement → do not let these patients leave the hospital without a complete baseline workup.
  ○ Clues: facial edema, fever, peripheral eosinophilia, lymphadenopathy, transaminitis, interstitial nephritis, myocarditis, interstitial pneumonitis, myositis, thyroiditis, encephalitis
- Eruption and internal manifestations may persist for months even with treatment
  ○ Can have late involvement of visceral organs even after tapering steroid => check thyroid profile for 2 years after DRESS
- Mortality 2–10%

Key DDx

- Infectious mononucleosis
- Exanthematous drug eruption
- Early SJS/TEN
- Viral exanthema
- Toxic shock syndrome
- Secondary syphilis
- Roseola
- Measles
- Parvovirus B19 infection

Work Up Pearls

- Onset: 2–6 weeks (first exposure), <2 weeks (re-exposure)
- Use RegiSCAR or J-SCAR criteria to aid in diagnosis and prognosis
- Check CBC with differential, renal function, hepatic function, urinalysis, TSH, free T4, ECG, CXR, MRI if indicated by symptoms
- Biopsy may show features of common drug eruptions, but may show keratinocyte necrosis indicative of EM or SJS/TEN
- N.B. Many drug-induced eruptions can show extravasation of RBCs which should not be confused with vasculitis

Treatment Ladder

- Discontinue offending drug
- Prednisone 0.5–2.0 mg/kg daily with taper over weeks to months
- Cyclosporine, 3–5 mg/kg, if steroids contraindicated
- Control of pruritus with topical and/or systemic agents

Outside the Box Treatment Options

- Consider NB-UVB phototherapy if eruption is slow to clear and if pruritus is difficult to control with topical or systemic agents

Cutaneous Small Vessel Vasculitis (CSVV) [3]

What Not To Miss

- Drugs: hydralazine, minocycline, propylthiouracil, levamisole-adulterated cocaine, penicillins, cephalosporins, sulfonamides, phenytoin, allopurinol, NSAIDs

- Cutaneous manifestations include urticaria, hemorrhagic blisters, pustules, digital necrosis, or ulcers
- Internal manifestations: arthritis, nephritis, peripheral neuropathy, GI bleeding

Key DDx

- Henoch-Schonlein purpura/IgA vasculitis
- Urticarial vasculitis
- ANCA-associated vasculitis
- Bacterial septic vasculitis
- Disseminated fungal infection
- Meningococcemia
- Rocky mountain spotted fever
- Capillaritis
- Thormboangiitis obliterans
- Disseminated intravascular coagulation

Work Up Pearls

- Onset: 7–21 days (first exposure), ≤3 days (re-exposure)
- Biopsy new lesions <24–48 h old
- Perform lesional DIF
- Must get urinalysis, urine sediment, and BMP to evaluate for renal involvement
- Need to rule out other underlying causes of CSVV like infection, neoplasms, autoimmune connective tissue disease via careful history taking and review of systems. See "Vasculitis" section below
  - Order tests as appropriate

Treatment Ladder

- Discontinue offending drug and rule out other causes of vasculitis (see "Vasculitis" section)
- Pruritus control with topical and/or systemic agents
- Patients without systemic involvement can be safely observed with symptomatic control
  - If cutaneous disease is refractory to topical therapies, consider colchicine 0.6 mg twice daily or dapsone 50 mg daily (up to 150 mg daily)
- If internal end-organ involvement is present, consider systemic immunosuppression with the following:
  - Prednisone 0.5 mg/kg daily
  - Methotrexate 10–25 mg once weekly
  - Mycophenolate mofetil 1–3 g daily
  - Azathioprine 1–3 mg/kg daily

Outside the Box Treatment Options

- May consider wet wraps if internal organ involvement is not present

Acute Generalized Exanthematous Pustulosis (AGEP) [6]

What Not To Miss

- Mucosal involvement in about 50% of patients
  - Systemic involvement uncommon, but can include kidney and liver
- Drugs: antibiotics (penicillins, cephalosporins, carbapenems, clindamycin, sulfonamides, metroniazaole, quinolones, macrolides), calcium channel blockers (esp. diltiazem), carbamazepine, hydroxychloroquine, NSAIDs, PPIs, terbinafine

Key DDx

- Pustular psoriasis/deficiency of the IL-36 receptor antagonist (DITRA)
- Folliculitis
- Sneddon–Wilkinson subcorneal pustular dermatosis
- Miliaria pustulosa
- Cutaneous candidiasis
- Dermatitis herpetiformis
- Exanthematous drug eruption

Work Up Pearls

- Onset: few hours to 4 days (first exposure)
- Use EuroSCAR criteria to aid in diagnosis
- May be preceded by high fevers and a neutrophilia that start within 4 days of exposure to a new drug
- Check CBC with differential and CMP to evaluate for internal involvement

Treatment Ladder

- Discontinue offending drug
- Topical corticosteroids
- Supportive care for fever, pruritus, exfoliation, and disrupted skin barrier

Acute Febrile Neutrophilic Dermatosis (Sweet Syndrome) [3]

What Not To Miss

- Can have neutrophilic infiltrates in muscles and lung
- Drugs: granulocyte growth factors, all-trans-retinoic acid, antibiotics (TMP-SMX, minocycline, quinolones), azathioprine, furosemide, hydralazine, NSAIDs, abacavir, imatinib, bortezomib, checkpoint inhibitors
- Associated inflammatory bowel disease or malignancy
    - PEARL: Most common malignancy is hematologic

Key DDx

- Pyoderma gangrenosum
- Neutrophilic eccrine hidradenitis
- Bowel-associated dermatosis-arthritis syndrome
- Wells syndrome
- Erythema multiforme
- Azathioprine hypersensitivity syndrome
- Urticarial vasculitis
- Erythema elevatum diutinum
- Cutaneous small vessel vasculitis
- Atypical mycobacterial infection

Work Up Pearls

- Onset: about 1 week after first exposure
- Consider workup to rule out infection-associated, IBD-associated, or malignancy-associated Sweet's syndrome

Treatment Ladder

- Discontinue offending drug
- Topical class I or II corticosteroids for mild cases
- For more severe cases
    - Prednisone 0.5–1.0 mg/kg daily
    - Colchicine 1.0–1.5 mg daily
    - Dapsone 100–200 mg daily
    - Potassium iodide 900–1500 mg daily

Linear IgA Bullous Dermatosis [3]

What Not To Miss

- Drugs: vancomycin (most common); beta-lactam antibiotics, captopril, NSAIDs, phenytoin, sulfonamide antibiotics, furosemide, lithium, rifampin, G-CSF

Key DDx

- Bullous drug eruption
- Bullous pemphigoid
- Mucous membrane pemphigoid
- Epidermolysis bullosa acquisita
- Sneddon-Wilkinson subcorneal pustular dermatosis
- Leukocytoclastic vasculitis

Work Up Pearls

- Onset: 24 h to 15 days after first exposure
- Lesions are often grouped in annular arrangements on the elbows, knees, and buttocks ("string of pearls")
- Oral involvement is common (~80% of cases) and favors the hard and soft palates
- Perform biopsy for H&E and DIF to demonstrate band-like deposition of IgA at DEJ

Treatment Ladder

- Discontinue offending drug
- For severe cases
  - Dapsone 50–150 mg daily
  - Sulfapyridine 1000–1500 mg daily
  - Sulfamethoxypyridazine 1000–1500 mg daily
  - Colchicine 0.6–1.0 mg twice to three times daily
  - Prednisone (high doses are often needed for treatment)

Stevens–Johnson Syndrome (SJS) and Toxic Epidermal Necrolysis (TEN) [7, 8]

What Not To Miss

- Drugs: allopurinol, aromatic anticonvulsants, sulfonamide antibiotics, lamotrigine, nevirapine, oxicam NSAIDs

- Risk factors: HIV infection, mycoplasma pneumoniae infection, underlying autoimmune disease, underlying hematologic malignancy, HLA-B*15:02 or HLA-A*31:01 for carbamazepine in South Asians and Asians, HLA-B*58:01 for allopurinol
- Early ophthalmology consult for ocular symptoms (seen in ~80%) like severe conjunctivitis with purulent discharge, bulla formation, corneal ulceration, anterior uveitis, panophthalmitis
  - Late sequelae include pain, dryness, synechiae development
- Early OB/GYN or urology consult for urogenital symptoms (seen in ~66%): urethritis, genital erosions/ulcerations, genital synechiae development

Key DDx

- Erythema multiforme
- Mycoplasma pneumonia-induced rash and mucositis
- Staphylococcal scalded skin syndrome
- Toxic shock syndrome
- Purpura fulminans/disseminated intravascular coagulation
- Acute GVHD
- Drug-induced hypersensitivity syndrome
- Generalized fixed drug eruption
- Bullous drug eruption
- Paraneoplastic pemphigus (for hemorrhagic crusting of lips)

Work Up Pearls

- Biopsy tips
  - Perform two punch biopsies from acutely involved skin
    - (1) Frozen section
    - (2) DIF
    - PEARL: Frozen section specimen should be in saline NOT formalin; at most institutions, the frozen section can be read very quickly
- Onset: 7–28 days after first exposure, <48 h with re-exposure; risk limited to 8 weeks after starting drug
- Prodrome of fevers, flu-like symptoms, malaise, myalgia, arthralgias precede eruption by 1–3 days
  - Photophobia, conjunctival itching/burning, odynophagia, dysuria may be early symptoms of mucosal involvement
- Nikolsky sign—sloughing of apparently uninvolved skin with gentle pressure
- Asboe-Hansen sign—lateral extension of bulla with pressure
- Check CBC, CMP, ESR, CRP, Mycoplasma Pneumoniae PCR or serologies; get baseline cultures (skin, blood, urine, and NG tube) and repeat every 48 h during the acute phase
- Prognosis: estimate BSA accurately; use SCORTEN system to gauge prognosis

Treatment Ladder

- Discontinue offending drug
- Roughly equivalent rates of survival and re-epithelialization when comparing surgical debridement versus "anti-shear" wound care designed to leave skin in place
- Consider nonadherent nanocrystalline gauze materials containing silver over petrolatum-impregnated gauze
- Order a fluidized air bed when the back is significantly denuded
- Increase room temp to 30–32 C or use a heated-air body-warmer to minimize caloric expenditures due to transepidermal heat loss
- Fluids: start with (2 mL) × (weight in kg) × (% BSA involved) in the first 24 h, then titrate to maintain good urine output
- Early gynecologic examination with use of intravaginal steroids or soft vagina molds as necessary
- Consult ophthalmology early for topical steroid, topical antibiotic, and possible amniotic membrane transplantation
- Medications
  - There is no universally agreed-upon treatment ladder for SJS/TEN and direct comparison studies are often lacking.
  - Cyclosporine 3–5 mg/kg daily early in disease course may slow disease progression, shorten time to re-epithelialization, and decrease mortality
    - PEARL: High rate of acute renal insufficiency in patients with SJS/TEN could limit or complicate the use of this medication
  - TNF-alpha inhibitors may halt the disease, shorten disease duration, improve mortality, and decrease SJS/TEN related adverse events.
    - Etanercept 50 mg subcutaneously once
    - Infliximab 5 mg/kg infusion once
    - Studies to date showing benefit from TNF-alpha inhibitors have had low numbers of patients
  - Some studies show a mortality benefit from high dose IVIG (>2 g/kg total dose) but other reviews showed no such benefit
    - A large U.S. multicenter retrospective cohort study recently demonstrated benefit for IVIG when used in conjunction with systemic steroids.
  - Some studies suggest potential benefit from the use of systemic steroids but there is much heterogeneity in dosage, frequency, pulse versus continuous, and adjunctive therapies used along with systemic steroids
    - Systemic steroids may increase risk of infection, create a hypercatabolic state, and decrease re-epithelialization rates
  - Equivocal evidence to support routine use of plasmapheresis
    - May be used to rapidly decrease blood levels of offending agents, especially if the agents have a long half life

Erythema Multiforme (EM) [9]

What Not To Miss

- Mucous membrane involvement in EM Major > Minor
  - Oral (70%), ocular (17%), or genital (25%)
- EM Major can have systemic symptoms: fever, malaise, myalgias
- Causative infections (about 90% cases): HSV 1 > 2 (usually EM Minor), mycoplasma (usually EM Major), histoplasmosis, hepatitis C, EBV, coxsackie virus
- Causative drugs (less than 10% cases): allopurinol, phenobarbital, phenytoin, valproic acid, sulfonamide antibiotics, penicillins, erythromycin, nitrofurantoin, tetracyclines, acetylsalicylic acid, statins, TNF-α inhibitors

Key DDx

- SJS/TEN
- Mycoplasma pneumonia-induced rash and mucositis
- Generalized fixed drug eruption
- Erythema annulare centrifugum

Work Up Pearls

- Onset: 3–5 days after offending agent/infection; occurs 2–17 days after HSV eruption
- Diagnosis is often clinical, may consider biopsy
- If HSV lesions present, swab for PCR/culture; may consider blood serologic testing for HSV; may consider HSV testing on biopsy for recurrent EM to establish diagnosis of HSV-related EM
- Obtain mycoplasma serologies/PCR in patients with respiratory symptoms

Treatment Ladder

- Topical corticosteroids and symptomatic control of cutaneous lesions
- High potency topical steroid gels/washes (e.g. fluocinonide gel or dexamethasone swish and spit) for painful oral lesions
  - If oral lesions are severe, may consider prednisone 40–60 mg daily with a 2–4 week taper
- For ocular involvement, start dexamethasone 0.1% eye drops and consult ophthalmology emergently
- Treatment for HSV and mycoplasma as indicated
  - Consider suppressive acyclovir/valacyclovir therapy if recurrent HSV-related EM; in antiviral-resistant cases of recurrent HSV-related EM, consider azathioprine, mycophenolate mofetil, or dapsone

Graft Versus Host Disease [10, 11]

What Not To Miss

- Risk factors: prior GVHD, unrelated donor, related donor with HLA mismatch, older age of recipient/donor, female donor with male recipient
- Early diagnosis of GVHD is lifesaving → must recognize early cutaneous clues and have LOW threshold for biopsy
  - Can begin as subtle perifollicular erythema
  - Early disease often appears on the acral surfaces (ears, palms, soles) and posterior neck/upper back; mucositis may be an early finding as well

Key DDx

- Acute GVHD
  - Viral exanthem
  - Toxic erythema of chemotherapy
  - Eruption of lymphocyte recovery
  - Exanthematous drug/viral eruption
  - Early SJS/TEN
  - Early DIHS
  - Engraftment syndrome

- Chronic GVHD
  - Lichen planus
  - Lichenoid drug eruption
  - Morphea
  - Lichen sclerosis
  - Scleroderma
  - Nephrogenic systemic fibrosis

Work Up Pearls

- Skin biopsy is necessary
  - Biopsy an acute lesion and send for normal H&E
  - PEARL: Consider checking short-tandem-repeats (STRs) on the tissue block as well as in peripheral blood for solid organ only
- Timing: <14 days (hyperacute GVHD), <100 days (classic GVHD), >100 days with features of acute GVHD (late-onset acute GVHD), ~4 months (chronic GVHD)
- Clinical findings: most commonly affects skin, GI tract, liver
  - Cutaneous eruption can have associated nausea, vomiting, diarrhea, abdominal pain and hyperbilirubinemia (cholestatic hepatitis)

Treatment Ladder

- High potency topical steroids for skin
- Medium-high potency topical steroids for mucosa (e.g. fluocinonide gel, dexamethasone swish and spit)
  - Consider topical lidocaine for mucositis
- Consult Bone Marrow Transplant team; they will guide systemic steroids, systemic calcineurin inhibitors, cyclosporine, TNF-α inhibitors, and extracorporeal photopheresis

Deep Fungal Infections

What Not To Miss

- Can present with cutaneous and/or systemic manifestations
- Consider in a patient with new papulonodular, sporotrichoid, or ulcerative skin lesions
- Risk factors for disseminated infection:
  - HIV/AIDS, solid organ/bone marrow transplant, hematologic malignancy, hyperglycemic states (diabetic ketoacidosis), immunosuppression, chemotherapy, neutropenia (<500 PMNs/mL for >10 days), severe burn, broad-spectrum antibiotic use (with continued fever), IV/urinary catheters

Key DDx

- Cutaneous tuberculosis
- Sarcoidosis
- Leishmaniasis
- Leprosy
- Squamous cell carcinoma

Work Up Pearls

- Punch biopsy (×2) for H&E and tissue culture
  - H&E: formalin-containing bottle
  - Tissue culture: sterile cup containing gauze soaked in **NON-BACTERIO-STATIC** saline
    - Order: aerobic/anaerobic bacteria, fungi, mycobacteria
    - PEARL: Inform the lab if suspect coccidioidomycosis (highly infectious)
- Fungal cell wall markers (serum)
  - Galactomannan—relatively specific to Aspergillus

- o 1,3-Beta-D-glucan—non-specific
- o Mannan—yeasts (Candida)
- Fungal DNA detection via PCR (high sensitivity and specificity)
  - o Tissue, blood, other bodily fluids
- Respiratory symptoms → CXR
- Ophthalmology consult in suspected disseminated candidiasis to rule out endophthalmitis

Treatment Ladder

- Systemic antifungals in conjunction with infectious diseases specialist

Outside the Box Treatment Ideas

- Consider decreasing duration of neutropenia (GM-CSF) and stopping immuno-suppressant if appropriate

Herpes Virus Infections [12–14]

What Not To Miss

- Any patient with erosions or grouped vesicles
  - o Symptoms including pain/tenderness/burning/tingling prior to onset
  - o Distribution can be localized or diffuse
- Risks: age, immunosuppression (zoster in 50% of immunocompromised pts)
- Common sites
  - o HSV: lips, gingivae, anogenital mucosa
  - o Zoster: face, scalp, trunk, thighs
  - o Primary varicella: prodrome followed by pruritic, erythematous clear vesicles with surrounding red halos ("dew drops on a rose petal") starting on the face and spreading downward to trunk + extremities

Key DDx

- Furunculosis
- Contact dermatitis
- Candidiasis
- Bullous fixed drug

Work Up Pearls

- DFA for VZV (institution/practice specific)
  - o Use #15 blade to collect vesicular fluid on glass slide (no coverslip)

- o Put in a cardboard slide carrier
- o Results in 1–2 days
- o High sensitivity
- Viral culture: high specificity, low sensitivity, results in 2–5 days
- HSV PCR
- Tzanck smear
- +/− Biopsy: if other blistering process is in the DDx

Treatment Ladder (**adult dosing guidelines provided)

- Start treatment at earliest sign of disease (tingling, burning, pain) and definitely within 72 h of onset to reduce viral shedding, time to healing, and pain
- Orolabial HSV, immunocompetent patients
  - o Initial episode: valacyclovir 2 g PO twice daily for one day –or– acyclovir 200 mg five times daily for 7–10 days –or– acyclovir 400 mg three times daily for 7–10 days
  - o Recurrent episodes: valacyclovir 2 g twice daily for one day –or– acyclovir 400 mg five times daily for 7–10 days
  - o Suppressive therapy: valacyclovir 500–1000 mg daily –or– acyclovir 400 mg twice daily

- Orolabial HSV, immunocompromised patients
  - o Initial or recurrent episodes: valacyclovir 1 g twice daily for 5–10 days –or– acyclovir 400 mg three times daily for 5–10 days –or– acyclovir 5 mg/kg every 8 h IV (for severe disease) with switch to oral once lesions regress
  - o Suppressive therapy: valacyclovir 500 mg twice daily –or– acyclovir 400 mg twice daily

- Genital HSV, immunocompetent patients
  - o Initial episode: valacyclovir 1 g PO twice daily 7–10 days –or– acyclovir 200 mg five times daily for 7–10 days –or– acyclovir 400 mg three times daily for 7–10 days –or– acyclovir 5–10 mg/kg every 8 h IV for 2–7 days (for severe disease) followed by oral therapy for a total antiviral course of 10 days or until lesion resolution
  - o Recurrent episodes: valacyclovir 500 mg PO twice daily for 3 days –or– valacyclovir 1 g daily for 5 days –or– acyclovir 400 mg three times daily for 5 days –or– acyclovir 800 mg twice daily for 5 days –or– acyclovir 800 mg PO three times daily for 3 days
  - o Suppressive dosing: valacyclovir 500–1000 mg daily for up to 12 months –or– acyclovir 400 mg twice daily for up to 12 months

- Genital HSV, immunocompromised patients
  - o Initial or recurrent episodes: valacyclovir 1 g twice daily for 5–10 days –or– acyclovir 400 mg three times daily for 7–10 days –or– acyclovir 5–10 mg/kg

every 8 h IV for 2–7 days (for severe disease) followed by oral therapy for a total antiviral course of 10 days
- o Suppressive dosing: valacyclovir 500 mg twice daily –or– acyclovir 400–800 mg two to three times daily

- Genital HSV, pregnant patients
  - o Consult OB/GYN in addition to starting therapy
  - o Initial episode: valacyclovir 1 g twice daily for 7–10 days –or– acyclovir 400 mg three times daily for 7–10 days
  - o Recurrent episodes: valacyclovir 500 mg twice daily for 3 days –or– valacyclovir 1 g daily for 5 days –or– acyclovir 400 mg three times daily for 5 days –or– acyclovir 800 mg twice daily for 5 days
  - o Suppressive therapy if a genital lesion occurs during pregnancy: valacyclovir 500 mg twice daily –or– acyclovir 400 mg three times daily beginning at 36 weeks gestation until onset of delivery

- Herpes Zoster (Shingles), immunocompetent patient
  - o Valacyclovir 1 g three times daily for 7 days

- Herpes Zoster (Shingles), immunocompromised patient
  - o Localized dermatomal: valacyclovir 1 g three times daily for 7–10 days
  - o Extensive cutaneous or visceral involvement: initial treatment with IV acyclovir with transition to valacyclovir 1 g three times daily orally for a total antiviral course of 10–14 days or until lesion resolution

- IV acyclovir: neonatal HSV, immunocompromised patients, severe eczema herpeticum, and visceral dissemination

- Immunocompromised patients: treat until the cutaneous lesions are healed

In the Context Of …

- Hutchinson's sign → ocular involvement
  - o Consult ophthalmology

- Eczema herpeticum (HSV in areas of eczema, Darier's, Hailey-Hailey)
  - o More common in children, can be severe with +/− systemic symptoms, lymphadenopathy
  - o Treat aggressively, usually as disseminated HSV

- HSV Encephalitis
  - o Fever, altered mental status, localized neurologic findings
  - o Mortality $\geq 70\%$ without treatment; residual neurologic defects in others
  - o Consult neurology

Ulcers [15–17]

What Not To Miss

- Obtain appropriate HPI: onset (including inciting factors) and clinical course, symptoms, associated edema or paresthesias, past history of wounds
- Response to therapy, history of healing, debridement
- PMH: HIV, sickle cell, Raynauds, scleroderma, chemotherapy, viral hepatitis, drug use, vasculopathy, neurologic disorders, malnutrition
- Medications: hydroxyurea, warfarin, heparin
- Social history: Smoker? Where do they live/who cares for them?
- Exam:
  - Look at the entire area
  - Depth, necrosis, "punched out" appearance, rolled margin, gun metal grey, purulence, bleeding, visible bone/tendon, geometric
  - Edema, hemosiderin, varicosities, capillary refill, adenopathy, diminished sensation
  - Measure and take photos

Key DDx

- Venous ulcers
- Neurogenic (diabetic) ulcers
- Infections
- Vasculitis
- Pyoderma gangrenosum
- Factitial ulcer
- Brown recluse spider bite

Work Up Pearls

- Review labs: CBC, albumin, HgbA1c, ESR/CRP, INR, ANA, ANCA, cryoglobulins, APS, protein C/S, factor V Leiden
- Obtain bacterial and viral cultures if indicated
- Consider biopsy
  - Deep wedge biopsies that include the ulcer margin and bed are preferred (punch is more realistic)

Treatment Ladder

- Moisture is essential for proper wound healing

- o Speeds re-epithelialization, stimulates collagen synthesis, promotes angiogenesis and reduces pain
- o Exception: Highly exudative wounds (may cause maceration which inhibits fibroblasts)
- Eliminate infection: culture and tailor coverage
- Debridement: conversion of a chronic to an acute wound
  - o May be considered for diabetic, venous ulcers and pressure ulcers
  - o Not advised for arterial ulcers: *eschar overlying heel wound* with vascular compromise should be left alone
  - o Watch out for pyoderma gangrenosum!

- Compression: 1st line treatment for venous ulcers
  - o Must rule out significant arterial disease prior to use
  - o If ABI is <0.5 → no compression

Vasculitis [18]

What Not To Miss

- Polymorphic clinical findings based on the size of the vessels involved:
  - o Small vessels (arterioles, capillaries, postcapillary venules)
    - Palpable purpura
    - Petechiae
    - Macular purpura
    - Targetoid papules and plaques
  - o Medium vessels (arteries and veins in the deep dermis or subcutis)
    - Livedo racemosa
    - Retiform purpura
    - Ulceration
    - Subcutaneous nodules
    - Digital necrosis
  - o Large vessels (aorta, other named arteries)
    - Cyanotic or necrotic skin
    - Hair loss or skin atrophy in affected limbs
    - Ulceration (pyoderma gangrenosum-like lesions on the lower legs)
- Etiologies
  - o Idiopathic (45–55%)
  - o Infection
    - Group A Streptococcus, mycobacterium leprae, TB, mycoplasma pneumonia, Hep B, Hep C, viral URI, HIV, parvo B19

- ○ Autoimmune
  - ▪ RA, SLE, Sjogren's, Behcet's, IBD
- ○ Drug
  - ▪ Allopurinol, cephalosporins, NSAIDs, OCPs, hydralazine, minocycline, G-CSF, PCN, MTX, phenytoin, quinolones, sulfa, thiazides, TNF-α, Levamisole
- ○ Neoplasm
  - ▪ Plasma cell dyscrasias, myelodysplasia, myeloproliferative dx, lymphoproliferative dx
- Systemic sx: fever, malaise, arthralgias, myalgias, GI/GU symptoms

Key DDx

- Coagulopathy
- Urticarial vasculitis
- Disseminated fungal infection
- Meningococcemia
- Rocky mountain spotted fever
- Capillaritis
- Disseminated intravascular coagulation

Work Up Pearls

- Punch biopsy ($\times 2$) for H&E and DIF
  - ○ H&E:
    - ▪ **CENTER** of well-established lesion, ideally >72 h
    - ▪ If lesion is an ulcer, biopsy the edge
  - ○ DIF: especially useful in small vessel vasculitis
    - ▪ New lesion, ideally <24 h
  - ○ PEARL: If suspecting medium or large vessel vasculitis—need deep incisional biopsy
- General Screening
  - ○ CBCd, CMP, ESR, CRP, stool guaiac, UA with microscopy, stool guaiac, +/−urine toxin screen
  - ○ Hematologic: SPEP, UPEP, serum immunofixation (for M-spike)
  - ○ Infectious: Hep B, Hep C, HIV, antistreptolysin Ab, EBV, CMV, B19, L2 serotype, urine/throat/blood culture
  - ○ Immunologic: RF, ANA, C3, C4, CH50, anti-dsDNA, anti-ENA (Ro/La/RNP/Sm +/−Scl70, Jo-1), ANCAs, cryoglobulins, antiphospholipid abs
  - ○ Malignancy: CT chest/abdomen/pelvis, bone marrow biopsy, age-appropriate malignancy screens

Treatment Ladder

- Topical corticosteroids
- Systemic corticosteroids
- Immunosuppressives (choice depends on etiology)

References

1. Nigwekar SU, Thadhani R, Brandenburg VM. Calciphylaxis. N Engl J Med. 2018;378(18):1704–14.
2. Bolognia JL, Cerroni L. Dermatology: 2-volume set. Elsevier; 2017. Chap. 122.
3. Bolognia JL, Cerroni L. Dermatology: 2-volume set. Elsevier; 2017. Chap. 21.
4. Husain Z, Reddy BY, Schwartz RA. DRESS syndrome: Part I. Clinical perspectives. J Am Acad Dermatol. 2013;68(5):693. e1–14.
5. Husain Z, Reddy BY, Schwartz RA. DRESS syndrome: Part II. Management and therapeutics. J Am Acad Dermatol. 2013;68(5):709. e1–9.
6. Szatkowski J, Schwartz RA. Acute generalized exanthematous pustulosis (AGEP): a review and update. J Am Acad Dermatol. 2015;73(5):843–8.
7. Schneider JA, Cohen PR. Stevens-Johnson syndrome and toxic epidermal necrolysis: a concise review with a comprehensive summary of therapeutic interventions emphasizing supportive measures. Adv Ther. 2017;34(6):1235–44.
8. Micheletti RG, Chiesa-fuxench Z, Noe MH, et al. Stevens-Johnson syndrome/toxic epidermal necrolysis: a multicenter retrospective study of 377 adult patients from the United States. J Invest Dermatol. 2018;138(11):2315–21.
9. Lerch M, Mainetti C, Terziroli beretta-piccoli B, Harr T. Current perspectives on erythema multiforme. Clin Rev Allergy Immunol. 2018;54(1):177–84.
10. Hymes SR, Alousi AM, Cowen EW. Graft-versus-host disease: Part I. Pathogenesis and clinical manifestations of graft-versus-host disease. J Am Acad Dermatol. 2012;66(4):515. e1–18.
11. Hymes SR, Alousi AM, Cowen EW. Graft-versus-host disease: Part II. Management of cutaneous graft-versus-host disease. J Am Acad Dermatol. 2012;66(4):535. e1–16.
12. Wanat KA, et al. Bedside diagnostics in dermatology: viral, bacterial, and fungal infections. JAAD. 2017;77(2):197–218.
13. Ahronowitz I, Fox LP. Herpes zoster in hospitalized adults: practice gaps, new evidence, and remaining questions. JAAD. 2018;78(1):223–30.
14. Fatahzadeh M, Schwartz RA. Human herpes simplex virus infections: epidemiology, pathogenesis, symptomatology, diagnosis, and management. JAAD. 2007;57(5):737–63.
15. Morton LM, Phillips TJ. Wound healing and treating wounds: differential diagnosis and evaluation of chronic wounds. JAAD. 2016;74(4):589–605.
16. Fonder MA, et al. Treating the chronic wound: a practical approach to the care of nonhealing wounds and wound care dressings. J Am Acad Dermatol. 2008;58(2):185–206.
17. Alavi A, et al. What's new: management of venous leg ulcers: treating venous leg ulcers. JAAD. 2016;74(4):643–64.
18. Elston DM, et al. Skin biopsy: biopsy issues in specific diseases. JAAD. 2016;74(1):1–16.

Phototherapy and PUVA

Tasneem F. Mohammad, Iltefat H. Hamzavi and Henry W. Lim

Phototherapy

What Not To Miss

- New medication with photosensitizing potential (e.g. thiazide diuretics, doxy-cycline, minocycline, retinoids):
  - Action spectrum is in the UVA range; therefore, it is relevant for patients on PUVA or UVA1
    - Decrease starting/current dose by 30%
  - Dose for NB-UVB does not need to be adjusted [1]
  - An exception is systemic retinoids, which decrease thickness of epidermis, hence enhancing erythemogenic response to UV

Pearls

- Post-phototherapy erythema:
  - Peaks at
    - 24 h: NB-UVB, excimer
    - 48 h: UVA, PUVA

T. F. Mohammad · I. H. Hamzavi
Department of Dermatology, Henry Ford Health System,
3031 West Grand Blvd, Suite 800, Detroit, MI 48202, USA

H. W. Lim (✉)
Department of Dermatology, Henry Ford Health System, 3031 West Grand Blvd, Suite 800, Detroit, MI 48202, USA
e-mail: hlim1@hfhs.org

© Springer Nature Switzerland AG 2020
H. W. Lim et al. (eds.), *Practical Guide to Dermatology,*
https://doi.org/10.1007/978-3-030-18015-7_9

- Treatment time for UVA1 in a stand-up unit is in 15–20 min range, and it becomes fairly warm inside the unit
  - This may be a limiting factor for patients
- Patient size may also be a limiting factor for UVA1 phototherapy as some morbidly obese patients may not comfortably fit inside the unit

In the Context Of ...

- New bulbs in phototherapy machine
  - Decrease dose by 20% [2]
- Insurance coverage
  - Provide patient with insurance verification information prior to scheduling
  - Medicare will cover 80% of cost; patient or secondary insurance is responsible for remaining 20%
  - Medicaid coverage is stage specific and may not be covered
  - Commercial insurance:
    - Recommend asking patients to contact their insurance companies to verify coverage of phototherapy using ICD-10 diagnosis and procedure codes

Individual Phototherapy Modalities

NB-UVB (Office Phototherapy)

In the Context Of ...

- CTCL
  - 2–3×/week until 1 month after clearance. Then taper as follows: 2×/week × 8 weeks, 1×/week × 8 weeks, then stop
- PMLE desensitization
  - 3×/week × 5 weeks, then 20–30 min/week of midday sun exposure (10AM–2PM, without sunscreen) for maintenance
- Vitiligo
  - 2–3×/week until maximal repigmentation then taper as follows: 2×/week × 1 month, 1×/week × 1 month, once every other week × 2 months, then stop [2]
- Psoriasis
  - 2–3×/week until >95% clearance then taper as follows: 1×/week × 1 month, once every other week × 1 month, once every 4 weeks × 1 month, then stop [3]
- Dosing orders for all cutaneous disorders based upon skin phototype:
  - Exception—vitiligo: use skin phototype I

Dosing of NBUVB Based on Skin Type

Skin type	Starting dose (mJ/cm^2)	Increase	Max
I	150	10–15% per session as tolerated	3 J/cm^2 body, 1 J/cm^2 face
II	150	10–15% per session as tolerated	3 J/cm^2 body, 1 J/cm^2 face
III	250	10–15% per session as tolerated	3 J/cm^2 body, 1 J/cm^2 face
IV	250	10–15% per session as tolerated	3 J/cm^2 body, 1 J/cm^2 face
V	400	10–15% per session as tolerated	3 J/cm^2 body, 1 J/cm^2 face
VI	400	10–15% per session as tolerated	3 J/cm^2 body, 1 J/cm^2 face

Henry Ford Health System in-office NBUVB phototherapy protocol [2]

Dose escalation	15% at each subsequent visit
Maximum dose	1000 mJ/cm^2 (face) 3000 mJ/cm^2 (body)
Dose adjustments for erythema	
No erythema	Increase dose as directed
Light pink erythema (desired response to phototherapy)	Maintain same dose
Moderate erythema	Decrease dose by 15%
Severe erythema/blisters	Physician evaluation
Dose adjustment for missed sessions	
1–2 sessions	Maintain previous dose
1–2 weeks	Decrease dose by 33%
2–4 weeks	Decrease dose by 66%
>4 weeks	Restart at initial dose
Assessment of response to treatment	3 months or 30 treatments PEARL: In vitiligo, may require up to 70–80 treatments to see response
Maintenance regimen	Physician discretion, consider tapering to prevent relapse
Face cover	Yes, if face is spared
Goggles	Yes, unless eyes are affected, then close eyes during treatment
Genital protection	Yes, protect areola in women with shields or sunscreen Yes, protect genitals in males if not involved
Use of topicals before treatment	Apply moisturizer prior to phototherapy No topical medications 4 h before phototherapy
Post exposure recommendation	Apply SPF 30 sunscreen on exposed areas

Excimer Laser

Pearls

- Ideal for localized lesions (<10% BSA), skin folds, scalp

In the Context Of…

- Vitiligo
  - Starting dose—150 mJ/cm^2
  - Increase by 5–15% per session if mild asymptomatic erythema
  - Max 3 J/cm^2 body and 1 J/cm^2 face
  - Can treat eyelids and genitals
- Psoriasis
  - Consider applying mineral oil for improved penetration

Dosing of Psoriasis with NBUVB Based on Skin Type

Skin type	Initial dose for thin plaques (mJ/cm^2)	Moderately thick plaques (mJ/cm^2)	Severely thick plaques (mJ/cm^2)
I	150	200	300
II	200	300	450
III	250	400	600
IV	300	500	750
V	350	600	900
VI	400	700	1050

NB-UVB (Home Phototherapy) [4]

Pearls

- Treatment regimen: 3 times weekly versus 6 times weekly phototherapy regimen depending upon the device
  - Single panel—6 days per week phototherapy regimen
    - Front/Back (Day 1, 3, and 5)
    - Left/Right Sides (Day 2, 4 and 6)
  - Three-panel—3 non-consecutive days per week phototherapy regimen (MWF; each day front/back)
  - Newer units: treatment can be set by dose; older units: set by time
  - Patient to stand 6–8 inches from light
  - Dose-based unit: same starting dose as office NB-UVB; increase by 10 mJ/cm^2 as indicated on the table that comes with the unit
  - Time-based unit: start with 30 s, increase by 15–30 s as tolerated.

- ○ Maximum: 8–10 min per side as tolerated (for both dose-based and time-based units)
  - ▪ Note: this maximum time is set for patient's comfort/tolerance.
- ○ Clinical follow-up should remain every 3–6 months

In the Context Of...

- Prescribing home phototherapy
  - ○ Home phototherapy (NBUVB)
    - ▪ Two major companies: Daavlin and National Biologic
    - ▪ Both will take care of prior authorization
      - • Daavlin: http://www.daavlin.com/physicians/prescribing-home-units/prescribing-home-phototherapy-units/
      - • National Biologic: http://www.natbiocorp.com/forms/papo-df105w.pdf
  - ○ Select the appropriate device to be ordered and give the patient the packet to complete his/her sections. The patient will email/fax this back to the company.
  - ○ Physician will fax their section to the company:
    - ▪ Device order forms:
      - • Usually prescribe 150 treatments if three panel device (75 front/back sessions) or 300 treatments if single panel (75 sessions of treating full body with 6-day regimen)
    - ▪ Recent clinical encounter note
    - ▪ The company will let you know if any additional information is required
  - ○ Renewing orders / Adding more sessions to a device:
    - ▪ A code will flash on the device's display when ~5 treatments remain
      - • Patient will need to provide this code and the manufacturer's name to you
    - ▪ Login to manufacturer's website and renew orders to collect the new code, which the patient is to input into his/her device

PUVA

What Not To Miss

- Contraindications
  - ○ Children <10 years
  - ○ Pregnancy
  - ○ Lactation
  - ○ XP
  - ○ SLE
  - ○ Personal or family history of melanoma

- Caution: history of NMSC, radiation exposure, arsenic, MTX, cyclosporine, photosensitizing meds, history of dysplastic nevi, uremia and hepatic failure, severe infirmity, photosensitivity disorder, young children [5]

Pearls

- Cover
  - o Males: genitals/eyes
  - o Females: eyes and, if nipples are exposed, apply sunscreen
- If eyelids are involved, treatment can be done by having the patient close their eyes

In the Context Of …

- Systemic (for psoriasis and MF)
  - o Check pre-PUVA eye exam, then yearly
  - o Dose of 8-methoxypsoralen (Oxsoralen-Ultra) is 0.4–0.5 mg/kg taken 1 h prior to treatment
    - ▪ Dose may be increased up to 0.6 mg/kg in resistant cases; max 70 mg per treatment
    - ▪ Available as 10 mg capsules
    - ▪ Taken with small meal at SAME TIME each day at the same time interval prior to phototherapy so psoralen levels are consistent
      - • Best absorption on empty stomach, but causes nausea
  - o Frequency: 2–3 × weekly, not on successive days
  - o MUST BE PHOTOPROTECTED following ingestion of psoralen on the day of treatment only

- PUVA therapy for vitiligo
  - o Initial dose of UVA is 0.25 J/cm^2, increase by 0.25–0.5 J/cm^2
  - o Once moderate erythema, hold dose

- Topical PUVA (hand/foot):
  - o 0.1% methoxypsoralen in Lubriderm lotion applied IN THE OFFICE 20–30 min before treatment to same areas
  - o Initial UVA dose to palms, soles, or dorsal feet/hands is 0.25–0.5 J/cm^2 (increased 0.25–0.5 J/cm^2 per treatment)
    - ▪ MAX dose: 8 J/cm^2
  - o Frequency: 3 × weekly → 2 × weekly for 4–8 weeks → once weekly for 4–8 weeks and stop when clear

- Side effects
  - o Acute: nausea, pruritus, erythema, blistering, tanning
  - o Subacute: lunula hyperpigmentation, melanonychia, photo-onycholysis

o Chronic: cataracts, NMSC (when >250 treatments), melanoma, genital tumors [5, 6]

Dosing of UVA for PUVA Based on Skin Type

Skin type	Initial UVA dose (J/cm^2)	Dosage increase per treatment (J/cm^2)	Maximum dose per treatment (J/cm^2)
I	1–1.5	0.5–1.5	8 (4-face)
II	2–2.5	0.5–1.5	8 (4-face)
III	3–3.5	1.0–2.5	12 (4-face)
IV	4–4.5	1.0–2.5	12 (4-face)
V	5–5.5	1.5–3.5	20 (4-face)
VI	6–6.5	1.5–3.5	20 (4-face)

Note Decrease UVA dosing by 30% when adding retinoids

UVA-1

In the Context Of …

- **Low Dose UVA-1 (<40 J/cm^2): Hardening for Solar Urticaria** [7]
  - o Start at 5 J/cm^2, increase by 5 J/cm^2 till a maximum of 20 J/cm^2; 3 × weekly
    - ▪ For exquisitely photosensitive patient, do minimal urticarial dose: 1/2/4/5 J/cm^2, and do immediate reading
  - o Schedule patient for re-evaluation by physician after 15–20 treatments.

- **Medium Dose UVA-1 (40–80 J/cm^2): For morphea and other scleroder-moid diseases** [8]
  - o Unless specifically indicated, all patients should be treated at the medium dose, 3 × weekly
  - o Patients without photosensitivity or photosensitizing medications:
    - ▪ Start at 30 J/cm^2, increase by 10 J/cm^2 at each visit until 50 J/cm^2 reached and then maintain at this dose
  - o Photosensitive patients: Before treatment, perform MED test at 5/10/20/40 J/cm^2 and read at 24 h
    - ▪ No erythema, proceed as above
    - ▪ If MED is low, start at 70% MED and increase by 10 J/cm^2 per treatment until 50 J/cm^2 reached
  - o Patient should be evaluated after 20–30 treatments at which point, physician may decide to stop treatment (without tapering of frequency)
  - o Improvement/softening may continue to occur even after discontinuation of treatment
  - o Treatment may be repeated in a few months as needed

- Side effects: Tanning, erythema (mild)

Photodynamic Therapy (PDT)

What Not To Miss

- **Screening questions:** [9, 10]
  - ○ Nut/soy allergies (both MAL PDT and Ameluz preparations are made with nut/soy oils)
    - ■ PEARL: The levulan kerastick is not made with nut oils and can be used in this population
  - ○ History of photosensitizing disorder, porphyria, allergy to ALA or MAL, planned sun exposure in the next 48 h, isotretinoin use within past 6 months, and pregnancy
  - ○ If history of HSV, consider pre-treatment with antivirals to prevent flares

- **Patient counseling:** [9]
  - ○ Must avoid excessive exposure to sunlight or artificial light sources for 36–48 h post-treatment
    - ■ Cover treated areas with opaque clothing or thick opaque layer of sunscreen
  - ○ Should expect erythema, edema, scaling for up to 1-week post-treatment
  - ○ Darker skin types should be counseled on risk of dyspigmentation

In the Context Of …

- **Acne** [9]
  - ○ Aminolevulinic acid (ALA) incubation time: 1–4 h with occlusion
    - ■ Incubation times of at least 3 h associated with long-term remission
  - ○ Can use either red light (more effective, but more side effects) or blue light
  - ○ Indicated for the treatment of inflammatory papules, not comedones
  - ○ Usually requires 2–3 treatments repeated monthly

- **Actinic Keratoses** [9]
  - ○ ALA-PDT more effective for treatment of head/neck AKs than for thicker lesions on the arms or trunk
  - ○ Perform curettage of thicker hypertrophic lesions prior to treatment
  - ○ One session of ALA-PDT results in 60–90% of reduction in AKs
  - ○ Can repeat treatments monthly, with ALA incubation times of: 1–4 h
  - ○ Blue light (FDA approved) or red light (more effective due to higher penetration but more SE's)
  - ○ Combination regimens
    - ■ 5-FU applied BID × 2 weeks followed by 1 session of ALA-PDT
    - ■ More effective than ALA-PDT alone but increased incidence of extensive erythema/peeling × 1 week

- **Superficial BCC, Bowen's** [9, 11]
  - ○ Red light PDT; typically 4–6 h of incubation of ALA. Duration of incubation up to overnight.
    - ■ Can occlude with Saran wrap to increase penetration
  - ○ Pain during irradiation is a significant limiting factor for some.
    - ■ Pain control by:
      - • Cold air cooling, but may decrease efficacy
      - • Nerve blocks or local anesthesia
      - • Pause treatment for three minutes of cooling and then resume treatment
      - • Daylight PDT (not billable) v. in-office "painless PDT" protocol

References

1. Kim WB, Shelley AJ, Novice K, Joo J, Lim HW, Glassman SJ. Drug-induced phototoxicity: a systematic review. J Am Acad Dermatol. 2018;79:1069–75.
2. Mohammad TF, Al-Jamal M, Hamzavi IH, et al. The Vitiligo Working Group recommendations for narrowband ultraviolet B light phototherapy treatment of vitiligo. J Am Acad Dermatol. 2017;76(5):879–88.
3. Menter A, Korman NJ, Elmets CA, Feldman SR, Gelfand JM, Gordon KB, et al. Guidelines of care for the management of psoriasis and psoriatic arthritis: Section 5. Guidelines of care for the treatment of psoriasis with phototherapy and photochemotherapy. J Am Acad Dermatol. 2010;62:114–35.
4. Mohammad TF, Silpa-Archa N, Griffith JL, Lim HW, Hamzavi IH. Home phototherapy in vitiligo. Photodermatol Photoimmunol Photomed. 2017;33(5):241–52.
5. Matz H. Phototherapy for psoriasis: what to choose and how to use: facts and controversies. Clin Dermatol. 2010;28(1):73–80.
6. Stern RS, Bagheri S, Nichols K. The persistent risk of genital tumors among men treated with psoralen plus ultraviolet A (PUVA) for psoriasis. J Am Acad Dermatol. 2002;47(1):33–9.
7. Dawe RS, Ferguson J. Prolonged benefit following ultraviolet A phototherapy for solar urticaria. Br J Dermatol. 1997;137(1):144–8.
8. Connolly KL, Griffith JL, McEvoy M, Lim HW. Ultraviolet A1 phototherapy beyond morphea: experience in 83 patients. Photodermatol Photoimmunol Photomed. 2015;31(6):289–95.
9. Ozog DM, Rkein AM, Fabi SG, et al. Photodynamic therapy: a clinical consensus guide. Dermatol Surg Off Publ Am Soc Dermatol Surg [et al]. 2016;42(7):804–27.
10. Kumar N, Warren CB. Photodynamic therapy for dermatologic conditions in the pediatric population: a literature review. Photodermatol Photoimmunol Photomed. 2017;33(3):125–34.
11. Varma S, Wilson H, Kurwa HA, Gambles B, Charman C, Pearse AD, et al. Bowen's disease, solar keratoses and superficial basal cell carcinomas treated by photodynamic therapy using a large-field incoherent light source. Br J Dermatol. 2001;144:567–74.

Systemic Drugs Used in Dermatology

Karlee Novice and Ellen N. Pritchett

Systemic Immunomodulatory and Anti-proliferative Drugs

Antimalarials [1, 2]

Conditions that Best Respond

- Lupus erythematosus
  - Especially widespread discoid lupus erythematosus and subacute cutaneous lupus erythematosus
- Dermatomyositis
- Lichen planus and its variants (e.g., lichen planopilaris)
- Sarcoidosis
- Polymorphous light eruption
- Porphyria cutanea tarda (PCT)

Latest Updates to Lab Monitoring

- Baseline: CBC and CMP
- Follow up:
  - CBC monthly for 3 months, then every 4–6 months
  - CMP after 1 month, 3 months and then every 4–6 months
- Baseline ophthalmology exam within the first year and then yearly after 5 years [3]

E. N. Pritchett (✉)
Henry Ford Health System, 3031 West Grand Blvd, Suite 800, Detroit, MI 48202, USA
e-mail: epritch1@hfhs.org

K. Novice
Department of Dermatology, Henry Ford Health System, 3031 West Grand Blvd, Suite 800, Detroit, MI 48202, USA

© Springer Nature Switzerland AG 2020
H. W. Lim et al. (eds.), *Practical Guide to Dermatology*,
https://doi.org/10.1007/978-3-030-18015-7_10

- G6PDH
  - Largest study to date evaluating G6PDH deficiency and the associated risk of hemolytic anemia with concurrent use of hydroxychloroquine (HCQ) does not support routine measurement of G6PDH levels or withholding HCQ therapy among African American patients with G6PDH deficiency [4]

Hydroxychloroquine (HCQ, Plaquenil)

How Long *does this medication take to work*

- 3–4 months
- American Academy of Ophthalmology 2016 guidelines recommend daily doses <5 mg/kg daily of real body weight [5]

What to do if this Medication is Not Working

- Consider combining with quinacrine 100 mg daily

Most Common Side Effects

- Blue-gray to black hyperpigmentation on shins, face, palate, nail beds can be seen >4 months of use
  - Stop therapy and discoloration generally fades in months to years
- Reversible bleaching of hair roots (achromotrichia)
- Exanthem (e.g. urticaria, lichenoid reactions, exfoliative erythroderma)
  - Increased risk in patients with dermatomyositis > lupus
- 5% develop reversible ocular toxicity that resolves with discontinuation of therapy
  - Ask about blurry vision, halos of colors around lights
- 0.5% develop irreversible ocular toxicity (e.g., changes in visual acuity)
- Induction or exacerbation of psoriasis
- Gastrointestinal upset: nausea, vomiting

Avoid

- Concomitant chloroquine use due to retinal toxicity

Chloroquine

How Long this Medication Takes to Work

- 3–4 months of 250 mg daily; maximum dosing 2.3 mg/kg daily of real body weight

Most Common Side Effects

- 90% of patients develop reversible ocular toxicity
  - 1% develop irreversible ocular toxicity (e.g., changes in visual acuity)

Quinacrine

How Long this Medication Takes to Work

- 3–4 months of 100 mg daily
- Available at compounding pharmacies only

What to do if this Medication is Not Working

- Can combine with either HCQ or chloroquine

Most Common Side Effects

- Yellow skin discoloration
  - Reversible upon discontinuation
- No ocular side effects

Azathioprine (Imuran) [1, 2]

Conditions that Best Respond

- Autoimmune bullous dermatoses
- Dermatomyositis
- Atopic and contact dermatitis
- Pyoderma gangrenosum

How Long this Medication Takes to Work

- 6–8 weeks
- Start 1 mg/kg daily (i.e., 50–100 mg) once daily or BID dosing for 6–8 weeks
  - Can increase by ~0.5 mg/kg daily every 4 weeks as needed to a max of 2.5 mg/kg daily
  - If GI symptoms occur, consider decreasing daily dose or switching to BID dosing

Latest Updates to Lab Monitoring

- Baseline: TPMT (thiopurine S-methyltransferase), CBC w/diff, CMP, TB testing, +/− serum beta-hCG for female, UA
  - TPMT
    - <6.3 U: contraindicated
    - 6.3–15 U: up to 1 mg/kg daily
    - 15.1–26.4 U: up to 2.0–2.5 mg/kg daily
- Follow up
  - CBC w/diff and LFTs biweekly for 2 months then every 2–3 months thereafter

Most Common Side Effects

- GI upset: nausea, vomiting, diarrhea
  - Seen between first and tenth day of therapy
  - Treatment: reduce dose, divide into BID doses, take medication with food
- Myelosuppression
  - Predictable risk in those with reduced or absent TPMT
  - Discontinue or at least temporarily discontinue drug if WBC < 3500–4000 K/uL, Hgb < 10 g/dL, and/or platelets < 100,000/mm^3
- Infections: HPV, herpes simplex, scabies
- Teratogenic
- NMSC (nonmelanoma skin cancer)
  - Azathioprine was associated with increased risk for high-frequency keratinocyte cancers, defined as 6 or more in a 10-year period [6]
  - Dermatology patients with adequate photoprotection practice, smaller doses, and less than 3 years of azathioprine treatment are less likely to develop skin cancer than are other high-risk patients [7]
- Possible increased risk of malignancies, especially lymphoproliferative disorders
  - Numerous studies of various patient populations present conflicting conclusions [7] but there are reports of patients with psoriasis and dermatomyositis who have been on azathioprine treatment for more than 5 years who have developed non-Hodgkin lymphoma [8]
- Rare drug induced hypersensitivity syndrome

Avoid

- Caution with allopurinol as allopurinol inhibits xanthine oxidase (XO)
  - XO is one of two metabolic pathways involved in the metabolism of azathioprine leading to an excess of active purine analog 6-thioguanine (6-TG), which leads to increased risk of myelosuppression [9]

Corticosteroids (CS) [1, 2]

Steroid Withdrawal Syndrome (SWS)

- Occurs with abrupt CS tapering with intermediate and chronic duration therapy; typically, when treated with systemic CS beyond 2–3 weeks
  - Fatigue, lethargy, depression, mood swings, headache, myalgias, arthralgias, flu like symptoms
- Treatment: return to higher CS doses with more gradual CS tapering
- More severe forms of HPA suppression including adrenal crisis is uncommon for dosing regimens used in dermatology

Osteonecrosis

- Majority of cases are with pharmacologic doses of prednisone for 2–3 months

Bone Health

- Calcium and vitamin D supplementation in any patient receiving pharmacologic doses of CS for at least 1 month
  - ○ Calcium 1000–1500 mg daily
  - ○ Vitamin D 600–800 U daily
- PEARL: Every other day CS dosing decreases risk of osteoporosis
- Bisphosphonates [10]
  - ○ Caution in women of child-bearing potential
    - ■ Animal studies have shown adverse effects on both the fetus and the mother including protracted parturition, maternal mortality, skeletal retardation of the fetuses, and small fetal weight [11]
  - ○ Start in adults with moderate-to-high risk of fracture beginning long-term glucocorticoid treatment (e.g. >6 months at a dose of >7.5 mg daily)
  - ○ Very rare side effects: fracture at shaft of femur, osteonecrosis of jaw

Intramuscular CS

- Debated amongst clinicians on its benefits due to concern for HPA suppression and other side effects, which may not be substantiated
  - ○ Severe adverse effects are rare with a single IM CS injection
  - ○ IM triamcinolone acetonide (e.g., Kenalog) appears safe with no HPA axis suppression when administered as 2 injections at 6-week intervals [12]
- Short to intermediate acting products (e.g., Celestone and Aristocort) are preferred for repeated use
- Long-acting forms (e.g., Kenalog) can still be safely used: 3–4 injections per year is a reasonable limit
- Particularly good option in subsets for inflammatory dermatoses, especially hand dermatitis
- Can be used in conjunction with other immunosuppressives

Cyclosporine (CsA) [1, 2]

Conditions that Best Respond

- Psoriasis
- Severe atopic dermatitis
- Pyoderma gangrenosum

How Long this Medication Takes to Work

- Fast acting, effects can be seen within days
- Start 2.5 mg/kg daily in 2 divided doses for 4 weeks, increase by 0.5 mg/kg daily every 2 weeks for a max up to 5 mg/kg daily

Latest Updates to Lab Monitoring

- Baseline: blood pressure (BP), CBC, CMP, serum Mg, Uric acid, Lipid profile
- Follow up
  - BP checked at each visit
  - CBC, CMP, Mg, uric acid, lipids every 2 weeks for 1–2 months, then monthly thereafter

Most Common Side Effects

- Neurologic: tremor, headache, paresthesia, hyperesthesia
  - Self-limiting after several weeks of treatment [13]
  - Reversible upon discontinuation
- Hypertension
  - Duration and dose-related
  - Develops in ¼ patients with psoriasis on cyclosporine
  - Management: reduce dose or treat with calcium channel blockers
- Nephrotoxicity

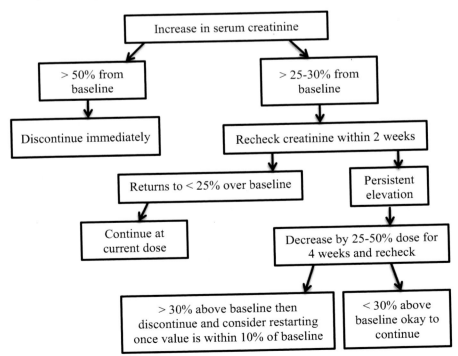

- Hyperlipidemia
  - Can consider treatment with fluvastatin (Lescol), rosuvastatin (Crestor) or pravastatin (Pravacol)
  - PEARL: Avoid lovastatin (Altoprev) due to risk of rhabdomyolysis [14]
- Increased risk of NMSC if treated for >2 years [15]
- Gingival hyperplasia
  - Improves with careful dental hygiene
- Hypomagnesium
  - May require replacement therapy
    - No clear consensus on when or how to replete hypomagnesium; however, repletion has shown protection against CsA induced hypertension and nephrotoxicity [16]
  - If tolerable to patient, consider starting with magnesium oxide 800 mg daily
    - Can cause diarrhea

Avoid

- Lovastatin ➔ increases risk of rhabdomyolysis [14]
- Diltiazem and verapamil can alter CsA blood levels
- Potassium-sparing diuretics increases serum K+ levels
- Caution with drugs that interact with hepatic CYP3A4
  - PEARL: Avoid grapefruit juice!
- Caution with phototherapy, especially PUVA, given possible risk of NMSC

Dapsone [1, 2]

Conditions that Best Respond

- Dermatitis herpetiformis
- Leprosy
- Linear IgA
- Bullous SLE
- Erythema elevatum diutinum

How Long this Medication Takes to Work

- Rapid improvement within 48 h for dermatitis herpetiformis

Latest Updates to Lab Monitoring

- Baseline labs: G6PD, CBC with diff, reticulocyte count, CMP
  - PEARL: If G6PD deficient, increased risk of hemolytic anemia and methemoglobinema
- Follow up

- o CBC with diff and reticulocyte count weekly for 4 weeks, followed by twice monthly for 8 weeks then CBC every 3–4 months
  - ■ Expect increase in reticulocyte count due to low grade hemolysis
- o CMP every 2 weeks for 3 months then every 3–6 months

Most Common Side Effects

- Hemolytic anemia
  - o Occurs to some degree in all patients
  - o G6PD deficient patients are more susceptible
  - o PEARL: May result in falsely low levels of HgbA1c in patients with poorly controlled diabetes [17]
- Methemoglobinemia
  - o Presents with excessive fatigue, headaches or increasing cardiac or pulmonary symptoms
  - o Not a clear relationship with hemolytic anemia
  - o <30%—treat with ascorbic acid or cimetidine
  - o >30% or symptomatic—treat with oral methylene blue (100–300 mg daily); however ineffective and contraindicated if patient is G6PD deficient, in which case consider plasma exchange
- Agranulocytosis
  - o Essentially all cases of agranulocytosis develop within first 12 weeks of therapy
  - o Present with fever and flu-like symptoms
  - o Management: discontinue immediately
    - ■ Recover after cessation of dapsone, typically within 7–14 days
- GI upset and anorexia
  - o Mostly mild, self-limited, improved by taking with meals
- Peripheral neuropathy is primarily a distal motor neuropathy +/− sensory neuropathy
  - o Unrelated to dose
  - o Recover completely with discontinuation within weeks but can take up to 2 years [18]
- Dapsone hypersensitivity syndrome
  - o Rare but serious
  - o Fever, generalized cutaneous eruption and hepatitis 3-12 weeks after therapy

Methotrexate (MTX) [1, 2]

Conditions that Best Respond

- Psoriasis
- Epidermal proliferative disease (e.g. PRP, PLEVA, PLC, reactive arthritis (Reiter's disease))

- Autoimmune bullous dermatoses
- Autoimmune connective diseases

How Long this Medication Takes to Work

- 4–8 weeks
- Test dose of 5–10 mg daily for one day with repeat CBC and LFTs 5–7 days later
  - ○ Dose escalation by 2.5–5.0 mg weekly until benefit achieved without toxicity, usually do not exceed 30 mg weekly
  - ○ PEARL: Check the CBC and LFTs 5 days later as this coincides with the normalization of any transient transaminitis
  - ○ PEARL: Can consider rheumatology dosing where MTX is started at 15 mg weekly, escalating with 5 mg monthly up to 25–30 mg weekly [19]
- 1 mg folic acid daily, or 6 days a week (except on day of MTX)
  - ○ Can decrease nausea or other GI effects
  - ○ Decreases risk of hematologic toxicity
  - ○ Does not affect efficacy of methotrexate
- IM or SubQ available if cannot tolerate oral MTX due to GI upset

Latest Updates to Lab Monitoring

- Baseline: CBC (include platelet counts), CMP, hepatitis screening panel
- Follow up
  - ○ CBC and LFTs
    - ■ 5–7 days after test dose, every 1–2 weeks for 2–4 weeks and 1–2 weeks after dose escalations then every 3–4 months on stable dose
    - ■ If WBC < 3500/mm^3, the platelet count is < 100,000/mm^3, or increase over twice the upper normal value for LFTs, discontinue or reduce dose of MTX
      - • If laboratory abnormality resolves, can restart at lower dose after 2–3 weeks
  - ○ Renal function one to two times yearly
    - ■ Aside from checking creatinine and BUN, check creatinine clearance in patients > 50 years old:
      - • If CrCl < 50 mL/min, use lower doses of MTX and much more cautiously [20]
- For patients without risk factors for hepatic fibrosis, liver biopsies may be recommended at lower frequency than previously reported; consider after 1.5–2.0 g in lower-risk patients
  - ○ Consider referral to Hepatology as there are new screening tools such as transient elastography [21] and amino terminal type III procollagen peptide (P3NP) [22] that may be valuable in monitoring for liver fibrosis in patients with psoriasis on MTX

Most Common Side Effects

- GI symptoms
  - Nausea and anorexia: very common
  - Diarrhea, vomiting and ulcerative stomatitis
  - Treatment: folic acid 1–5 mg daily or consider IM or SubQ MTX
- Pancytopenia
  - Occurs early in therapy
  - Increased risk factor with renal disease
  - For significant myelosuppression, treat with leucovorin (folinic acid)
- Hepatic fibrosis and cirrhosis
  - Takes years to develop
- Teratogen
  - Recommend females wait one month after stopping treatment to attempt pregnancy and men wait three months prior to conception [1]; however, studies are needed to help elucidate the unclear evidence of MTX effects on male fertility and pregnancy outcomes [23]
- Sunburn recall

Avoid

- Bactrim
  - Increased risk of myelosuppression
  - PEARL: This can be life-threatening! [24]
- Be mindful with NSAIDs
  - Increased risk of myelosuppression and acute renal failure has been reported [25]; however, recent studies suggest safety when co-administered in patients with rheumatoid arthritis on MTX with the exception of aspirin [26]
  - PEARL: Avoid Aspirin!
- Caution in pregnancy and in women of childbearing potential

Mycophenolate Mofetil (Cellcept, MMF) [1, 2]

Conditions that Best Respond

- Multiple inflammatory dermatologic diseases
- Autoimmune connective tissue disease
- Autoimmune bullous dermatoses
- PEARL: An effective, corticosteroid-sparing agent in patients who cannot tolerate other medications secondary to comorbid disease

How Long this Medication Takes to Work

- 6–8 weeks
- Initiate dose with 500 mg daily for 1 week, increase to 500 mg BID every 2–4 weeks until a maximum dose of 1.5 mg BID or once patient develops intolerance
- Alternative
  - Enteric-coated mycophenolate sodium formulation (EC-MPS/Myfortic ©) 180 mg is equivalent to 250 mg MMF
  - May decrease GI side effects

Latest Updates to Lab Monitoring

- Baseline: CBC, CMP, hepatitis screening panel, tuberculosis (TB) testing, serum beta-hCG in women with childbearing potential
  - PEARL: Optimal screening strategy for TB is not clear with disagreement on whether to use an interferon gamma release assay (IGRAs, e.g. QuantiF-ERON ©—TB gold blood test) or tuberculin skin test (TST) or both [27]
  - PEARL: IGRAs have a higher specificity than TST in patients with Bacillus Calmette-Guerin (BCG) vaccination [28]
- Follow up
  - CBC and CMP every 2–4 weeks following dose escalation and then 2–3 months with stable dosing

Most Common Side Effects

- GI upset
  - Most common side effects
    - Nausea, diarrhea, soft stools, anorexia, abdominal cramps, frequent stools, vomiting and tenderness
  - Improves with time
  - Treatment
    - Take with food
    - Switch from BID to TID dosing
    - Switch to Myfortic ©
- GU
  - Urgency, frequency, dysuria, burning and sterile pyuria
  - Decreases in frequency after first year
- Hematologic
  - 2–11% develop agranulocytosis, neutropenia, anemia and thrombocytopenia
  - Dose dependent and reversible
- Infectious
  - More common in transplant patients and with doses >2 g daily

- o Infection risk in dermatologic patients is less clear but cases of herpes zoster, herpes simplex, bacterial, atypical mycobacterial and fungal infections have been reported
- Neurologic
  - o Weakness, fatigue, headache, tinnitus, and insomnia
- Teratogen
  - o Pregnancy category D
- Peripheral edema, especially lower extremities
- Malignancy potential is controversial
  - o Most evidence for carcinogenesis is seen in transplant populations on multiple immunosuppressive drugs for long duration of times

Avoid

- Azathioprine
  - o Used together increases risk of bone marrow suppression
- May decrease serum levels of levonorgestrel
  - o Caution if this is a component of oral contraceptive
- PPIs, antacids and calcium channel blockers at least 1 h from MMF ingestion
  - o Decrease serum levels of active drug

Systemic Retinoids [1, 2]

Acitretin (Soriatane)

Conditions that Best Respond

- Psoriasis
  - o Monotherapy for erythrodermic, pustular psoriasis or palmoplantar psoriasis
  - o As a combination treatment for chronic plaque psoriasis
- Disorders of cornification (e.g., Darier disease, adult onset pityriasis rubra pilaris, non-syndromic autosomal recessive congenital ichthyosis)
- At low doses (10–25 mg), as chemoprevention of keratinocyte carcinomas in high-risk individuals (e.g. solid organ transplant recipients, basal cell nevus syndrome, xeroderma pigmentosum) [29, 30]

How Long this Medication Takes to Work

- 2–3 months of 25–50 mg daily
  - o Fewer side effects at doses <25 mg
- Take with food

Latest Updates to Lab Monitoring

- Baseline: CBC, CMP, Lipid profile, serum beta-hCG
- Follow up
  - Lipid profile monthly for 3 months, then every 2–3 months
    - 50% of patients develop elevated triglycerides; 30% elevated cholesterol
    - Treatment for elevated lipids
      - Recommend dietary and lifestyle modifications
      - Decrease dose
      - Discontinue if fasting TGs > 800 mg/dL
  - PEARL: Risk of pancreatitis at TGs levels > 800 mg/dL
  - Liver function tests monthly for 3 months, then every 2–3 months
    - Mild elevation between 2–8 weeks after starting therapy, typically return to normal within another 2–4 weeks despite continued therapy
    - Discontinue at > 3-fold elevations
  - CBC and renal function test every 3 months
- X-ray in setting of worsening arthritis or skeletal symptoms to rule out diffuse idiopathic skeletal hyperostosis (DISH)
  - If DISH involves the posterior longitudinal ligament, spinal cord compression leading to neurologic deficits can occur and consideration should be given to discontinuing the retinoid [31]
  - PEARL: In the most common clinical settings used in dermatology (short courses of relatively high-dose isotretinoin for acne and long-term courses of low-to-moderate doses of acitretin for psoriasis), there does not appear to be any significant risk of skeletal effects

What to do if this Medication is Not Working

- For psoriasis
  - Combine with methotrexate (monitor LFTs closely), cyclosporine (monitor serum triglycerides closely), biologics, and/or phototherapy

Most Common Side Effects:

- Palmoplantar peeling with fissuring
- "Sticky skin"—especially the palms
- Retinoid dermatitis
- Diffuse hair loss (telogen effluvium)
  - Dose related
  - Reversible approximately two months after either discontinuation of therapy or significant dose reduction
- Cheilitis, nasal dryness, and xerosis
- Blepharoconjunctivitis
- Nail fragility

- Teratogenic
  - ○ Do not donate blood while on therapy and for 3 years afterwards
  - ○ Requires contraception for 3 years after cessation of therapy due to re-esteri-fication to etretinate, which has a long half-life of 80–160 days
    - ■ PEARL: Higher rate of re-esterification with alcohol ingestion
- Elevated triglycerides

Avoid

- Alcohol—causes reverse metabolism to etretinate
- In women of childbearing potential

Bexarotene (Targretin)

Conditions that Best Respond

- CTCL

How Long this Medication Takes to Work

- 4 weeks
- Start at 150 mg/m^2, increase to 300 mg/m^2 after 4 weeks

Latest Updates to Lab Monitoring

- Baseline: CBC, CMP, TSH, free T4, fasting lipid panel, creatinine kinase, +/− serum beta-hCG
- Follow up
  - ○ Free T4 and fasting lipid panel every 1–2 weeks until in target range, then every 1–2 months
  - ○ CBC, CMP, lipid panel monthly for 3–6 months, then every 3 months

What to do if this Medication is Not Working

- Combine with narrowband UVB, PUVA, MTX, or interferon-alpha

Most Common Side Effects

- Hyperlipidemia
  - ○ 79% develop elevated serum triglycerides and/or cholesterol within 1–2 weeks of therapy [32]
    - ■ Triglycerides >300–500 mg/dL → manage with lifestyle and dietary mod-ifications

- Triglycerides >500 mg/dL → start fenofibrate 145–200 mg daily to achieve triglycerides <200 mg/dL
  - ○ +/− statin to achieve LDL level <160 mg/dl
  - ○ Do NOT use gemfibrozil (Lopid)
    - ■ PEARL: Inhibits CYP3A4 which increases bexarotene levels and toxicity
- Central hypothyroidism [33]
  - ○ Occurs in 80% of patients with decrease in thyroid hormones
  - ○ Start levothyroxine 50 mcg at beginning of therapy, adjust as required
- Teratogen

Avoid

- Gemfibrozil (Lopid)—inhibits CYP 3A4 and increases risk of bexarotene toxicity

Isotretinoin

Conditions that Best Respond

- Severe cystic acne
- Dissecting cellulitis
- Gram negative folliculitis

How Long this Medication Takes to Work

- 1–3 months
- 0.5–1.0 mg/kg daily in 2 divided doses for ~15–20 weeks
- Goal is cumulative dose of 120–150 mg/kg for acne
- No taper necessary when ready to discontinue

Latest Updates to Lab Monitoring

- Baseline: CBC with diff, CMP, fasting lipids, beta-hCG
- In healthy patients with normal baseline lipid panel and LFTs, can repeat these studies after 2 months of isotretinoin therapy and if normal, no further testing required
  - ○ No need for CBC monitoring [34]

What to do if this Medication is Not Working

- 1/3 of patients require second course for acne

Most Common Side Effects

- Dry mucous membranes and skin
  - Treatment: apply topical emollients regularly
- Transient headaches
  - PEARL: If accompanied by nausea, vomiting and visual changes → evaluate for pseudotumor cerebri
  - PEARL: If mild, divide dose by taking higher dose in the evening
- 10–15% develop myalgias
  - Associated with increased creatine phosphokinase levels but not rhabdomyolysis
- Acne fulminans [35]
  - Dose reduction or discontinue
  - Start systemic corticosteroids
- Teratogenicity
  - Register with iPledge
  - Women of childbearing potential need
    - Two negative pregnancy tests before starting
    - Two forms of birth control (the mini-pill is not acceptable)
  - Do not donate blood while on medication or within one month of discontinuing treatment
- Photosensitivity—caution patients during summer or sunny vacations
- Staphylococcus aureus colonization → overt cutaneous infections
  - PEARL: Avoid treating with tetracyclines due to increased risk of pseudotumor cerebri
- Decreased night vision
  - Returns to normal following cessation of therapy
- Exuberant granulation tissue at sites of previous acne lesions, around nail folds and sites of trauma
  - Treatment: reduce dose or discontinue, curettage, silver nitrate and pulse dye laser
- Pyogenic granulomas, including periungual
- Data regarding isotretinoin use as a cause of inflammatory bowel disease is conflicting
  - If personal or family history of inflammatory bowel disease, monitor with gastroenterologist
- No large studies that have definitively proved or disproved that isotretinoin causes or worsens depression
  - If a history of anxiety or depression, monitor closely with psychiatric consultants

Avoid

- Tetracyclines secondary to risk of pseudotumor cerebri

Biologics [36]

Dupilumab [1, 2]

Conditions that Best Respond

- Atopic dermatitis

How Long this Medication Takes to Work

- 4 weeks
- 600 mg subcutaneously initially then 300 mg subcutaneously once every other week

Latest Updates to Lab Monitoring

- No baseline or laboratory monitoring described to date

Most Common Side Effects [37]

- Local injection site reaction
- Ocular symptoms
  - Conjunctivitis, keratitis, xeropthalmia, eye pruritus
  - Consider treatment with fluorometholone 0.1% eye drops, dexamethasone 0.1% eye drops, or off-label use of tacrolimus 0.03% eye ointment [38]
  - Further studies are needed to confirm risk factors for development and effective treatment [39]
- No significant association was found for dupilumab compared to placebo in terms of herpesvirus infections and overall infections [40]

Avoid

- Administration of live vaccines

Tumor Necrosis Factor (TNF) Inhibitors [1, 2]

Latest Updates to Lab Monitoring

- Baseline: CBC, CMP, hepatitis screening panel, TB testing (IGRAs or TST)
- Follow up: CBC and CMP every 2–3 months and yearly TB testing

Most Common Side Effects

- Injection site reactions
- Infections

- o Monitor closely in patients with underlying conditions that predispose to infection (e.g., diabetes)
  - o Reasonable to temporarily withdraw therapy in patients with active infections
  - o Tuberculosis
    - Increased risk for reactivation of latent TB
    - Increased risk of active TB infections
  - o Reactivation of hepatitis B
- Demyelinating diseases
  - o Relationship has not been well established
- New-onset heart failure and worsening of heart failure
  - o PEARL: Caution in patients with CHF—particularly for infliximab, as it is an infusion.
- Positive ANA and anti-dsDNA
  - o Some associated with drug induced lupus
  - o Resolve after discontinuation
- Autoimmune hepatitis
- Conflicting results regarding malignancy risk including lymphomas and skin cancers

Avoid

- Caution in patients with congestive heart failure
- Caution in patients with demyelinating diseases (optic neuritis, Guillain-Barre, multiple sclerosis)
- Administration of live vaccines

Adalimumab (Humira)

Conditions that Best Respond

- Psoriasis
- Psoriatic arthritis
- Hidradenitis suppurativa
- Pyoderma gangrenosum

How Long this Medication Takes to Work

- ~71% reached PASI-75 by 16 weeks, which was maintained through week 24 with 80 mg subcuatneously on week 0; then 40 mg subcutaneously every 2 weeks starting on week 1 [41, 42]
- Psoriasis Dose: 80 mg subcutaneously on week 0 then 40 mg subcutaneously every 2 weeks
- HS Dose: 160 mg subcutaneously on week 0; 80 mg subcutaneously on week 2, then starting on week 4 with 40 mg subcutaneously weekly thereafter
- Can lose efficacy over time due to production of anti-adalimumab antibodies

- o PEARL: Minimize with addition of low-dose (5.0–7.5 mg) weekly methotrexate

Additional Side Effects

- The prefilled syringe needle covers contain latex
  - o PEARL: Pens are latex free

Etanercept (Enbrel)

Conditions that Best Respond

- Plaque psoriasis (children and adult)
- Psoriatic arthritis
- SJS/TEN [43]

How Long this Medication Takes to Work

- Psoriasis
  - o 49% reached PASI-75 by 12 weeks on 50 mg twice weekly [44]
  - o Dose: 50 mg subcutaneously twice weekly for 3 months, then once weekly for maintenance
  - o 2% of patients develop autoantibodies, but these are not neutralizing, nor have they been found in association with ineffective treatment or adverse events
- SJS/TEN
  - o Dose: 50 mg subcutaneously once [43]

Infliximab (Remicade)

Conditions that Best Respond

- Psoriasis
- Psoriatic arthritis
- Hidradenitis suppurativa
- Pyoderma gangrenosum

How Long this Medication Takes to Work

- May see improvement after 1–2 infusions
- 80% reached PASI-75 at week 10 with 5 mg/kg at weeks 0, 2, and 6 and 71% continued to have PASI-75 until week 50 with maintenance infusions every 8 weeks [45]
- Dose: IV 5–10 mg/kg at weeks 0, 2, and 6, then every 4–8 weeks thereafter

Most Common Side Effects

- Infusion reactions
  - ○ Seen in ~20% of patients
  - ○ Occur during infusion or up to 3 h post infusion
    - ■ Headache, flushing, nausea, dyspnea, injection site infiltration and taste perversion
    - ■ Treatment: decrease infusion rate, adjunctive medications including acetaminophen and antihistamines
  - ○ <1% with serious reactions including hypotension and anaphylaxis
    - ■ Treatment: epinephrine and systemic corticosteroids
- Anti-drug antibodies
  - ○ Correspond to increased clearance rate of infliximab, an increased incidence of infusion reactions and reduced efficacy
  - ○ Patients who developed these antibodies were less likely to, but not entirely precluded from, maintaining a PASI-75 response at week 50 [46]
  - ○ Measurement of serum human anti-chimeric antibodies (HACA) and infliximab concentrations can impact management and can be clinically useful [47]
    - ■ Increasing infliximab dose in patients who have HACAs is ineffective; should consider switching to another biologic

Avoid

- Doses >5 mg/kg contraindicated in patients with congestive heart failure

---

Interleukin 12/23 Inhibitor [1, 2]

Latest Updates to Lab Monitoring

- Baseline: CBC, CMP, hepatitis screening panel, TB testing
- Follow up: CBC and CMP every 2–3 months, yearly TB testing

Ustekinumab (Stelara)—inhibits IL-12 and IL-23

Conditions that Best Respond

- Psoriasis (approved age > 12)
- Approved but not as effective for psoriatic arthritis:
  - ○ 42% of patients receiving 90 mg injections reached ACR20 (i.e. minimum 20% improvement in the American College of Rheumatology criteria) at week 12: 25% reached ACR50 and 11% reached ACR70 at week 12 [48]

How Long this Medication Takes to Work

- ~65% reached PASI-75 at week 12 with both 45 and 90 mg dosing which was maintained for at least a year in most patients [49]

- Dose
  - <100 kg: 45 mg subcutaneously on weeks 0 and 4 then every 12 weeks thereafter
  - >100 kg: 90 mg subcutaneously on weeks 0 and 4 then every 12 weeks thereafter
  - PEARL: Ideal for patients who prefer infrequent administration of medication

Most Common Side Effects

- Long-term side effects are unknown but the safety and tolerability over several years appears excellent [50]
  - In PHOENIX 1 and 2 clinical trials, side effects were mild and did not require treatment adjustment
- Infections
  - Mucocutaneous candidiasis
  - Reactivation of latent tuberculosis
- Major cardiac events were found in early trials but not confirmed in larger studies

Avoid

- Administration of live vaccines

Interleukin 23 Inhibitors [1, 2]

Guselkumab (Tremfya), Tildrakizumab (Ilumya)

Conditions that Best Respond

- Psoriasis
  - Highly effective, well-tolerated maintenance therapy including in adalimumab non-responders [51]
  - Works well for scalp and nail psoriasis
  - Achieved PASI 90
- Phase II trials underway regarding efficacy in psoriatic arthritis

How Long this Medication Takes to Work

- 12–16 weeks
- Dose
  - Guselkumab100 mg subcutaneously at weeks 0 and 4, then every 8 weeks
  - Tildrakizumab 100 mg subcutaneously at weeks 0 and 4, then every 12 weeks

Most Common Side Effects

- Infections
  - Upper respiratory tract infections, gastroenteritis, tinea, HSV, candidiasis

Avoid

- Administration of live vaccines

Interleukin 17 Inhibitors [1, 2, 52]

Conditions that Best Respond

- Plaque psoriasis
- Nail and scalp psoriasis
- Psoriatic arthritis

Latest Updates to Lab Monitoring

- Baseline: CBC, CMP, hepatitis screening panel, TB testing (IGRAs or TST)
- Follow up: CBC and CMP every 2–3 months, yearly TB testing

Most Common Side Effects

- Infections
  - Mucocutaneous candidiasis: oral or vulvovaginal most commonly
  - Nasopharyngitis
  - Upper respiratory tract infections
- Injections-site reactions
- New onset or exacerbation of Crohn's disease and ulcerative colitis

Avoid

- Patients with inflammatory bowel disease
- Caution in those with chronic/recurrent infections
- Administration of live vaccines

Ixekizumab (Taltz)

How Long this Medication Takes to Work

- ~85–90% reached PASI-75 within 12 weeks of treatment [53]
- Dose: 160 mg subcutaneously once, then 80 mg at weeks 2, 4, 6, 8, 10 and 12, then 80 mg every 4 weeks

Secukinumab (Cosentyx) [54]

How Long this Medication Takes to Work

- ~77 and 81% reached PASI-75 within 12 weeks of treatment with 300 mg dosing in two phase 3, doubled blinded studies [55]
- Dose: 300 mg subcutaneously on weeks 0, 1, 2, 3 and 4, then 300 mg subcutaneously monthly starting on week 8
  - ○ Each 300 mg dose is given as 2 subcutaneous injections of 150 mg
  - ○ For patients who weigh < 90 kg, consider 150 mg subcutaneous dosing

Brodalumab (Siliq)

Note

- This is an IL17 **receptor** inhibitor

How Long this Medication Takes to Work

- ~80–85% and 60–70% reached PASI-75 with 210 and 140 mg respectively after 12 weeks
- Dose: 210 mg subcutaneously at weeks 0, 1 and 2, then 210 mg once every 2 weeks.
  - ○ Consider discontinuing if inadequate response after 12–16 weeks

Avoid

- Patients with a history of depression or suicide
  - ○ Black Box Warning: Suicidal Ideation and Behavior—medication only available under restricted program: RILIQ REMS
- Contraindicated in patients with Crohn's disease

JAK Inhibitors [1, 2]

Conditions that Best Respond

- FDA approved for psoriatic arthritis (tofacitanib only)
- Psoriasis
- Alopecia areata
- Atopic dermatitis
- Vitiligo
  - ○ May require concomitant light exposure [56]

Latest Updates to Lab Monitoring

- Baseline: CBC, CMP, lipid profile, hepatitis screening panel, TB testing (IGRAs or TST)
- Follow up: CBC, CMP, lipid profile 1 month after starting then every 3 months thereafter; yearly TB testing

Most Common Side Effects

- Infections
  - Nasopharyngitis
- Headaches
- GI effects
  - Diarrhea
  - Elevated LFTs
- Malignancy
  - Lymphoma has developed in patients with rheumatoid arthritis
  - NMSC
- Bone marrow suppression
  - Neutropenia, lymphopenia (tofacitinib mostly), anemia and thrombocytopenia (ruxolitinib)
- Hyperlipidemia

Avoid

- Severe hepatic impairment
- Serious active infection
- Lymphopenia, neutropenia, anemia
- Caution in patients at increased risk of gastrointestinal perforation
- Administration of live vaccines

Tofacitinib (Xeljanz, Jakvinus)—JAK1/3 inhibitor

How Long this Medication Takes to Work

- Psoriasis [57]
  - 65% and 45% treated with 10 mg or 5 mg BID respectively reached PASI-75 at week 16 with efficacy maintained in most through 24 months
- Alopecia areata (AA)
  - Oral: 32% had >50% improvement in Severity of Alopecia Tool (SALT) score with 5 mg BID for 3 months; however, drug cessation led to disease relapse with a median of 8 weeks
  - Topical: 1 and 2% BID

- Used between 3–18 months in 6 patients with AA, 4 with hair regrowth [58]
- Atopic dermatitis
  - Topical
    - Improvement across all endpoints with 2% ointment BID vs placebo within 4 weeks [59]
- Dosing, oral
  - Immediate release (IR) 5 mg BID, extended release (ER) 11 mg once daily
  - In moderate renal or liver impairment, IR 5 mg once daily only

Ruxolitinib—JAK1/2 inhibitor

How Long this Medication Takes to Work

- Alopecia Areata
  - Oral: 75% had >50% improvement in their SALT score with 20 mg BID for 3–6 months; during the 3 months following drug discontinuation, responders had increased shedding with marked hair loss in 33% [60]
- Vitiligo
  - Topical: 76% had improvement in facial Vitiligo Area Scoring Index with 1.5% cream BID at week 20 [61]

Miscellaneous Systemic Drugs

Apremilast (Otezla) [2]

Conditions that Best Respond

- Chronic plaque psoriasis
- Psoriatic arthritis

How Long this Medication Takes to Work

- 30 mg BID after starter kit
  - Starter kit (to reduce risk of GI symptoms) titrate in one week to recommended dose of 30 mg twice daily

Latest Updates to Lab Monitoring

- Consider baseline CMP to assess renal function and if CrCl < 30 mL/min, then reduce dose to 30 mg once daily
- No lab monitoring required

Most Common Side Effects

- GI intolerance
  - Treatment: slow titration, give promethazine or loperamide
- Headache
- Upper respiratory tract infections
- Depression
- Weight loss

Avoid

- Caution when co-administrating with strong cytochrome P450 enzyme inducers including rifampin, phenobarbital, carbamazepine, and phenytoin as they may significantly diminish apremilast levels

---

Antiandrogens and Androgen Inhibitors [1, 2]

Spironolactone

Conditions that Best Respond

- Acne vulgaris
- Androgenic alopecia in women
- Hidradenitis suppurativa
- Hirsutism

How Long this Medication Takes to Work

- 2–3 months
- 50–200 mg daily

Latest Updates to Lab Monitoring

- Routine K+ monitoring is unnecessary for healthy women taking spironolactone for acne [62]
  - Monitor for muscle cramps or weakness

Most Common Side Effects

- Menorrhagia or other menstrual dysfunction
  - Typically resolves after 2–3 months of therapy
  - Treatment: reduce dose to 50–75 mg daily, give spironolactone for 21 days on and 7 days off, add oral contraceptives
- Hyperkalemia
  - Most likely to occur in severe renal insufficiency

- The rate of hyperkalemia in healthy young women taking spironolactone for acne is equivalent to the baseline rate of hyperkalemia in this population.
- No definitive evidence linking spironolactone use to estrogen-dependent malignancies
  - Benign adenomas of the thyroid and testes, malignant mammary tumors and proliferative changes in the liver were found in chronic toxicity studies of rats in which 25–250 times the usual human dose was given to rats
  - Caution in giving to women with a genetic predisposition to breast cancer [63]

Avoid

- Pregnancy
  - Feminization of male fetus
- Other agents that increase the risk of hyperkalemia, (e.g., angiotensin-converting enzyme inhibitors, aliskiren (direct renin inhibitor), angiotensin II receptor blockers and aldosterone inhibitors)

Finasteride (Propecia)

Conditions that Best Respond

- Male and female pattern androgenic alopecia
  - Can trial up to 5 mg daily in postmenopausal women with no clinical or laboratory signs of hyperandrogenism [64]
- Hirsutism
- Frontal fibrosing alopecia [65]

How Long this Medication Takes to Work

- 3 months
- Dosing varies based on conditions being treated, typically 1–5 mg daily

Latest Updates to Lab Monitoring

- Consider baseline PSA in men >50 years prior to starting
- Men need to inform their physician as finasteride will suppress PSA level

Most Common Side Effects

- Sexual dysfunction
  - 2% of men receiving 1 mg daily reported decreased libido, erectile dysfunction or decreased volume of ejaculate
  - Post-finasteride syndrome
    - Reports of long-standing sexual dysfunction but incidence is unknown
- Teratogen

- o No teratogenic effects from trace amounts of finasteride detected in the semen of men who took 1 mg daily; however, rare cases of teratogenicity have been reported to FDA Adverse Events Reporting System.
  - o Do not donate blood for at least 6 months after last dose of medication to prevent blood donation to a pregnant female transfusion recipient, which may harm the male fetus
- Decrease serum PSA
  - o Adjust measured serum PSA concentrations upwards by 40–50% for the purposes of prostate cancer screening [66]
- Prostate Cancer
  - o Cochrane review of men with a mean age of 64 years and PSA 2.1 taking finasteride found 26% relative risk reduction in prostate cancer but a greater number of high-grade Gleason score tumors [67]
  - o Uncertain significance of these findings in younger men, but all men should be counseled regarding this finding

Avoid

- Women of childbearing potential, category X
- Children

Colchicine [1, 2]

Conditions that Best Respond

- Neutrophilic dermatoses (e.g., Behcet's disease)
- Recurrent aphthous stomatitis
- Chronic cutaneous leukocytoclastic vasculitis

How Long this Medication Takes to Work

- 4–6 weeks
- 0.6 mg BID or TID
  - o Consider starting once daily and increasing gradually over a few weeks to decrease side effects
- Taper dose as disease activity allows

Latest Updates to Lab Monitoring

- CBC and CMP every 3 months

Most Common Side Effects

- GI effects
  - Abdominal cramping and watery diarrhea often occur with TID dosing
  - Treatment for diarrhea: aluminum containing antacids (Amphojel), loperamide
- Chronic intoxication
  - Leukopenia, aplastic anemia, myopathy and alopecia
  - Can occur after prolonged therapy with at least 1 mg daily

IVIg [1, 2]

Conditions that Best Respond

- Dermatomyositis
- Scleroderma
- Autoimmune bullous dermatoses
- SJS/TEN
- Pyoderma gangrenosum
- Scleromyxedema
- IVIg can induce long-term remission of various dermatoses and allow the reduction or discontinuation of concomitant immunosuppressive treatments

How Long this Medication Takes to Work

- Monthly infusion cycles until effective disease control
  - 2 g/kg per cycle divided into 3 equal doses, given on each of 3 consecutive days
- Peak serum concentrations immediately
- Serum half-life is 3–5 weeks

Latest Updates to Lab Monitoring

- Baseline: IgA, CBC, CMP, hepatitis screening panel, HIV, rheumatoid factor, cryoglobulins
  - If low or no IgA, confirm that the IVIg product has no IgA to avoid anaphylaxis
  - PEARL: Patients with rheumatoid factor and cryoglobulins are at an increased risk of renal failure
- No specific follow-up laboratory testing required
- Assess for fluid overload at follow up visits

Most Common Side Effects

- Infusion related general effects
  - Headache, myalgia, chills, flushing, fever, nausea, vomiting, low back pain, wheezing, chest pain, blood pressure changes and tachycardia
  - Generally mild
  - Occur 30–60 min after infusion
  - Treatment: slow dose infusion rate, pretreatment with analgesics, NSAIDs, antihistamines or low dose IV corticosteroids
    - For adults can consider the following regimen 30 min prior to infusion:
      - Acetaminophen 650–1000 mg orally
      - Ibuprofen 400 or 800 mg orally
      - Diphenhydramine 25–50 mg orally, intravenously or intramuscularly
      - For patients with severe adverse reactions such as headaches, consider methylprednisolone 40–60 mg intravenously
- Risk of fluid overload
  - Monitor closely in those with significant cardiac and kidney disease
- Aseptic meningitis
  - Headache and photophobia that are self-limiting and resolve without sequelae
  - Treatment: analgesics and anti-emetics
- Thromboembolic events
  - Decrease risk by lowering IVIg dose and slowing rate of infusion
- Hematologic effects
  - Neutropenia and hemolysis seen in those with autoantibodies against blood group antigens of ABO and Rhesus (Rh) system
- Anaphylaxis
  - Few cases reported, particularly in those with IgA deficiency having anti-IgA antibodies
- Renal failure
  - Increased risk in patients with rheumatoid factor and cryoglobulins

Avoid

- In patients with IgA deficiency

Naltrexone [68]

Conditions that Best Respond

- Pruritus
  - Associated with psoriasis, atopic dermatitis, lichen simplex chronicus and prurigo nodularis
- Hailey-Hailey disease

- Lichen planopilaris (LPP)

How Long this Medication Takes to Work

- ~2 months
- No standard dosing guidelines exist but consider the following
  - High-dose naltrexone at 50–100 mg daily
    - Pruritus
    - Alcohol and opioid addiction
  - Low dose naltrexone (LDN) at 1.5–5.0 mg daily
    - Used in a variety of cutaneous conditions including Hailey-Hailey, LPP, Grover's and Darier's disease

Latest Updates to Lab Monitoring

- None

Most Common Side Effects

- Low dose naltrexone has proven to be safe without serious adverse events
- High dose naltrexone
  - GI upset: abdominal cramps, nausea, vomiting, anorexia
  - Dizziness
  - Fatigue
  - Insomnia

Avoid

- Caution in patients on opioids as high dose naltrexone will decrease efficacy and may induce withdrawal symptoms

Nicotinamide (Vitamin B3) [69]

Conditions that Best Respond

- Autoimmune bullous dermatoses
- NMSC chemoprevention in high risk patients
- Pellagra

How Long this Medication Takes to Work

- 2–3 months of 500 mg BID-TID
  - Usually given in combination with tetracycline for treatment of autoimmune bullous dermatoses

- 500 mg BID for NMSC chemoprevention with effects noticed within 3 months of use
  PEARL: Chemoprevention effect is lost after discontinuation of medication

Latest Updates to Lab Monitoring

- None

Most Common Side Effects

- Headache
- GI complaints

Avoid

- PEARL: Do not confuse with niacin (or nicotinic acid), which will cause a flushing reaction

---

Rituximab [1, 2]

Conditions that Best Respond

- Autoimmune bullous dermatoses
- Autoimmune connective tissue diseases
- GVHD
- Vasculitis
- Cutaneous B cell lymphoma

How Long this Medication Takes to Work

- Dosing adopted from rheumatoid arthritis guidelines
  - 1000 mg IV infusions given 2 weeks apart (i.e. day 0 and day 14)
  - Infusion cycle can be repeated at 4–6-month intervals
- CD20 + B cell depletion within 2–3 weeks, which is sustained for ~6 months
  - B cell numbers return to normal levels within the first year after treatment

Latest Updates to Lab Monitoring

- Baseline labs: CBC w/diff, CMP, hepatitis screening panel, TB testing (IGRAs or TST)
- Follow up
  - CBC w/diff every 2 weeks during treatment then 1-3 months thereafter

  ○ Consider monitoring CD 19 + and CD20 + B cells, which may help serve as a
    tool to predict relapses [70]

Most Common Side Effects

- Infusion reactions
  ○ Generally mild and occur only with the first infusion
  ○ If severe reactions occur, they typically do so within 30–120 min
- Infections
  ○ Bacterial, viral and fungal infections during treatment and up to 12 months
    afterwards
  ○ Significant increased risk of reactivation of hepatitis B virus
- Cytopenias
- Human anti-chimeric antibodies (HACA)
  ○ Higher levels seen in patients treated for autoimmune disease (up to 30% in
    SLE patients)
  ○ Unclear whether they affect rituximab levels or the efficiency of B cell
    depletion
- Arrhythmias
- Tumor lysis syndrome
- Intestinal perforation

Avoid

- Patients with active infections
- Administration of live vaccines
  ○ Non-live vaccines can be administered 4 weeks prior to treatment

References

1. Wolverton S. Comprehensive dermatologic drug therapy, 3rd ed. Philadelphia: Elsevier
   Saunders; 2013.
2. Bolognia J, Schaffer J, Cerroni L. Dermatology. Philadelphia: Elsevier Saunders; 2017.
3. Marmor MF, et al. Revised recommendations on screening for chloroquine and hydroxychloroquine retinopathy. Ophthalmology. 2011;118(2):415–22.
4. Mohammad S, et al. Examination of hydroxychloroquine use and hemolytic anemia in
   G6PDH-Deficient patients. Arthritis Care Res (Hoboken). 2018;70(3):481–5.
5. Melles RB, Marmor MF. The risk of toxic retinopathy in patients on long-term hydroxychloroquine therapy. JAMA Ophthalmol. 2014;132(12):1453–60.
6. Cho HG, et al. Azathioprine and risk of multiple keratinocyte cancers. J Am Acad Dermatol.
   2018;78(1): 27–28. e1.
7. Patel AA, Swerlick RA, McCall CO. Azathioprine in dermatology: the past, the present, and
   the future. J Am Acad Dermatol. 2006;55(3):369–89.
8. Phillips T, et al. Non-Hodgkin's lymphoma associated with long-term azathioprine therapy.
   Clin Exp Dermatol. 1987;12(6):444–5.

9. Snow JL, Gibson LE. The role of genetic variation in thiopurine methyltransferase activity and the efficacy and/or side effects of azathioprine therapy in dermatologic patients. Arch Dermatol. 1995;131(2):193–7.
10. Buckley L, et al. 2017 American College of Rheumatology guideline for the prevention and treatment of glucocorticoid-induced osteoporosis. Arthritis Rheumatol. 2017;69(8):1521–37.
11. Stathopoulos IP, et al. The use of bisphosphonates in women prior to or during pregnancy and lactation. Hormones (Athens). 2011;10(4):280–91.
12. Reddy S, Ananthakrishnan S, Garg A. A prospective observational study evaluating hypothalamic-pituitary-adrenal axis alteration and efficacy of intramuscular triamcinolone acetonide for steroid-responsive dermatologic disease. J Am Acad Dermatol. 2013;69(2):226–31.
13. Maza A, et al. Oral cyclosporin in psoriasis: a systematic review on treatment modalities, risk of kidney toxicity and evidence for use in non-plaque psoriasis. J Eur Acad Dermatol Venereol. 2011;25(Suppl 2):19–27.
14. Neuvonen PJ, Niemi M, Backman JT. Drug interactions with lipid-lowering drugs: mechanisms and clinical relevance. Clin Pharmacol Ther. 2006;80(6):565–81.
15. Paul CF, et al. Risk of malignancies in psoriasis patients treated with cyclosporine: a 5 y cohort study. J Invest Dermatol. 2003;120(2):211–6.
16. Pere AK, et al. Dietary potassium and magnesium supplementation in cyclosporine-induced hypertension and nephrotoxicity. Kidney Int. 2000;58(6):2462–72.
17. Serratrice J, et al. Interference of dapsone in HbA1c monitoring of a diabetic patient with polychondritis. Diabetes Metab. 2002;28(6 Pt 1):508–9.
18. Tack CJ, Wetzels JF. Decreased HbA1c levels due to sulfonamide-induced hemolysis in two IDDM patients. Diabetes Care. 1996;19(7):775–6.
19. Visser K, van der Heijde D. Optimal dosage and route of administration of methotrexate in rheumatoid arthritis: a systematic review of the literature. Ann Rheum Dis. 2009;68(7):1094–9.
20. Fairris GM, et al. Methotrexate dosage in patients aged over 50 with psoriasis. BMJ. 1989;298(6676):801–2.
21. Cheng HS, Rademaker M. Monitoring methotrexate-induced liver fibrosis in patients with psoriasis: utility of transient elastography. Psoriasis (Auckl). 2018;8:21–9.
22. Khan S, Subedi D, Chowdhury MM. Use of amino terminal type III procollagen peptide (P3NP) assay in methotrexate therapy for psoriasis. Postgrad Med J. 2006;82(967):353–4.
23. Gutierrez JC, Hwang K. The toxicity of methotrexate in male fertility and paternal teratogenicity. Expert Opin Drug Metab Toxicol. 2017;13(1):51–8.
24. Cudmore J, et al. Methotrexate and trimethoprim-sulfamethoxazole: toxicity from this combination continues to occur. Can Fam Physician. 2014;60(1):53–6.
25. Frenia ML, Long KS. Methotrexate and nonsteroidal antiinflammatory drug interactions. Ann Pharmacother. 1992;26(2):234–7.
26. Colebatch AN, Marks JL, Edwards CJ. Safety of non-steroidal anti-inflammatory drugs, including aspirin and paracetamol (acetaminophen) in people receiving methotrexate for inflammatory arthritis (rheumatoid arthritis, ankylosing spondylitis, psoriatic arthritis, other spondyloarthritis). Cochrane Database Syst Rev. 2011;11:CD008872.
27. Hewitt RJ, et al. Screening tests for tuberculosis before starting biological therapy. BMJ. 2015;350:h1060.
28. Dobler CC. Biologic agents and tuberculosis. Microbiol Spectr 2016;4(6).
29. Bavinck JN, et al. Prevention of skin cancer and reduction of keratotic skin lesions during acitretin therapy in renal transplant recipients: a double-blind, placebo-controlled study. J Clin Oncol. 1995;13(8):1933–8.
30. DiGiovanna JJ. Retinoid chemoprevention in the high-risk patient. J Am Acad Dermatol. 1998;39(2 Pt 3):S82–5.
31. DiGiovanna JJ. Isotretinoin effects on bone. J Am Acad Dermatol. 2001;45(5):S176–82.
32. Gniadecki R, et al. The optimal use of bexarotene in cutaneous T-cell lymphoma. Br J Dermatol. 2007;157(3):433–40.
33. Sherman SI, et al. Central hypothyroidism associated with retinoid X receptor-selective ligands. N Engl J Med. 1999;340(14):1075–9.

34. Hansen TJ, et al. Standardized laboratory monitoring with use of isotretinoin in acne. J Am Acad Dermatol. 2016;75(2):323–8.
35. Chivot M. Acne flare-up and deterioration with oral isotretinoin. Ann Dermatol Venereol. 2001;128(3 Pt 1):224–8.
36. Menter A, Strober B, Kaplan DH, Kivelevitch D, et al. Guidelines of care for the management and treatment of psoriasis with biologics. J Am Acad Dermatol In preparation.
37. Ou Z, et al. Adverse events of Dupilumab in adults with moderate-to-severe atopic dermatitis: a meta-analysis. Int Immunopharmacol. 2018;54:303–10.
38. Wollenberg A, et al. Conjunctivitis occurring in atopic dermatitis patients treated with dupilumab-clinical characteristics and treatment. J Allergy Clin Immunol Pract. 2018;6(5):778–1780. e1.
39. Treister AD, Kraff-Cooper C, Lio PA. Risk factors for dupilumab-associated conjunctivitis in patients with atopic dermatitis. JAMA Dermatol. 2018;154(10):1208–11.
40. Fleming P, Drucker AM. Risk of infection in patients with atopic dermatitis treated with dupilumab: a meta-analysis of randomized controlled trials. J Am Acad Dermatol. 2018;78(1):62–69. e1.
41. Menter A, et al. Adalimumab therapy for moderate to severe psoriasis: a randomized, controlled phase III trial. J Am Acad Dermatol. 2008;58(1):106–15.
42. Gordon K, et al. Long-term efficacy and safety of adalimumab in patients with moderate to severe psoriasis treated continuously over 3 years: results from an open-label extension study for patients from REVEAL. J Am Acad Dermatol. 2012;66(2):241–51.
43. Paradisi A, et al. Etanercept therapy for toxic epidermal necrolysis. J Am Acad Dermatol. 2014;71(2):278–83.
44. Papp KA, et al. A global phase III randomized controlled trial of etanercept in psoriasis: safety, efficacy, and effect of dose reduction. Br J Dermatol. 2005;152(6):1304–12.
45. Reich K, et al. Infliximab induction and maintenance therapy for moderate-to-severe psoriasis: a phase III, multicentre, double-blind trial. Lancet. 2005;366(9494):1367–74.
46. Menter A, et al. A randomized comparison of continuous vs. intermittent infliximab maintenance regimens over 1 year in the treatment of moderate-to-severe plaque psoriasis. J Am Acad Dermatol. 2007;56(1):31. e1–15.
47. Afif W, et al. Clinical utility of measuring infliximab and human anti-chimeric antibody concentrations in patients with inflammatory bowel disease. Am J Gastroenterol. 2010;105(5):1133–9.
48. Gottlieb A, et al. Ustekinumab, a human interleukin 12/23 monoclonal antibody, for psoriatic arthritis: randomised, double-blind, placebo-controlled, crossover trial. Lancet. 2009;373(9664):633–40.
49. Leonardi CL, et al. Efficacy and safety of ustekinumab, a human interleukin-12/23 monoclonal antibody, in patients with psoriasis: 76-week results from a randomised, double-blind, placebo-controlled trial (PHOENIX 1). Lancet. 2008;371(9625):1665–74.
50. Emer JJ, Frankel A, Zeichner JA. A practical approach to monitoring patients on biological agents for the treatment of psoriasis. J Clin Aesthet Dermatol. 2010;3(8):20–6.
51. Blauvelt A, et al. Efficacy and safety of guselkumab, an anti-interleukin-23 monoclonal antibody, compared with adalimumab for the continuous treatment of patients with moderate to severe psoriasis: Results from the phase III, double-blinded, placebo- and active comparator-controlled VOYAGE 1 trial. J Am Acad Dermatol. 2017;76(3):405–17.
52. Gomez-Garcia F, et al. Short-term efficacy and safety of new biological agents targeting the interleukin-23-T helper 17 pathway for moderate-to-severe plaque psoriasis: a systematic review and network meta-analysis. Br J Dermatol. 2017;176(3):594–603.
53. Gordon KB, et al. Phase 3 trials of ixekizumab in moderate-to-severe plaque psoriasis. N Engl J Med. 2016;375(4):345–56.
54. van de Kerkhof PC, et al. Secukinumab long-term safety experience: a pooled analysis of 10 phase II and III clinical studies in patients with moderate to severe plaque psoriasis. J Am Acad Dermatol. 2016;75(1):83–98. e4.

55. Langley RG, et al. Secukinumab in plaque psoriasis–results of two phase 3 trials. N Engl J Med. 2014;371(4):326–38.
56. Liu LY, et al. Repigmentation in vitiligo using the Janus kinase inhibitor tofacitinib may require concomitant light exposure. J Am Acad Dermatol. 2017;77(4): 675–682. e1.
57. Papp KA, et al. Tofacitinib, an oral Janus kinase inhibitor, for the treatment of chronic plaque psoriasis: long-term efficacy and safety results from 2 randomized phase-III studies and 1 open-label long-term extension study. J Am Acad Dermatol. 2016;74(5):841–50.
58. Bayart CB, et al. Topical Janus kinase inhibitors for the treatment of pediatric alopecia areata. J Am Acad Dermatol. 2017;77(1):167–70.
59. Bissonnette R, et al. Topical tofacitinib for atopic dermatitis: a phase IIa randomized trial. Br J Dermatol. 2016;175(5):902–11.
60. Mackay-Wiggan J, et al. Oral ruxolitinib induces hair regrowth in patients with moderate-to-severe alopecia areata. JCI Insight. 2016;1(15):e89790.
61. Rothstein B, et al. Treatment of vitiligo with the topical Janus kinase inhibitor ruxolitinib. J Am Acad Dermatol. 2017;76(6):1054–1060. e1.
62. Plovanich M, Weng QY, Mostaghimi A. Low usefulness of potassium monitoring among healthy young women taking spironolactone for acne. JAMA Dermatol. 2015;151(9):941–4.
63. Biggar RJ, Andersen EW, Wohlfahrt J, Melbye M. Spironolactone use and the risk of breast cancer. J Am Acad Dermatol. 2016:AB72.
64. Oliveira-Soares R, et al. Finasteride 5 mg/day treatment of patterned hair loss in normo-androgenetic postmenopausal women. Int J Trichology. 2013;5(1):22–5.
65. Danesh M, Murase JE. Increasing utility of finasteride for frontal fibrosing alopecia. J Am Acad Dermatol. 2015;72(6):e157.
66. Zakhem GA, Motosko CC, Mu EW, Ho RS. Infertility and teratogenicity after paternal exposure to systemic dermatologic medications: A systematic review. J Am Acad Dermatol. 2019;80(4):957–69.
67. D'Amico AV, Roehrborn CG. Effect of 1 mg/day finasteride on concentrations of serum prostate-specific antigen in men with androgenic alopecia: a randomised controlled trial. Lancet Oncol. 2007;8(1):21–5.
68. Wilt TJ, et al. Five-alpha-reductase Inhibitors for prostate cancer prevention. Cochrane Database Syst Rev. 2008(2);CD007091.
69. Ekelem C, et al. Utility of naltrexone treatment for chronic inflammatory dermatologic conditions: a systematic review. JAMA Dermatol. 2018.
70. Chen AC, et al. A phase 3 randomized trial of nicotinamide for skin-cancer chemoprevention. N Engl J Med. 2015;373(17):1618–26.
71. Trouvin AP, et al. Usefulness of monitoring of B cell depletion in rituximab-treated rheumatoid arthritis patients in order to predict clinical relapse: a prospective observational study. Clin Exp Immunol. 2015;180(1):11–8.

Pigmentary Disorders

Bhavnit K. Bhatia, Richard H. Huggins and Alison Tisack

Ashy Dermatosis/Erythema Dyschromicum Perstans (EDP) [1, 2] Lichen Planus Pigmentosus (LPP) [1, 3]

What Not To Miss

- Other mucocutaneous features of lichen planus

Key DDx

- Post-inflammatory hyperpigmentation

Work Up Pearls

- Frequently a clinical diagnosis
  - Most commonly seen in adults with skin types III–V
  - Erythema dyschromicum perstans (EDP) is most commonly found on trunk and upper extremities and may have a rim of erythema in active lesions
  - Lichen planus pigmentosus (LPP) is most commonly found in photodistributed or intertriginous pattern (this is usually referred to as lichen planus pigmentosus inversus)

B. K. Bhatia · A. Tisack
Department of Dermatology, Henry Ford Health System,
3031 West Grand Blvd, Suite 800, Detroit, MI 48202, USA

R. H. Huggins (✉)
Henry Ford Health System, 3031 West Grand Blvd, Suite 800, Detroit, MI 48202, USA
e-mail: rhuggin1@hfhs.org

© Springer Nature Switzerland AG 2020
H. W. Lim et al. (eds.), *Practical Guide to Dermatology*,
https://doi.org/10.1007/978-3-030-18015-7_11

- Biopsy
  - Erythema dyschromicum perstans (EDP) and lichen planus pigmentosus (LPP) often cannot be distinguished on histology. Both show epidermal atrophy, vacuolar degeneration of the basal layer, and a variable lichenoid lymphocytic infiltrate

Treatment Ladder

- Photoprotection
  - Broad-brimmed hats, sunglasses, photoprotective clothing
  - Sunscreen with PHYSICAL filters (i.e. zinc oxide, titanium dioxide) and broad-spectrum UVA/UVB sunscreens with SPF 30–50+
- Topicals
  - Hydroquinone 4% (can prescribe higher potency via compounding pharmacies)
  - Topical retinoids such as adapalene 0.1–0.3% or tretinoin 0.025–1%
  - Triple combination depigmentation cream consisting of a topical retinoid (adapalene 0.1–0.3% or tretinoin 0.025–0.1%), a low potency topical steroid (hydrocortisone 1–2.5%, desonide 0.05%, fluocinolone 0.01%) and hydroquinone 4% (such as Kligman's formula)
  - Topical tacrolimus 0.1% ointment [4]
- Systemics
  - Minocycline 100 mg BID
  - Dapsone 100 mg daily [5]
  - Hydroxychloroquine 200 mg BID (or 5 mg/kg daily)

Outside the Box Treatment Options

- Chemical peels [6], including glycolic acid and salicylic acid (safer for skin of color)
- Oral retinoids [7]
- Q-switched Nd:YAG laser—safe for use in skin of color
  - Multiple treatments necessary and recurrence has been reported [8–10]
- 1550 nm non-ablative fractional laser with topical tacrolimus [11]
- Single case series showing efficacy of clofazimine in decreasing inflammation in EDP, however all patients experienced temporary orange skin discoloration and length of follow up was not reported [12]

Melasma [1, 2]

What Not To Miss

- Exogenous hyperestrogenism including OCPs, hormone replacement therapy
- Role of visible light

- Exogenous ochronosis
  - Look for stippled blue appearance

Key DDx

- Post-inflammatory hyperpigmentation
- Riehl's melanosis
- Atypical periorbital acanthosis nigricans
- Drug related hyperpigmentation (HCTZ, calcium channel blockers)

Work Up Pearls

- Look for typical acanthosis nigricans at other sites if considering periorbital acanthosis nigricans
- Post-pregnancy, melasma may fade in lighter skin types but persist in skin of color

Treatment Ladder

- Photoprotection as in ashy dermatosis
  - Tinted sunscreens are preferred [13]
- Topicals
  - Similar to ashy dermatosis (above)
  - 20% azelaic acid
  - Glycolic acid
  - 2–6% kojic acid
    - Avoid if penicillin or mushroom allergy
  - Vitamin C
- Chemical peels
  - 30–70% αHA glycolic acid
  - Salicylic acid
  - Jessner's peel: salicylic acid (14 g), resorcinol (14 g), lactic acid 85% (14 g), ethanol
    - Consider modified Jessner's with citric acid rather than resorcinol as resorcinol can cross react with hydroquinone potentially sensitizing these patients
  - Tricholoracetic acid (TCA) 10–25%—use with caution in skin of color and consider a test spot
    - Can combine with Jessner's peel applied first then TCA
- Laser therapies [8, 14]
  - Non-ablative fractional resurfacing lasers, 1550 and 1927 nm
    - Caution with higher fluences and higher densities in Fitzpatrick IV–VI

- Low fluence Q-switch Nd:Yag or Q-switch Alexandrite
  - Fitzpatrick I–III
- Consider pulse dye laser as adjunctive treatment in melasma with prominent vascularity [15]

Outside the Box Treatment Options

- Tranexamic acid 325 mg BID
  - Caution if history of thromboembolism or renal impairment
- Compounds with higher concentration hydroquinone (8–12%) with additions of: kojic acid, vitamin C, azelaic acid, niacinamide, and/or topical retinoids
  - PEARL: Previously, higher percentage hydroquinone was avoided due to risk of ochronosis, but now more widely used. Recommend close monitoring for ochronosis, especially in darker phototypes and in locations with sunny climate
- Microneedling [16]
- *Polypodium leucotomos* 240 mg BID to TID [17]

Post-inflammatory Hyperpigmentation [1, 2]

What Not To Miss

- Underlying dermatosis causing PIH
- Drug induced pigmentation

Key DDx

- Erythema dyschromicum perstans
- Lichen planus pigmentosus
- Melasma

Treatment Ladder

- Photoprotection as in ashy dermatosis

- Topicals
  - Similar to ashy dermatosis
  - Glycolic acid
  - 2–6% kojic acid

- Chemical peels
  - 30–70% αHA glycolic acid
  - Salicylic acid for skin of color
  - Jessner's peel: salicylic acid (14 g), resorcinol (14 g), lactic acid 85% (14 g), ethanol
    - PEARL: Great for combination of mild acne + PIH

Outside the Box Treatment Options

- Low energy low density non-ablative fractional 1927 nm thulium laser [18]
  - Can also add topical drug delivery of hydroquinone or tranexamic acid
  - Caution: risk of adverse reactions to topicals

Points to Consider When Using Lasers in Skin of Color [19–21]

Pre-Procedure

- Do not treat if ongoing inflammatory process—disease must be stable
- Limit sun exposure as much as possible
- Consider hydroquinone 2–4% for 2–4 weeks prior to treatment

During Procedure

- Reduce fluence and density, increase number of treatments

Post-Procedure

- Consider systemic agents including a short course of oral steroids (prednisone 10 mg × 3 days) [19] or tranexamic acid [20]
- Consider topicals including steroids [21] or hydroquinone

Vitiligo

For vitiligo, a multifaceted approach is key. This includes topicals, phototherapy, and addressing psychosocial needs, in addition to cosmetic agents, systemic agents, and surgery when appropriate. Emerging treatments for vitiligo include oral and topical janus kinase inhibitors

What Not To Miss

- Concomitant autoimmune conditions, including thyroid disorders, alopecia areata, pernicious anemia

- Rapidly progressive disease
  - o Signs include confetti-like macules or trichrome vitiligo

Key DDx

- Post-inflammatory hypopigmentation
- Pityriasis alba
- Progressive macular hypomelanosis
- Idiopathic guttate hypomelanosis
- Nevus depigmentosus

Work Up Pearls

- Check baseline TSH; then PRN if symptomatic

Treatment Ladder

- Medical Management [22, 23]
  - o Topicals
    - Repigmentation: topical corticosteroids, calcineurin inhibitors for head/neck [24]
    - Depigmentation: monobenzyl ether of hydroquinone 20–40% [25]
  - o Antioxidants
    - Alpha lipoic acid 100 mg daily [26] (PEARL: best when combined with UVB)
    - Gingko biloba 60 mg BID [27] (PEARL: best for slowly spreading disease)
    - Foods with high levels of antioxidants, such as blueberries and dark green vegetables
  - o Phototherapy [28–32]
    - Excimer laser 2–3 times weekly for localized lesions (BSA < 10%)
    - NB-UVB 2–3 times weekly for more generalized over 6–9 months
    - Increased efficacy when used in combination with topical calcineurin inhibitors and corticosteroids
- Surgical
  - o Melanocyte-keratinocyte transplantation procedure (MKTP) [33, 34]
    - Indications:
      - ≤10% BSA
      - Stable vitiligo for 6–24 months
      - Segmental > focal > generalized > acrofacial

- Psychosocial [35–37]
  - Refer to support groups, behavioral health/social work PRN
  - List of US vitiligo support groups/Facebook groups: https://www.globalvitiligofoundation.org/support-groups
  - Books and camps for children with vitiligo: https://www.globalvitiligofoundation.org/global-vitiligo-support-community
- Cosmetics [38, 39]
  - Concealers: Dermablend®, CoverBlend®, Cover FX®, Microskin™, Zanderm Vitiligo Concealer™
  - Self-tanning products containing dihydroxyacetone (water-resistant, last longer, but may have more of an orange tone)

Outside the Box Treatment Options

- Tofacitanib cream and ruxolitinib cream (2%) are available can be obtained at compounding pharmacies
- Systemics
  - If rapidly spreading:
    - Minocycline 100 mg BID for 3–6 months [40, 41]
    - Dexamethasone 2.5–4 mg daily on weekends only for 3–6 months [41, 42]
    - Prednisone 20 mg daily or every other day dosing
  - Afamelanotide (subcutaneous injection; FDA approval pending) + NB-UVB
  - Tofacitinib 5 mg daily to BID [43]
    - PEARL: best for face > other sun-exposed areas [44]

In the Context Of…

- Head/neck lesions
  - Topical calcineurin inhibitors equivalent but safer than topical steroids
- Psychosocial Morbidity
  - Be vigilant in higher-risk patients, such as females, younger patients, darker skin types, and those with vitiligo on exposed sites
- Recalcitrant disease
  - Systemics can be used in combination with NB-UVB

Photoprotection [1, 2, 45]

- Sunscreens
  - Apply broad-spectrum (UVA/UVB) SPF 30–50+ and reapply every 2–4 h
- Self-tanner (dihydroxyacetone)
  - SPF 3
  - Adequate for Soret band (400–410 nm) coverage

- Iron oxide (3%)
  - Good photoprotection to blue visible light (Soret band)
  - Useful in porphyrias, melasma, and PIH—particularly for darker-complexioned individuals
- Photoprotective clothing, wide-brimmed hats, sunglasses

UVB filters	UVA filters	UVA + UVB filters
Cinoxate	Avobenzone (Parsol 1789)	Titanium dioxide
Ensulizole	Dioxybenzone	Zinc oxide
Homosalate	Meradimate	
Octinoxate	Oxybenzone	
Octisalate	Sulisobenzone	
Octocrylene		
Para-Aminobenzoic acid		
Padimate O		
Trolamine salicylate		

References

1. Molinar VE, Taylor SC, Pandya AG. What's new in objective assessment and treatment of facial hyperpigmentation? Dermatol Clin. 2014;32(2):123–35.
2. Pandya AG, Guevara IL. Disorders of hyperpigmentation. Dermatol Clin. 2000;18(1):91–8. ix.
3. Robles-Méndez JC, Rizo-Frías P, Herz-Ruelas ME, Pandya AG, Ocampo Candiani J. Lichen planus pigmentosus and its variants: review and update. Int J Dermatol. 2018;57(5):505–14.
4. Mahajan VK, Chauhan PS, Mehta KS, Sharma AL. Erythema dyschromicum perstans: response to topical tacrolimus. Indian J Dermatol. 2015;60(5):525.
5. Bahadir S, Cobanoglu U, Cimsit G, Yayli S, Alpay K. Erythema dyschromicum perstans: response to dapsone therapy. Int J Dermatol. 2004;43(3):220–2.
6. Wolff M, Sabzevari N, Gropper C, Hoffman C. A case of lichen planus pigmentosus with facial dyspigmentation responsive to combination therapy with chemical peels and topical retinoids. J Clin Aesthet Dermatol. 2016;9(11):44–50.
7. Wang F, Zhao YK, Wang Z, Liu JH, Luo DQ. Erythema dyschromicum perstans response to isotretinoin. JAMA Dermatol. 2016;152(7):841–2.
8. Aurangabadkar SJ. Optimizing q-switched lasers for melasma and acquired dermal melanoses. Indian J Dermatol Venereol Leprol. 2019;85:10–17. 2018 Jul 16.
9. Shah DSD, Aurangabadkar DS, Nikam DB. An open-label non-randomized prospective pilot study of the efficacy of Q-switched Nd-YAG laser in management of facial lichen planus pigmentosus. J Cosmet Laser Ther. 2019;21:108–15 Epub 2018 May 16.
10. Han XD, Goh CL. A case of lichen planus pigmentosus that was recalcitrant to topical treatment responding to pigment laser treatment. Dermatol Ther. 2014;27(5):264–7.
11. Wolfshohl JA, Geddes ER, Stout AB, Friedman PM. Improvement of erythema dyschromicum perstans using a combination of the 1,550-nm erbium-doped fractionated laser and topical tacrolimus ointment. Lasers Surg Med. 2017;49(1):60–2.
12. Barranda L, Torres-Alvarez B, Cortes-Franco R, et al. Involvement of cell adhesion and activation molecules in the pathogenesis of erythema dyschromicum perstans (ashy dermatitis). The effect of clofazamine therapy. Arch Dermatol. 1997;133:325–9.

13. Castanedo-Cazares JP, Hernandez-Blanco D, Carlos-Ortega B, Fuentes-Ahumada C, Torres-Álvarez B. Near-visible light and UV photoprotection in the treatment of melasma: a double-blind randomized trial. Photodermatol Photoimmunol Photomed. 2014;30(1):35–42.

14. Trivedi MK, Yang FC, Cho BK. A review of laser and light therapy in melasma. Int J Womens Dermatol. 2017;3(1):11–20.

15. Geddes ER, Stout AB, Friedman PM. Retrospective analysis of the treatment of melasma lesions exhibiting increased vascularity with the 595-nm pulsed dye laser combined with the 1927-nm fractional low-powered diode laser. Lasers Surg Med. 2017;49(1):20–6.

16. Lima EVA, Lima MMDA, Paixão MP, Miot HA. Assessment of the effects of skin microneedling as adjuvant therapy for facial melasma: a pilot study. BMC Dermatol. 2017;17(1):14.

17. Ahmed AM, Lopez I, Perese F, Vasquez R, Hynan LS, Chong B, Pandya AG. A randomized, double-blinded, placebo-controlled trial of oral Polypodium leucotomos extract as an adjunct to sunscreen in the treatment of melasma. JAMA Dermatol. 2013;149(8):981–3.

18. Brauer JA, Alabdulrazzaq H, Bae YS, Geronemus RG. Evaluation of a low energy, low density, non-ablative fractional 1927 nm wavelength laser for facial skin resurfacing. J Drugs Dermatol. 2015;14(11):1262–7.

19. Cho SB, Lee SJ, Kang JM, Kim YK, Chung WS, Oh SH. The efficacy and safety of 10,600-nm carbon dioxide fractional laser for acne scars in Asian patients. Dermatol Surg. 2009;35(12):1955–61.

20. Kim MS, Bang SH, Kim JH, Shin HJ, Choi JH, Chang SE. Tranexamic acid diminishes laser-induced melanogenesis. Ann Dermatol. 2015;27(3):250–6.

21. Cheyasak N, Manuskiatti W, Maneeprasopchoke P, Wanitphakdeedecha R. Topical corticosteroids minimise the risk of postinflammatory hyper-pigmentation after ablative fractional CO_2 laser resurfacing in Asians. Acta Derm Venereol. 2015;95(2):201–5.

22. Felsten LM, Alikhan A, Petronic-Rosic V. Vitiligo: a comprehensive overview Part II: treatment options and approach to treatment. J Am Acad Dermatol. 2011;65(3):493–514.

23. Rodrigues M, Ezzedine K, Hamzavi I, Pandya AG, Harris JE, Vitiligo Working Group. Current and emerging treatments for vitiligo. J Am Acad Dermatol. 2017;77(1):17–29.

24. Ho N, Pope E, Weinstein M, Greenberg S, Webster C. A double-blind, randomized, placebo-controlled trial of topical tacrolimus 0.1% vs. clobetasol propionate 0.05% in childhood vitiligo. Br J Dermatol. 2011;165(3):626–32.

25. Tan ES, Sarkany R. Topical monobenzyl ether of hydroquinone is an effective and safe treatment for depigmentation of extensive vitiligo in the medium term: a retrospective cohort study of 53 cases. Br J Dermatol. 2015;172(6):1662–4.

26. Dell'Anna ML, Mastrofrancesco A, Sala R, et al. Antioxidants and narrow band-UVB in the treatment of vitiligo: a double-blind placebo controlled trial. Clin Exp Dermatol. 2007;32(6):631–6.

27. Parsad D, Pandhi R, Juneja A. Effectiveness of oral Ginkgo biloba in treating limited, slowly spreading vitiligo. Clin Exp Dermatol. 2003;28(3):285–7.

28. Passeron T, Ostovari N, Zakaria W, et al. Topical tacrolimus and the 308-nm excimer laser: a synergistic combination for the treatment of vitiligo. Arch Dermatol. 2004;140(9):1065–9.

29. Mehrabi D. A randomized, placebo-controlled, double-blind trial comparing narrowband UV-B Plus 0.1% tacrolimus ointment with narrowband UV-B plus placebo in the treatment of generalized vitiligo. Arch Dermatol. 2006;142(7):927–9.

30. Nordal EJ, Guleng GE, Ronnevig JR. Treatment of vitiligo with narrowband-UVB (TL01) combined with tacrolimus ointment (0.1%) vs. placebo ointment, a randomized right/left double-blind comparative study. J Eur Acad Dermatol Venereol JEADV. 2011;25(12):1440–3.

31. Bae JM, Hong BY, Lee JH, Lee JH, Kim GM. The efficacy of 308-nm excimer laser/light (EL) and topical agent combination therapy versus EL monotherapy for vitiligo: a systematic review and meta-analysis of randomized controlled trials (RCTs). J Am Acad Dermatol. 2016;74(5):907–15.

32. Bae JM, Jung HM, Hong BY, Lee JH, Choi WJ, Lee JH, Kim GM. Phototherapy for vitiligo: a systematic review and meta-analysis. JAMA Dermatol. 2017;153(7):666–74.

33. Huggins RH, Henderson MD, Mulekar SV, et al. Melanocyte-keratinocyte transplantation procedure in the treatment of vitiligo: the experience of an academic medical center in the United States. J Am Acad Dermatol. 2012;66(5):785–93.

34. Silpa-Archa N, Griffith JL, Huggins RH, Henderson MD, Kerr HA, Jacobsen G, Mulekar SV, Lim HW, Hamzavi IH. Long-term follow-up of patients undergoing autologous noncultured melanocyte-keratinocyte transplantation for vitiligo and other leukodermas. J Am Acad Dermatol. 2017;77(2):318–27.

35. Sampogna F, Raskovic D, Guerra L, et al. Identification of categories at risk for high quality of life impairment in patients with vitiligo. Br J Dermatol. 2008;159(2):351–9.

36. Linthorst Homan MW, Spuls PI, de Korte J, Bos JD, Sprangers MA, van der Veen JP. The burden of vitiligo: patient characteristics associated with quality of life. J Am Acad Dermatol. 2009;61(3):411–20.

37. Ezzedine K, Sheth V, Rodrigues M, et al. Vitiligo is not a cosmetic disease. J Am Acad Dermatol. 2015;73(5):883–5.

38. Rajatanavin N, Suwanachote S, Kulkollakarn S. Dihydroxyacetone: a safe camouflaging option in vitiligo. Int J Dermatol. 2008;47(4):402–6.

39. Hossain C, Porto DA, Hamzavi I, Lim HW. Camouflaging agents for vitiligo patients. J Drugs Dermatol JDD. 2016;15(4):384–7.

40. Parsad D, Kanwar A. Oral minocycline in the treatment of vitiligo–a preliminary study. Dermatol Ther. 2010;23(3):305–7.

41. Singh A, Kanwar AJ, Parsad D, Mahajan R. Randomized controlled study to evaluate the effectiveness of dexamethasone oral minipulse therapy versus oral minocycline in patients with active vitiligo vulgaris. Indian J Dermatol Venereol Leprol. 2014;80(1):29–35.

42. Kanwar AJ, Mahajan R, Parsad D. Low-dose oral mini-pulse dexamethasone therapy in progressive unstable vitiligo. J Cutan Med Surg. 2013;17(4):259–68.

43. Craiglow BG, King BA. Tofacitinib citrate for the treatment of vitiligo: a pathogenesis-directed therapy. JAMA Dermatol. 2015;151(10):1110–2.

44. Liu LY, Strassner JP, Refat MA, Harris JE, King BA. Repigmentation in vitiligo using the Janus kinase inhibitor tofacitinib may require concomitant light exposure. J Am Acad Dermatol. 2017;77(4):675–82 e1.

45. Kullavanijaya P, Lim HW. Photoprotection. J Am Acad Dermatol. 2005;52(6):937–58. quiz 959–62.

General Dermatology

Samantha L. Schneider and Holly Kerr

Acanthosis Nigricans [1]

What Not To Miss

- Malignancy
    - Can be a sign of internal malignancy if new/abrupt onset and/or atypical locations (i.e. face, hands)
        - Most common = gastric adenoma
- Medications
    - Common: nicotinic acid, insulin, pituitary extract, systemic corticosteroids, diethylstilbestrol and protease inhibitors
    - Rarely: oral contraceptives, fusidic acid, and heroin

- HAIR-AN (hyperandrogenism, insulin resistance, and acanthosis nigricans) [2]
    - Commonly affects women
    - Considered a sub-type of polycystic ovarian syndrome (PCOS)

- Facial "hyperpigmentation" can be AN→ especially on the zygomatic cheeks, dorsal nose and mental chin

S. L. Schneider · H. Kerr (✉)
Department of Dermatology, Henry Ford Health System, 3031 West Grand Blvd, Suite 800, Detroit, MI 48202, USA
e-mail: hkerr1@hfhs.org

S. L. Schneider
e-mail: samantha.schneider@gmail.com

© Springer Nature Switzerland AG 2020
H. W. Lim et al. (eds.), *Practical Guide to Dermatology*,
https://doi.org/10.1007/978-3-030-18015-7_12

Key DDx

- Confluent and reticulated papillomatosis
- Terra firma-forme dermatosis

Work Up Pearls

- Associated with obesity and metabolic syndrome
  - Check fasting glucose and A1C +/− fasting plasma insulin
  - Calculate BMI

Treatment Ladder

- Most important: counsel on lifestyle modifications
- Topical
  - Keratolytics: topical lactic acid, urea, retinoids and combinations of above [3]
  - Triple combination depigmentation cream (Kligman's bleaching formula: tretinoin 0.05%, hydroquinone 4%; fluocinolone 0.01%) nightly with daily photoprotection [4]
  - Topical calcipotriol, podophyllin and salicylic acid

- Systemic
  - Metformin
  - Acitretin
  - Isotretinoin

Outside the Box Treatment Options

- PUVA
- Laser dermabrasion with long-pulsed alexandrite laser [5]

In the Context Of …

- Extensive palmar involvement or "tripe palms" work up for a possible internal malignancy, especially gastrointestinal carcinoma

Acne Vulgaris [6]

What Not To Miss

- Hyperandrogenism

- ○ Consider in patient with other signs of hyperandrogenism (i.e. abnormal hair growth patterns, deepening voice, irregular menses)
- Medication induced
  - ○ Common medications include EGFR inhibitors and prednisone
- Rosacea

Key DDx

- Iododerma and bromoderma
- Chloracne
- Follicular mycosis fungoides
- Perioral dermatitis
- Demodex folliculorum

Work Up Pearls

- Consider checking free and total testosterone, sex-hormone binding globulin, follicle stimulating hormone (FSH), luteinizing hormone (LH) and dehydroepi-androsterone (DHEA) (see below)

Treatment Ladder

- Topical Therapies
  - ○ Antibiotics: clindamycin, erythromycin
  - ○ Retinoids: tretinoin, adapalene, tazarotene
  - ○ Dapsone 5% gel for women with inflammatory acne
  - ○ Azalaic acid 20% cream
- Oral Therapies (in combination with topical therapies)
  - ○ Antibiotics: doxycycline, minocycline
  - ○ Systemic retinoids: isotretinoin
  - ○ Hormonal therapies (women): OCPs, spironolactone
- Make sure patients are using noncomedogenic products
- Discontinue hair grease that may migrate to forehead and other potential occlusive agents

Outside the Box Treatment Options

- Topical 5% zinc sulfate for mild-moderate acne [7]
- Oral zinc sulfate or zinc gluconate in moderate to severe acne [7]
- Light therapy [8]
  - ○ Blue light (1–2 times per week for 4 weeks)
  - ○ Red+blue light (15 min daily for 12 weeks)
- PDT [8]

- o ALA + red light or blue light
- Chemical Peels (e.g. salicylic acid, glycolic)
- Ampicillin 500 mg daily
- 1450 nm diode laser [8]
  - o Fluence 10–14 J/cm^2, 6 mm spot size, 250 ns pulse duration and cooling at 35 ms with 2 passes
  - o Treatments monthly for 3–6 months

In the Context Of …

- Hyperandrogenism
  - o Order free and total testosterone levels
  - o If elevated testosterone: sex hormone binding globulin level, DHEAs, androstenedione, LH, FSH, prolactin, 17-hydroxyprogesterone level, 24-hour urinary free cortisol

- Pregnancy
  - o Consider treatment with erythromycin solution (pregnancy category B) or azelaic acid (pregnancy category B)
  - o Can use erythromycin stearate or azithromycin as oral therapies in pregnancy
  - o PEARL: Use erythromycin stearate, NOT estolate due to risk of hepatotoxicity/cholestasis
  - o Glycolic acid peels (category B/C) are likely safe; may be used in conjunction with manual extraction

- Acne Scarring
  - o Chemical peels (i.e. glycolic, salicylic acid, pyruvic)
    - Can be helpful in skin of color
  - o TCA-CROSS [9]
    - CROSS = chemical reconstruction of skin scars
    - Use a 30-gauge needle to draw up 100% trichloracetic acid (TCA). Place the needle into the ice pick acne scars repeatedly until the lesion starts to frost
    - Treatments done monthly and need at least 4–6 to see any improvement
  - o Fractional ablative laser resurfacing [8]
  - o Needle-derived radiofrequency [8]

- Pre-adolescent children
  - o Topical adapalene
  - o Topical tretinoin
  - o Benzoyl peroxide wash
  - o Tetracycline antibiotics (i.e. minocycline or doxycycline) can be used with caution in children older than 8 years of age

- Post-inflammatory dyspigmentation
  - Azelaic acid
  - Topical retinoids
  - Chemical peels
  - Hydroquinone

- Concomitant seborrheic dermatitis or pityrosporum folliculitis (monomorphic papules near hairline)
  - Add sodium sulfaceamide wash (i.e. Plexion), SAL3 (salicylic acid sulfur soap bar) or fluconazole 200 mg daily for 2 weeks

- Acne that "doesn't go away" or monomorphic papules that are not inflamed or comedonal → biopsy

Atopic Dermatitis, Adult [10–12]

What Not To Miss

- Atopic triad: atopic dermatitis, allergies and asthma
  - Often associated with elevated serum IgE
- Longstanding dermatitis with no recent biopsies that could be mycosis fungoides or chronic actinic dermatitis
- Acute flares of a chronic dermatitis could be eczema herpeticum or other virus superinfection or a change in immune status

Key DDx

- Irritant contact dermatitis
- Allergic contact dermatitis
- Chronic actinic dermatitis
- Acute presentation of HIV

Work Up Pearls

- If impetiginized, can consider bacterial culture
- If punched out erosions, consider a viral culture

Treatment Ladder

- Moisturization
  - "Soak and Grease" with gentle (fragrance-free) soap and moisturizers
  - Emollients (i.e. glycol, glyceryl stereate, soy sterols): lubricate skin
  - Occlusive agents (i.e. petrolatum, dimethicone, mineral oil): form layer to prevent water evaporation

- o Humectants (i.e. glycerol, lactic acid, urea): attract water
- o Apply moisturizers immediately after lukewarm baths/showers

- Decolonization
  - o Bleach baths
    - ▪ ¼–½ cup of bleach in full-sized bath tub
    - ▪ Soak for at least 10 min
    - ▪ Recommend three times weekly
  - o If impetiginized, can consider topical or oral antibiotic → only if clinical evidence of infection per the AAD Choosing Wisely campaign

- Topical agents
  - o Corticosteroids
    - ▪ Use 1-2x/day for acute flares
    - ▪ Can suggest maintenance on weekends
  - o Calcineurin inhibitors
    - ▪ Better SE profile than corticosteroids
    - ▪ May cause burning sensation on skin with initial applications that should resolve with repeated use
  - o Crisaborole (Eucrisa) cream
  - o Wet wraps at home for severe flares
    - ▪ Topical steroid covered by wet layer (i.e. towels or pajamas), then put dry layer on top

- Phototherapy/Photochemotherapy
  - o First line: NB-UVB, followed by UVA-1, or PUVA

- Systemic Immunomodulators
  - o Cyclosporine 2–5 mg/kg daily
  - o Azathioprine 1–3 mg/kg daily
  - o Methotrexate 7.5–25 mg weekly
  - o Mycophenolate mofetil 1.0–1.5 g twice daily
  - o Dupilumab 600 mg (two 300 mg injections) then 300 mg every other week [13]
    - • Human monoclonal antibody against IL4 and IL13 [13]

Outside the Box Treatment Options

- Oral probiotic supplementation in pregnant and breastfeeding mothers with atopic dermatitis [14]
  - o Decreases risk of atopic dermatitis in the infant

In the Context Of...

- Impetiginization
  - ○ Treat with bleach baths +/− topical or oral antibiotics
- Refractory disease
  - ○ Can consider interferon-gamma
- Pediatric patients (see pediatric section)
- Pruritus
  - ○ Consider anti-pruritics
    - Hydroxyzine up to 50 mg nightly for pruritus interfering with sleep
    - Consider non-sedating antihistamines for day time (i.e. loratadine, cetirizine)
  - ○ Melatonin can be helpful particularly in pediatric patients

Brittle Nails [15] (Onychorrhexis)

What Not To Miss

- Underlying etiologies such as hypothyroid, anorexia, bulimia, oral retinoids, or anemia

Key DDx

- Early lichen planus
- 20 nail dystrophy

Work Up Pearls

- Can be idiopathic or due to nail plate trauma
- Risk Factors: wet working conditions, trauma, excessive manicures

Treatment Ladder

- Reduce exposure of nails to chemicals (wear rubber gloves)
- Apply petrolatum, lanolin, glycerin, or propylene glycol to moisturize
- Can use daily nail strengthening lacquer with 16% polyureathane
- Biotin 5–10 mg daily (for at least 6 months but should see improvement at 2 months)
  - ○ *PEARL:* Biotin can affect thyroid testing and also cardiac markers so be cautious [16]
- Replenish iron if ferritin < 10 ng/mL

Outside the Box Treatment Ideas

- Cysteine (amino acid) can also be helpful
- Can take zinc 20 mg daily
- One proposed treatment regimen
  - Glycerin soaks for 5 min once daily; ammonium lactate to proximal nail fold directly afterwards + biotin 2.5 mg daily

---

Chronic Urticaria [17, 18]

What Not To Miss

- Definition of chronic urticaria: occurring at least twice weekly for >6 weeks
- Common causes: idiopathic, autoimmune, drug-induced, infection-related
  - Can also include physical urticarias such as cold, delayed pressure, solar, heat, vibratory and cholinergic
- Chronic urticaria associated with autoimmune thyroid disease and other autoimmune conditions
- Certain medications can make urticaria worse
  - Notably aspirin and NSAIDs
- Urticarial vasculitis
  - Painful or burning lesions lasting >24 h
  - Leaves post-inflammatory hyperpigmentation

Key DDx

- Urticarial vasculitis
- Serum sickness
- Still's disease
- Mastocytosis
- Sweet's Syndrome
- Urticarial bullous pemphigoid

Work Up Pearls

- First line
  - History and physical
- Lab testing should be based on patient's signs/symptoms and history but often recommend CBC with differential, ESR/CRP, TSH and thyroid autoantibodies and liver function tests
- Controversial → checking chronic urticaria (CU) index (Fc-εR1α Ab or Ab to IgE)
- Consider tryptase for severe, chronic recalcitrant disease
- Consider BP antibodies (BP180) or DIF in an older patient
- Biopsy also not considered necessary (unless concern for vasculitis or urticarial BP)

Treatment Ladder

- Avoid triggers such as ASA and NSAIDs
- First line for idiopathic
  - ○ H1-antihistamines (cetirizine, levocetirizine, desloratadine)
    - • Can increase dosage up to 4-fold [19, 20]

- Second line
  - ○ Add another H1-antihistamine (cetirizine, levocetirizine, desloratadine)
  - ○ 1st generation H1 antihistamine nightly (diphenhydramine, hydroxyzine)
  - ○ Add H2 antihistamine (ranitidine)
  - ○ Consider leukotriene antagonist

In the Context Of...

- Physical urticaria (i.e. heat, pressure, water, cold)
  - ○ Avoidance of triggering factors if possible
- Recalcitrant idiopathic urticaria (third line therapy, after increasing dosage of H1 antihistamines) [20]
  - ○ NB-UVB
  - ○ Omalizumab 150–300 mg every 4 weeks [21, 22]
    - • IgG monoclonal antibody against Fc portion of IgE
  - ○ Cyclosporine 1–5 mg/kg daily [22]
  - ○ Montelukast + short course of oral corticosteroids
  - ○ Doxepin 10 mg three times daily, up to 50 mg nightly [23]
  - ○ Dapsone 100 mg daily [24]
  - ○ Sulfasalazine 500 mg daily, increased by 500 mg each weak until clinical response [25]
    - • Max dose of 2–4 g daily
  - ○ Mycophenolate mofetil (1–3 g) divided into twice daily dosing [26]
  - ○ Methotrexate 15–25 mg weekly
  - ○ Cyclosporine 3–5 mg/kg daily [22]
  - ○ Intravenous immunoglobulin 0.4 g/kg daily for 5 days, 0.15 g/kg monthly or high dose (2 g/kg over 2 days every 4–6 weeks) [27]
- Elderly patients
  - ○ Be wary of over-sedation, interactions with other medications and cardiac toxicity with doxepin
  - Be wary of anticholinergic affects

Solar Urticaria [28, 29]

What Not To Miss

- PEARL: Frequently triggered by visible light or by UVA
- Systemic urticaria reaction including possible angioedema and anaphylaxis

- Associated Diseases (uncommon):
  - PMLE, atopic disorders, other forms of urticaria, cystic fibrosis, eosinophilic granulomatosis with polyangiitis (formerly known as Churg-Strauss), hyper-eosinophilic syndrome

Key DDx

- Photo-eruption of lupus erythematosus
  - Usually a few days after exposure rather than immediate
- Erythropoietic protoporphyria
  - Presents with burning rather than pruritus

Work Up Pearls

- Phototesting
  - Minimal urticarial dose (MUD)
  - Must do immediate read (for MUD) and a second read at 24 h (for minimal erythema dose (MED))
  - Test for visible light, UVA and UVB

- CBC
- Complete Metabolic Panel
- ANA
- Plasma and red cell porphyrins

Treatment Ladder

- Oral Antihistamines = First Line
  - Require higher doses than other entities
- Phototherapy with UVA or UVB for hardening
  - To minimize risk of anaphylaxis, start with low dose and treat only sites that patients would normally expose to sunlight. Consider adding prednisone 40 mg daily for the first 7–10 days of hardening.

Outside the Box Treatment Options

- Cyclosporine
- Omalizumab [29]
- IVIg

Allergic Contact Dermatitis [30]

What Not To Miss

- Contact Urticaria
  - Can be due to latex, bacitracin (can be anaphylactic), ammonium persulfate (hair bleach), penicillin, paraphenylenediamine, chalk and others

Key DDx

- Irritant contact dermatitis
- Atopic dermatitis
- Cutaneous T cell lymphoma
- Mycosis fungoides
- Chronic actinic dermatitis

Work Up Pearls

- Patch testing can help identify relevant triggers
  - Importance is determining the relevance of any positive tests

Treatment Ladder

- Allergen/irritant avoidance
  - With membership, www.contactderm.org will provide patient specific codes to generate a "safe list" for patients to use in their application (ACDS CAMP)
    - Membership to ACDS is free for residents
  - Before patch testing, one can try a "skin diet"
    - Avoid the top 10 most common allergens (www.dermatitisacademy.com)
- For metal allergies
  - Use the dimethyglyoxime test for nickel-containing products
    - Will turn pink
  - Use the cobalt allergy spot test kit containing disodium-1-nitroso-2-naphthol-3,6-disulfonate to identify cobalt in jewelry/metals
  - Consider putting tape or clear nail polish over belt buckles or buttons
    - Need to re-apply the nail polish every few months
    - NIK-L-BLOK™ is a branded product that chelates nickel and cobalt, should be applied topically on a daily basis to affected areas
- Barrier cream
  - Recommend dimethicone as active ingredient for best barrier
  - Over the counter examples include Tetrix© or Gloves in a Bottle© to be used 2–3 times per day
- Topical corticosteroids
- Topical calcineurin inhibitors

Outside the Box Treatment Option

- Cyclosporine

Poison Ivy Dermatitis

Caused by

- *Toxicodendron* (i.e. poison oak, poison ivy, poison sumac)

What Not To Miss

- Pet fur can harbor the allergen
  - Pets who were exposed need a bath to prevent re-exposure

Work Up Pearls

- History and physical is generally sufficient
  - Black marks on the lesions can help with diagnosis as it represents urushiol on the skin

Treatment Ladder

- Recommend future avoidance by wearing protective clothing and gloves
  - Wash immediately after contact
- Wash with soap and water
  - Earlier the better
  - Unidirectional washing with dawn soap in hot water [31]
- Prednisone 1 mg/kg with a 3-week taper
- Cyclosporine 4 mg/kg with a 3-week taper

Outside the Box Treatment Options

- (Ivy Block) bentoquatam 5% applied 15 min before potential exposure can neutralize resin

Irritant Contact Dermatitis

Key DDx

- Dyshidrotic eczema
- Allergic contact dermatitis
- Chronic actinic dermatitis
- Erosio interdigitalis blastomycetica (if finger webspaces are involved)

Work Up Pearls

- Often history and physical examination are sufficient
- Consider patch testing to rule out allergic contact dermatitis if not improving

Treatment Ladder

- Avoid irritation from excess moisture or chemicals
- Use gloves when doing dishes or other wet works

- Barrier cream
  - ○ Recommend dimethicone as active ingredient for best barrier
  - ○ Over the counter examples include Tetrix© or Gloves in a Bottle© to be used 2–3 times per day

- Can also combine a barrier cream with a topical steroid
  - ○ 2.5% hydrocortisone powder compounded in 40% zinc oxide cream

Chronic Actinic Dermatitis (CAD) [32]

What Not To Miss

- HIV
  - ○ Associated with CAD in younger patients

- Contact allergy to *Compositae* oleoresins
  - ○ More common in United Kingdom

- CAD in skin of color
  - ○ Affects all Fitzpatrick skin types—particularly types V and VI

- CAD can disseminate to photoprotected sites over time → does not preclude diagnosis

Key DDx

- Allergic contact dermatitis
- Photoallergic contact dermatitis
- Cutaneous T cell lymphoma
- Systemic lupus erythematosus

Work Up Pearls

- Phototesting for UVA, UVB and visible light
  - ○ Patients demonstrated decreased mean erythema dosing (MED) most frequently for UVB and UVA, but can have reaction to UVB or UVA alone or to combination with visible light

- ANA
- HIV
- Biopsy

Treatment Ladder

- Photoprotection
  - ○ Broad-brimmed hat, sunglasses and photoprotective clothing
  - ○ Sunscreens
  - ○ Clear museum films or UVA filters can be applied to windows

Topical corticosteroids or topical calcineurin inhibitors

Oral corticosteroids (prednisone 0.5–1.0 mg/kg daily for several weeks)

Other oral agents
  - ○ Cyclosporine 3–5 mg/kg daily
  - ○ Azathioprine 1–2.5 mg/kg daily
  - ○ Mycophenolate mofetil 25–40 mg/kg daily or 1–2 g daily

Outside the Box Treatment Options

- Low-dose thalidomide
- Interferon—alpha

Dissecting Cellulitis [33]

What Not To Miss

- Tinea capitis
- Kerion
- Follicular occlusion triad—look for other signs/areas affected

Key DDx

- Folliculitis decalvans

Work Up Pearls

- Consider bacterial culture and fungal culture

Treatment Ladder

- First line
  - ○ Minocycline 100 mg twice daily
  - ○ Bactrim DS twice daily
  - ○ Ciprofloxacin 250–500 mg twice daily
  - ○ Minocycline + antiandrogens

- ○ Minocycline + clindamycin
- ○ Clindamycin and rifampin 300 mg twice daily
- ○ Hair removal
  - ▪ 1064 nm for skin types 3–6 and 694 or 800 nm laser for skin types 1–2
- Second line
  - ○ Isotretinoin 0.5–1.0 mg/kg daily for 3–12 months
  - ○ Isotretinoin + dapsone 50–100 mg
  - ○ Rifampin then isotretinoin
  - ○ Acitretin with oral prednisone
  - ○ Zinc sulfate 135 mg three times daily, then decrease to 135 mg 1–2 times daily [34]
- Third line
  - ○ Adalimumab 80 mg loading, then 40 mg at week 1, then 40 mg every other week
  - ○ Infliximab 5 mg/kg every 8 weeks

Outside the Box Treatment Options

- Intralesional triamcinolone (kenalog) 5–10 mg/ml
- Avoiding oils on the scalp
- Oral steroid taper starting at 60 mg

Drug-Induced Photosensitivity [35, 36]

What Not To Miss

- Divided into either: phototoxicity (exaggerated sunburn) or photoallergy (eczematous)
- Common medications causing *phototoxic* reactions by class:
  - ○ Antiarrhythmic: amiodarone
  - ○ Antifungal: voriconazole
  - ○ Antipsychotic: chlorpromazine
  - ○ ARBS: losartan, valsartan, olmesartan
  - ○ Diuretics: furosemide, thiazides
  - ○ NSAIDS: nabumetone, naproxen
  - ○ Oncologic: capecitabine, dabrafenib, nafoxidine, vandetanib, vinblastine
  - ○ Quinolone antibiotics: clindafloxacin
  - ○ Tetracycline antibiotics: doxycycline > minocycline
- Common medications causing *photoallergic* reactions:
  - ○ Sunscreens: oxybenzone
  - ○ Fragrances: sandalwood oil, musk ambrette
  - ○ Topical antimicrobials: chlorhexidine
  - ○ NSAIDS: celecoxib, diclofenac

Key DDx

- Sunburn
- Airborne contact dermatitis (will typically involve upper eyelids, submental region and postauricular sites unlike drug induced phototoxicity)
- Lupus
- Dermatomyositis
- Porphyria cutanea tarda or pseudoporphyria
- Chronic actinic dermatitis

Work Up Pearls

- Biopsy
- Take a careful medication history in patients presenting with photodistributed rash
- Phototesting can confirm the diagnosis
  ○ Positive phototest will show decreased minimal erythema dose (MED) to UVA, UVB or both

Treatment Ladder

- Eliminating or reducing dose of drug (if able)
- Photoprotection
- Symptomatic relief with cool compresses
- Topical corticosteroids
- Oral corticosteroids for severe flares

In the Context Of ...

- Pseudoporphyria can be seen in patients taking NSAIDS, undergoing renal dialysis, furosemide, tetracyclines and retinoids

Granuloma Annulare [37]

What Not To Miss

- Associated diseases: diabetes mellitus, malignancy, dyslipidemia
- Different subtypes: localized, generalized, subcutaneous, perforating, and patch
- TNFα inhibitors may trigger GA in some cases

Work Up Pearls

- Biopsy can be helpful

Treatment Ladder

- Localized disease
  - ○ Topical treatments
    - High potency topical steroids +/− occlusion
    - Tacrolimus or pimecrolimus
  - ○ Intralesional steroids (triamcinolone (kenalog) 5 mg/mL)
  - ○ Cryotherapy
  - ○ Phototherapy
    - NB-UVB, UVA1, PUVA
  - ○ Pulse dye laser, PDT
  - ○ Systemic treatments (ROM Therapy)
    - Rifampin 600 mg
    - Ofloxacin 400 mg
    - Minocycline 100 mg
    - All three given once monthly × 6 months

- Generalized Disease
  - ○ Phototherapy
  - ○ Systemic treatments
    - Hydroxycholoroquine 3–5 mg/kg daily
    - Isotretinoin 0.5 mg/kg daily
    - Dapsone 100 mg daily
    - Cyclosporine 3–4 mg/kg daily

Outside the Box Treatment Options

- Adalimumuab 40 mg every other week
- Subcutaneous GA: may consider excision

Hirsutism [38, 39]

What Not To Miss

- Hyperandrogenism/PCOS
  - ○ Consider in patient with other signs of hyperandrogenism (i.e. abnormal hair growth patterns, deepening voice, irregular menses)
- Adrenal or ovarian tumors

Key DDx

- Drug-induced hypertrichosis

- Paraneoplastic hypertrichosis

Work Up Pearls

- Order free and total testosterone levels
- If elevated testosterone: sex hormone binding globulin level, DHEAs, Andros-tenedione, LH, FSH, prolactin, 17-hydroxyprogesterone level, 24-h urinary free cortisol
- PEARL: Remember the severity of hirsutism does not correlate with androgen excess

Treatment Ladder

- Topical therapies
  - Vaniqa (Eflornithine) 13.9% cream BID
- Systemics
  - OCPs
  - Flutamide 25 mg twice daily (pregnancy category D)
  - Finasteride 5 mg daily (pregnancy category X)
  - Spironolactone 100 mg daily
- Laser hair removal
  - Nd:YAG for darker skin types
  - Diode laser for lighter skin/thin hair
    - Most effective in fair skin with dark hair
  - PEARL: Prior to laser hair removal, no waxing, plucking, hair removal lotions or hair bleach for 4 weeks. No retinoids or glycolics for 1 week

Outside the Box Treatment Ideas

- Combine eflornithine with laser therapy
- Metformin (but not as effective)

In the Context Of…

- Pregnancy
  - Do not give any anti-androgen therapies due to risk of feminization of the male fetus

Hyperhidrosis [40–42]

What Not To Miss

- Hyperthyroidism

- Pheochromocytoma
- Occult malignancy

Work Up Pearls

- Starch-iodine test can define hyperhidrotic area

Treatment Ladder

- 20% Aluminum chloride (Drysol)
  - Apply 3 times/week at bed time and use regular deodorant in the morning
  - Make sure site is completely dry to minimize irritation ($AlCl + H_2O \rightarrow HCl$)
- Glycopyrrolate (Robinul)
  - Start at 1 mg daily, increase to 1 mg twice daily over 2 weeks, continue to titrate up to 2 mg twice daily as needed
  - Do not exceed 2 mg three times daily
- Glycopyrrolate wipes (Qbrexza)
- Neurotoxin
  - Covered by some health insurance
  - Typically 25–50 units per axilla (at dilution of 100 units abotulinum toxin to 4 cc bacteriostatic saline)
  - Can use starch-iodine test to define areas of increased perspiration
  - Good for about 6–8 months
- Laser therapy (MiraDry)
- Iontophoresis

Outside the Box Treatment Options

- Oxybutynin (off-label) 2.5 mg once daily, titrate up to 7.5–10 mg daily (can do twice daily)
  - No tachyphylaxis

Keratosis Pilaris [43]

What Not To Miss

- Associated with atopic dermatitis, ichthyosis vulgaris, keratosis pilaris atrophicans, erythromelanosis folicularis faciei et colli, Graham Little-Piccardi-Lassueur syndrome

Key DDx

- Follicular eczema (especially in children)

Treatment Ladder

- Counsel patient of chronicity of disease (goal is improvement not cure).
  o May improve with age
- Keratolytics (lactic acid 12%, urea 20–40%, salicylic acid 4–12%)
- Topical retinoids
- Brief use of low- to mid-potency topical corticosteroid if substantial erythema

Outside the Box Treatment Options

- Vascular laser (i.e. KTP or PDL)

Lichen Planus [44, 45]

What Not To Miss

- Risk Factors: viruses (HCV, influenza), contact allergens (i.e. metals (amalgam, copper, gold), dental restorative material)

- Lichenoid drug eruption
  o Culprits: HBV vaccine, ACEi, thiazides, antimalarials, quinidine, gold
- Can affect any mucosa (oral or genital)
  o Can limit oral intake or bodily functions
  o Esophageal involvement
    ▪ One case series had 20/32 (62.5%) patients affected [46]
  o Can be present with cutaneous lesions
  o Can affect external auditory meatus/tympanic membrane causing otorrhea and hearing loss → 10-year Mayo clinic study showed topical tacrolimus best treatment [47]
- Malignant transformation of lesions—increased risk with mucosal and/or erosive lichen planus
- Lichen planopilaris
  o See skin of color section on alopecia for more information

Key DDx

- Consider nail matrix biopsy if no other evidence of lichen planus besides nails

Work Up Pearls

- Biopsy can be diagnostic—particularly for mucosal or nail
- Hepatitis C
- May need upper endoscopy to evaluate esophagus in symptomatic patients

Treatment Ladder

- Cutaneous
  - Topicals
    - Topical corticosteroids
    - Topical calineurin inhibitors
  - Intralesional corticosteroids
  - Phototherapy
    - NB-UVB, PUVA
  - Systemic treatment (used for extensive disease or resistance to above):
    - Metronidazole 250 mg every 8 h or 500 mg twice daily for 2–3 months
    - Sulfasalazine 1 g daily and increased by 0.5 g every 3 days until a dose of 2.5 g daily
    - Systemic steroids
    - Isotretinoin
    - Acitretin 30 mg daily [48]
    - Hydroxychloroquine 5 mg/kg daily
    - Methotrexate 10–25 mg weekly [49]
    - Itraconazole pulse therapy 200 mg twice daily for 1 week each month for 3 months [50]
    - Adalimumab 80 mg induction, followed by 40 mg every other week for 3 months [51]
      - PEARL: Be cautious because adalimumab can induce lichenoid drug reactions and/or psoriasis
- Mucosal
  - Fix any ill-fitting dental work (trauma can precipitate lesions)
  - Optimize oral hygiene
  - Topical corticosteroids as oral rinses, gels, or in orabase ®
  - Topical calcineurin inhibitors
  - Orals
    - Systemic corticosteroids—prednisone 1 mg/kg daily
    - Mycophenolate mofetil 500–1000 mg twice daily (max dose 1500 mg twice daily) [52]
    - Azathioprine
    - Methotrexate 10–25 mg weekly [49]
- Nail
  - Potent topical steroid to nail folds
  - Intralesional triamcinolone to matrix
  - Oral
    - Steroids
    - Retinoids

In the Context Of …

- Recalcitrant disease
  - Consider acitretin 30 mg daily [48]

Lichen Sclerosis et Atrophicus [53]

What Not To Miss

- Malignancy in longstanding lesions
- Scarring and dysfunction are a possibility
- Genital lesions (W > M)
- Psychological component, longstanding dyspareunia and sexual dysfunction

Key DDx

- Vaginal LP
- Atrophic vaginitis
- Candida infection
- Vitiligo

Treatment Ladder

- Topical
  - Ultrapotent corticosteroids
    - Clobetasol ointment BID ×4 weeks to twice daily for 4 weeks, then 1–2 times weekly as maintenance (M-F low potency topical or calcineurin inhibitor and weekend class 1 steroid)
    - Clobetasol for 2 weeks, triamcinolone for 2 weeks, then desonide for 2 weeks as needed
  - Topical calcineurin inhibitors (tacrolimus or pimecrolimus)
- Phototherapy
  - NB-UVB, PUVA or PDT (anecdotal evidence)
- Systemic
  - Consider methotrexate (up to 15–25 mg weekly) for extensive lesions.

Outside the Box Treatment Options

- Topical or intravaginal estrogen/progesterone cream or suppository
- Topical lidocaine may be necessary short term for focal tender areas
- Intralesional triamcinolone

In the Context Of …

- A non-healing ulceration ➔ biopsy
- Biopsy to rule out squamous cell carcinoma

Morphea (in Immune-mediated disorders chapter)

Notalgia Paresthetica [54]

Work Up Pearls

- Consider imaging or referral for evaluation of cervical and/or thoracic spine depending on symptoms

Treatment Ladder

- Topical
  - Capsaicin 0.025% cream 5 times daily for 1 week then three times daily
    - Caution patient about burning sensation preceding relief
    - If partial response, consider trial of 0.075% or 0.1%
  - Topical anesthetics (lidocaine, pramoxine, EMLA)
  - Topical calcineurin inhibitors

- Injections
  - Intralesional triamcinolone
  - Abotulinum toxin subcutaneous injections 4 units every 2 cm

- Oral
  - Low-dose amitriptyline at 10 mg nightly [55]
  - Gabapentin 300–900 mg daily (three times daily)
    - In many states, this is now considered a controlled substance

Periorificial Dermatitis [56]

What not to miss

- Risk Factors: medications (topical steroids, inhaled corticosteroids, systemic corticosteroids), cosmetics, ultraviolet light, heat/cold, *Candida spp., Demodex folliculorum*, toothpaste

Key DDx

- Acne
- Rosacea
- Seborrhea

Treatment Ladder

- Withdrawal of topical corticosteroids (if used)
- Topicals

- o Metronidazole
- o Erythromycin or clindamycin
- o Pimecrolimus
- o Sulfacetamide or sulfur
- o Azelaic acid
- o Poor evidence for adapalene
- Systemics
  - o Tetracycline (has best evidence)
  - o Poor evidence for erythromycin, doxycycline, minocycline, isotretinoin 0.5–1.0 mg/kg daily (or even lower dose) tapered over 6 months

Outside the Box Treatment Option

- If suspect toothpaste as cause, switch to a non-peppermint and non-cinnamon flavored toothpaste

Psoriasis (in Immune-mediated disorders chapter)

Photoprotection (in Immune-mediated disorders chapter)

Polymorphous Light Eruption (PMLE) [57, 58]

What Not To Miss

- PMLE can affect all races and ethnicities
- Systemic lupus erythematosus (SLE)
  - o The eruption seen with PMLE can be identical to photosensitivity seen in patients with systemic lupus erythematosus
  - o May need a biopsy to differentiate

PEARL: PMLE can be due to UVA (MC), UVB or both

Key DDx

- SLE

Work Up Pearls

- ANA

    ○ ANA is to rule out SLE. It should be noted, however, that patient with PMLE can have a positive ANA without other symptoms of lupus
- Phototesting must be done over several days
  - ○ Patients with PMLE often have normal mean erythema dosing (MED) for UVA and UVB when given a single test
  - ○ Patients require repeated exposures to localized UVA or UVB to induce localized PMLE reactions
  - ○ Best done in early spring before possible hardening over the summertime
- Biopsy

Treatment Ladder

- Photo-hardening
  - ○ NB-UVB or PUVA—suberythema dosing
  - ○ Treat 3 times per week for 15–20 treatments
  - ○ Prednisone 40 mg daily for first 5–7 days of treatment in exquisitely photosensitive patients.

- Photoprotection
  - ○ Broad-brimmed hats, sunglasses, and photoprotective clothing
  - ○ Sunscreens

  Topical corticosteroids

  Oral
  - ○ Prednisone 0.6–1 mg/kg for 7–10 days
  - ○ Hydroxychloroquine 5 mg/kg daily—unclear efficacy

Outside the Box Treatment Options

- Oral *Polypodium leucotomos* [59]
- Nutritional supplement with lycophene, β-carotene, and *Lactobacillus johnsonii)* [60]
- Topical vitamin D3 analogs (i.e. calcipotriol)

In the Context Of…

- Upcoming travel
  - ○ For patients with a known diagnosis, consider prednisone 40 mg daily for 7–10 days to take during wintertime vacations to warm/sunny locations to prevent severe flares

- Young adolescent boys
  - ○ Juvenile spring eruption frequently affects young boys with papulovesicular lesions on the ears. Resolves spontaneously
  - ○ Variant of PMLE

- Severe disease
  - Consider azathioprine

Primary Pruritus [61]

What Not To Miss

- Underlying malignancy

Key DDx

- Asteatosis/xerosis
- Drug induced/exacerbated: statins, opioids

Work Up Pearls

- CBC w/diff, ESR, CRP, CMP, TSH, +/− HIV, CXR, Hepatitis screen
- Age appropriate malignancy screening

Treatment Ladder

- Topical
  - Soak and grease
  - Topical corticosteroids or calcineurin inhibitors
  - Topical menthol, camphor, or anesthetics
  - Topical capsaicin or ketamine
  - Topical doxepin or amitriptyline

- Phototherapy: NB-UVB

- Systemics
  - Non-sedating antihistamines during day and sedating antihistamines at night
  - Gabapentin up to 300 mg three times daily or pregabalin
    - Considered to be controlled substance in some states
  - SSRI (fluoxetine, paroxetine, sertraline)
  - Amitriptyline (25–150 mg daily) or doxepin (up to 50 mg nightly)
  - Naltrexone 25–50 mg daily [62]
    - PEARL: Ensure that patients are not on opioid medications to avoid inducing withdrawal symptoms
  - Butorphanol nasal spray, 10 mg/ml. 1 puff (mg) each nostril nightly
    - Another opioid antagonist
  - Mycophenolate mofetil 1 g twice daily
  - Thalidomide 100 mg nightly
  - N-acetylcysteine 600–1000 mg daily (OTC)

- For prurigo nodularis
  - In development
    - Serlopitant (neurokinin receptor antagonis), nemolizumab (anti IL31)

In the Context Of...

- Uremic pruritus
  - Phototherapy (UVB)
  - Capsaicin 0.03% cream
  - Gabapentin/pregabalin
  - Naltrexone 25–50 mg daily [62]
- Cholestatic pruritus
  - Rifampin 300 mg once to twice daily [63]
  - Naltrexone 12.5–50 mg daily [62, 64]
  - Cholestyramine one 4 g sachet 1 h before and 1 h after breakfast [64]
    - Can increase to 16 g daily
  - Ursodeoxycholic acid 13–15 mg/kg daily [64]
  - Sertraline
  - Bezafibrate 400 mg daily [64]

Porphyria Cutanea Tarda [65]

What Not To Miss

- Risk factors: HCV, HIV, estrogen exposure, alcohol
- Hemochromatosis
  - Screen patients

Key DDx

- Drug-induced phototoxicity
- Pseudoporphyria
- Epidermolysis bullosa aquisita
- Bullous pemphigoid

Work Up Pearls

- HIV
- CBC with diff
- Complete metabolic panel
- Hepatitis panel
- Iron studies
- Plasma porphyrins (best screening test for all cutaneous porphyrias)

- RBC porphyrins
- If suspected associated hemochromatosis: C282Y and H63D mutation analyses

Treatment Ladder

- Phlebotomy 1 U (250–500 mL) weekly, stop when hematocrit = 30, or if patient has dyspnea with excertion; +/− epoetin alfa (Epogen) to cause increase iron uptake in RBCs
  - Usually takes 10–15 weekly treatments for decreased skin fragility
  - If there is renal failure, small volume (100 mL weekly) phlebotomy
- Plaquenil 100–200 mg weekly or twice weekly to increase excretion of porphyrins
  - Not effective in patients with end stage renal failure
  - Should NOT use daily doseage as it will cause chemical hepatitis
- Chloroquine 125 mg twice weekly
- Physical photoprotection to protect against Soret Band (400–410 nm)
  - Can consider self-tanner (dihydroxyacetone) or tinted sunscreens for same reason

Pseudoporphyria [65, 66]

What Not To Miss

- Porphyria cutanea tarda
  - Need to check porphyrin levels to rule it out
- Risk factors: hemodialysis/peritoneal dialysis, tanning beds/ultraviolet light
- Medications: NSAIDs, antibiotics (nalidixic acid, tetracycline, oxytetracycline, ampicillin-sulbactam, cefepime, fluoroquinolones), voriconazole, diuretics (loop diuretics), retinoids, antiarrhythmics, antineoplastic drugs (5 fluorouracil), sulfones, immunosuppressants (cyclosporine)

Key DDx

- Porphyria cutanea tarda

Work Up Pearls

- Negative serum and urine porphyrins

Treatment Ladder

- Discontinue offending drugs
- Photoprotection

Outside the Box Treatment Option

- N-acetylcysteine for the treatment of hemodialysis-associated pseuoporphyria [67, 68]

In the Context Of …

- Continued NSAID use
  - ○ NSAIDS that are safe to use:
    - ■ Diclofenac (Voltaren)
    - ■ Indomethacin (Indocin)
    - ■ Sulindac (Clinoril)

Pyoderma Gangrenosum (in Immune-mediated disorders chapter)

Rosacea [69, 70]

What Not To Miss

- Ocular rosacea

Key DDx

- Lupus
- Periorificial dermatitis
- Lupus miliaria disseminata facei
- Sarcoidosis

Treatment Ladder

- Lifestyle Changes
  - ○ Trigger avoidance (spicy foods, heat, etc.)
  - ○ Photoprotection—physical/inorganic sunscreens may be less irritating than chemical/organic sunscreens
  - ○ Facial moisturizers
    - ■ Dimethicone (Cetaphil moisturizing lotion, etc.)
- Transient erythema
  - ○ Alpha adrenergics (topical)
  - ○ Oral beta blockers
- Persistent erythema
  - ○ Brimonidine 0.5% gel (Mirvaso®)—may cause rebound erythema

- ■ Can use ophthalmologic gel three times daily off label
  - ○ Oxymetazoline 1% cream (Rhofade®)
  - ○ Intense pulsed light or PDL laser
- Inflammatory (i.e. papules/pustules)
  - ○ Topical
    - Azelaic acid
    - Ivermectin, (Soolantra®)
    - Metronidazole
    - Triple cream compound: azelaic acid 20%/metronidazole 1%/ivermectin 1%
    - Sodium Sulfacetamide (Plexion, Clenia, Rosanil)
  - ○ Systemic
    - Doxycycline 40 mg daily or 50–100 mg daily
    - Minocycline 50–100 mg daily
    - Isotretinoin 10–40 mg daily
- Phymatous
  - ○ Surgical excision
  - ○ Electrosurgery
  - ○ CO2 laser
- Ocular
  - ○ Needs systemic treatments (oral tetracycline/doxycycline) and close ophthalmologic follow up

Outside the Box Treatment Option

- Oral zinc sulfate 100 mg three times daily [7]

Sarcoidosis [71]

What Not To Miss

- Systemic involvement
  - ○ May need multidisciplinary approach for evaluation and management
  - ○ Recommend evaluation by pulmonology and baseline chest x-ray

- Clinical Variants
  - ○ Lofgren syndrome (EN, hilar adenopathy, fever, arthritis)
  - ○ Heerfordt syndrome (parotid gland enlargement, uveitis, fever, cranial nerve palsy)
  - ○ Darier-Roussy disease (subcutaneous sarcoidosis)

Work Up Pearls

- Diagnosis often requires biopsy

○ Demonstrates non-caseating granulomas
- Labs to consider include CBC with differential, CMP and ACE level

Treatment Ladder

- Topical
  ○ Corticosteroids
  ○ Calcineurin inhibitor (tacrolimus)

- Intralesional
  ○ Corticosteroids

- Systemic treatment
  ○ Oral corticosteroids 0.5–1 mg/kg/day
  ○ Hydroxychloroquine 200–400 mg daily (weight dosing)
    ▪ Can dose twice daily
  ○ Chloroquine 250–750 mg daily
  ○ Methotrexate—up to 25 mg weekly
  ○ Doxycycline and minocycline 200 mg daily
  ○ Thalidomide—50–400 mg daily

In the Context Of …

- Rapidly progressive lesions
  ○ Oral corticosteroids are the treatment of choice

- Recalcitrant disease
  ○ TNF alpha inhibitors
    ▪ Infliximab 3–7 mg/kg IV at 0, 2 and 6 weeks, then every 8 weeks
    ▪ Adalimumab 40 mg every 1–2 weeks

References

1. Kutlubay Z, Engin B, Bairamov O, Tuzun Y. Acanthosis nigricans: a fold (intertriginous) dermatosis. Clin Dermatol. 2015;33(4):466–70.
2. Melibary YT. Hidradenitis suppurativa in a patient with hyperandrogenism, insulin-resistance and acanthosis nigricans (HAIR-AN syndrome). Dermatol Rep. 2018;10(1):7546.
3. Blobstein SH. Topical therapy with tretinoin and ammonium lactate for acanthosis nigricans associated with obesity. Cutis. 2003;71(1):33–4.
4. Adigun CG, Pandya AG. Improvement of idiopathic acanthosis nigricans with a triple combination depigmenting cream. J Eur Acad Dermatol Venereol. 2009;23(4):486–7.
5. Rosenbach A, Ram R. Treatment of Acanthosis nigricans of the axillae using a long-pulsed (5-msec) alexandrite laser. Dermatol Surg. 2004;30(8):1158–60.
6. Greywal T, Zaenglein AL, Baldwin HE, et al. Evidence-based recommendations for the management of acne fulminans and its variants. J Am Acad Dermatol. 2017;77(1):109–17.
7. Gupta M, Mahajan VK, Mehta KS, Chauhan PS. Zinc therapy in dermatology: a review. Dermatol Res Pract. 2014;2014:709152.
8. Alexiades M. Laser and light-based treatments of acne and acne scarring. Clin Dermatol. 2017;35(2):183–9.

9. Agarwal N, Gupta LK, Khare AK, Kuldeep CM, Mittal A. Therapeutic response of 70% trichloroacetic acid CROSS in atrophic acne scars. Dermatol Surg. 2015;41(5):597–604.
10. Eichenfield LF, Tom WL, Berger TG, et al. Guidelines of care for the management of atopic dermatitis: section 2. Management and treatment of atopic dermatitis with topical therapies. J Am Acad Dermatol. 2014;71(1):116–32.
11. Eichenfield LF, Tom WL, Chamlin SL, et al. Guidelines of care for the management of atopic dermatitis: section 1. Diagnosis and assessment of atopic dermatitis. J Am Acad Dermatol. 2014;70(2):338–51.
12. Sidbury R, Davis DM, Cohen DE, et al. Guidelines of care for the management of atopic dermatitis: section 3. Management and treatment with phototherapy and systemic agents. J Am Acad Dermatol. 2014;71(2):327–49.
13. Beck LA, Thaci D, Hamilton JD, et al. Dupilumab treatment in adults with moderate-to-severe atopic dermatitis. N Engl J Med. 2014;371(2):130–9.
14. Rautava S, Kainonen E, Salminen S, Isolauri E. Maternal probiotic supplementation during pregnancy and breast-feeding reduces the risk of eczema in the infant. J Allergy Clin Immunol. 2012;130(6):1355–60.
15. Iorizzo M. Tips to treat the 5 most common nail disorders: brittle nails, onycholysis, paronychia, psoriasis, onychomycosis. Dermatol Clin. 2015;33(2):175–83.
16. Saenger AK, Jaffe AS, Body R, et al. Cardiac troponin and natriuretic peptide analytical interferences from hemolysis and biotin: educational aids from the IFCC Committee on Cardiac Biomarkers (IFCC C-CB). Clin Chem Lab Med. 2018.
17. Antia C, Baquerizo K, Korman A, Bernstein JA, Alikhan A. Urticaria: a comprehensive review: epidemiology, diagnosis, and work-up. J Am Acad Dermatol. 2018;79(4):599–614.
18. Antia C, Baquerizo K, Korman A, Alikhan A, Bernstein JA. Urticaria: a comprehensive review: treatment of chronic urticaria, special populations, and disease outcomes. J Am Acad Dermatol. 2018;79(4):617–33.
19. Sharma M, Bennett C, Carter B, Cohen SN. H1-antihistamines for chronic spontaneous urticaria: an abridged Cochrane Systematic Review. J Am Acad Dermatol. 2015;73(4):710–716. e714.
20. Tonacci A, Billeci L, Pioggia G, Navarra M, Gangemi S. Omalizumab for the treatment of chronic idiopathic urticaria: systematic review of the literature. Pharmacotherapy. 2017;37(4):464–80.
21. Pinto Gouveia M, Gameiro A, Pinho A, Goncalo M. Long-term management of chronic spontaneous urticaria with omalizumab. Clin Exp Dermatol. 2017;42(7):735–42.
22. Koski R, Kennedy KK. Treatment with omalizumab or cyclosporine for resistant chronic spontaneous urticaria. Ann Allergy Asthma Immunol. 2017;119(5):397–401.
23. Adhya Z, Karim Y. Doxepin may be a useful pharmacotherapeutic agent in chronic urticaria. Clin Exp Allergy. 2015;45(8):1370.
24. Morgan M, Cooke A, Rogers L, Adams-Huet B, Khan DA. Double-blind placebo-controlled trial of dapsone in antihistamine refractory chronic idiopathic urticaria. J Allergy Clin Immunol Pract. 2014;2(5):601–6.
25. McGirt LY, Vasagar K, Gober LM, Saini SS, Beck LA. Successful treatment of recalcitrant chronic idiopathic urticaria with sulfasalazine. Arch Dermatol. 2006;142(10):1337–42.
26. Zimmerman AB, Berger EM, Elmariah SB, Soter NA. The use of mycophenolate mofetil for the treatment of autoimmune and chronic idiopathic urticaria: experience in 19 patients. J Am Acad Dermatol. 2012;66(5):767–70.
27. Bulkhi A, Cooke AJ, Casale TB. Biologics in chronic urticaria. Immunol Allergy Clin North Am. 2017;37(1):95–112.
28. Morgado-Carrasco D, Fusta-Novell X, Podlipnik S, Combalia A, Aguilera P. Clinical and photobiological response in eight patients with solar urticaria under treatment with omalizumab, and review of the literature. Photodermatol Photoimmunol Photomed. 2018;34(3):194–9.
29. Goetze S, Elsner P. Solar urticaria. J Dtsch Dermatol Ges. 2015;13(12):1250–3.

30. Bolognia JL, Schaffer JV, Cerroni L. Dermatology. 4th ed. Elsevier; 2018.
31. Neill BC, Neill JA, Brauker J, Rajpara A, Aires DJ. Post-exposure prevention of toxicodendron dermatitis with early forceful unidirectional washing. J Am Acad Dermatol. 2018.
32. Paek SY, Lim HW. Chronic actinic dermatitis. Dermatol Clin. 2014;32(3):355–61. viii–ix.
33. Scheinfeld N. Dissecting cellulitis (Perifolliculitis Capitis Abscedens et Suffodiens): a comprehensive review focusing on new treatments and findings of the last decade with commentary comparing the therapies and causes of dissecting cellulitis to hidradenitis suppurativa. Dermatol Online J. 2014;20(5):22692.
34. Kobayashi H, Aiba S, Tagami H. Successful treatment of dissecting cellulitis and acne conglobata with oral zinc. Br J Dermatol. 1999;141(6):1137–8.
35. Kim WB, Shelley AJ, Novice K, Joo J, Lim HW, Glassman SJ. Drug-induced phototoxicity: a systematic review. J Am Acad Dermatol. 2018;79(6):1069–75.
36. Moore DE. Drug-induced cutaneous photosensitivity: incidence, mechanism, prevention and management. Drug Saf. 2002;25(5):345–72.
37. Piette EW, Rosenbach M. Granuloma annulare: pathogenesis, disease associations and triggers, and therapeutic options. J Am Acad Dermatol. 2016;75(3):467–79.
38. Escobar-Morreale HF, Carmina E, Dewailly D, et al. Epidemiology, diagnosis and management of hirsutism: a consensus statement by the Androgen Excess and Polycystic Ovary Syndrome Society. Hum Reprod Update. 2012;18(2):146–70.
39. van Zuuren EJ, Fedorowicz Z, Carter B, Pandis N. Interventions for hirsutism (excluding laser and photoepilation therapy alone). Cochrane Database Syst Rev. 2015;(4):CD010334.
40. de Almeida AR, Montagner S. Botulinum toxin for axillary hyperhidrosis. Dermatol Clin. 2014;32(4):495–504.
41. Cruddas L, Baker DM. Treatment of primary hyperhidrosis with oral anticholinergic medications: a systematic review. J Eur Acad Dermatol Venereol. 2017;31(6):952–63.
42. Pariser DM, Ballard A. Topical therapies in hyperhidrosis care. Dermatol Clin. 2014;32(4):485–90.
43. Hwang S, Schwartz RA. Keratosis pilaris: a common follicular hyperkeratosis. Cutis. 2008;82(3):177–80.
44. Alrashdan MS, Cirillo N, McCullough M. Oral lichen planus: a literature review and update. Arch Dermatol Res. 2016;308(8):539–51.
45. Sharma A, Bialynicki-Birula R, Schwartz RA, Janniger CK. Lichen planus: an update and review. Cutis. 2012;90(1):17–23.
46. Kern JS, Technau-Hafsi K, Schwacha H, et al. Esophageal involvement is frequent in lichen planus: study in 32 patients with suggestion of clinicopathologic diagnostic criteria and therapeutic implications. Eur J Gastroenterol Hepatol. 2016;28(12):1374–82.
47. Sartori-Valinotti JC, Bruce AJ, Krotova Khan Y, Beatty CW. A 10-year review of otic lichen planus: the Mayo Clinic experience. JAMA Dermatol. 2013;149(9):1082–6.
48. Guenther LC, Kunynetz R, Lynde CW, et al. Acitretin use in dermatology. J Cutan Med Surg. 2017;21(3_suppl):2S–12S.
49. Lajevardi V, Ghodsi SZ, Hallaji Z, Shafiei Z, Aghazadeh N, Akbari Z. Treatment of erosive oral lichen planus with methotrexate. J Dtsch Dermatol Ges. 2016;14(3):286–93.
50. Khandpur S, Sugandhan S, Sharma VK. Pulsed itraconazole therapy in eruptive lichen planus. J Eur Acad Dermatol Venereol. 2009;23(1):98–101.
51. Hollo P, Szakonyi J, Kiss D, Jokai H, Horvath A, Karpati S. Successful treatment of lichen planus with adalimumab. Acta Derm Venereol. 2012;92(4):385–6.
52. Deen K, McMeniman E. Mycophenolate mofetil in erosive genital lichen planus: a case and review of the literature. J Dermatol. 2015;42(3):311–4.
53. Murphy R. Lichen sclerosus. Dermatol Clin. 2010;28(4):707–15.
54. Howard M, Sahhar L, Andrews F, Bergman R, Gin D. Notalgia paresthetica: a review for dermatologists. Int J Dermatol. 2018;57(4):388–92.

55. Yeo B, Tey HL. Effective treatment of notalgia paresthetica with amitriptyline. J Dermatol. 2013;40(6):505–6.
56. Lee GL, Zirwas MJ. Granulomatous rosacea and periorificial dermatitis: controversies and review of management and treatment. Dermatol Clin. 2015;33(3):447–55.
57. Gruber-Wackernagel A, Byrne SN, Wolf P. Polymorphous light eruption: clinic aspects and pathogenesis. Dermatol Clin. 2014;32(3):315–34. viii.
58. Epstein JH. Polymorphous light eruptions: phototest technique studies. Arch Dermatol. 1962;85:502–4.
59. Tanew A, Radakovic S, Gonzalez S, Venturini M, Calzavara-Pinton P. Oral administration of a hydrophilic extract of Polypodium leucotomos for the prevention of polymorphic light eruption. J Am Acad Dermatol. 2012;66(1):58–62.
60. Marini A, Jaenicke T, Grether-Beck S, et al. Prevention of polymorphic light eruption by oral administration of a nutritional supplement containing lycopene, beta-carotene, and Lactobacillus johnsonii: results from a randomized, placebo-controlled, double-blinded study. Photodermatol Photoimmunol Photomed. 2014;30(4):189–94.
61. Steinhoff M, Cevikbas F, Ikoma A, Berger TG. Pruritus: management algorithms and experimental therapies. Semin Cutan Med Surg. 2011;30(2):127–37.
62. Ekelem C, Juhasz M, Khera P, Mesinkovska NA. Utility of naltrexone treatment for chronic inflammatory dermatologic conditions: a systematic review. JAMA Dermatol. 2018.
63. Tandon P, Rowe BH, Vandermeer B, Bain VG. The efficacy and safety of bile Acid binding agents, opioid antagonists, or rifampin in the treatment of cholestasis-associated pruritus. Am J Gastroenterol. 2007;102(7):1528–36.
64. Dull MM, Kremer AE. Management of chronic hepatic itch. Dermatol Clin. 2018;36(3):293–300.
65. Handler NS, Handler MZ, Stephany MP, Handler GA, Schwartz RA. Porphyria cutanea tarda: an intriguing genetic disease and marker. Int J Dermatol. 2017;56(6):e106–17.
66. Green JJ, Manders SM. Pseudoporphyria. J Am Acad Dermatol. 2001;44(1):100–8.
67. Massone C, Ambros-Rudolph CM, Di Stefani A, Mullegger RR. Successful outcome of haemodialysis-induced pseudoporphyria after short-term oral N-acetylcysteine and switch to high-flux technique dialysis. Acta Derm Venereol. 2006;86(6):538–40.
68. Cooke NS, McKenna K. A case of haemodialysis-associated pseudoporphyria successfully treated with oral N-acetylcysteine. Clin Exp Dermatol. 2007;32(1):64–6.
69. Gallo RL, Granstein RD, Kang S, et al. Standard classification and pathophysiology of rosacea: the 2017 update by the National Rosacea Society Expert Committee. J Am Acad Dermatol. 2018;78(1):148–55.
70. Schaller M, Almeida LM, Bewley A, et al. Rosacea treatment update: recommendations from the global ROSacea COnsensus (ROSCO) panel. Br J Dermatol. 2017;176(2):465–71.
71. Haimovic A, Sanchez M, Judson MA, Prystowsky S. Sarcoidosis: a comprehensive review and update for the dermatologist: part I. Cutaneous disease. J Am Acad Dermatol. 2012;66(5):699. e691–618. quiz 717-698.

Infectious Disease

Samantha L. Schneider and Laurie L. Kohen

Cellulitis [1]

Caused by

- Most commonly *Streptococcus*

What Not To Miss

- Erysipelas
  - Most commonly caused by beta-hemolytic streptococci
  - Common in pediatric patients
  - Type of superficial cellulitis on face, hands, or scalp
  - Treat with penicillin
- Preseptal or periorbital cellulitis
  - Limited to deeper infection by the orbital septum
- Orbital cellulitis
  - Can cause vision loss and cavernous sinus thrombosis
  - Need ophthalmology consultation
  - Look for proptosis, conjunctival edema, opthalmoplegia (weakness/paralysis of eye muscles), and decreased visual acuity

S. L. Schneider
Department of Dermatology, Henry Ford Health System,
3031 West Grand Blvd, Suite 800, Detroit, MI 48202, USA
e-mail: samantha.schneider@gmail.com

L. L. Kohen (✉)
Henry Ford Health System, 3031 West Grand Blvd, Suite 800, Detroit, MI 48202, USA
e-mail: lkohen1@hfhs.org

© Springer Nature Switzerland AG 2020
H. W. Lim et al. (eds.), *Practical Guide to Dermatology*,
https://doi.org/10.1007/978-3-030-18015-7_13

257

- *Pseudomonas*
  - ○ If there is involvement of the pinna, you must consider pseudomonas and cover with ciprofloxacin or equivalent
- Group A strep (GAS) intertrigo
  - ○ Seen in infants
  - ○ Particularly common in the neck folds with an erosive or "beefy red" appearance
  - ○ If you are concerned, you must culture
- Concomitant tinea pedis
  - ○ Maceration can cause skin breakdown which predisposes patients to bacterial infection

Key DDx

- Venous stasis dermatitis
  - ○ Do not use antibiotics in the case of venous stasis unless there is clear evidence of infection (per AAD "Choosing Wisely" guidelines) [2]
- Candidal intertrigo

Work Up Pearls

- Look for risk factors such as trauma, tinea pedis, onychomycosis, lymphatic or vascular compromise, peripheral vascular disease, lymph node dissection, liposuction, and/or radiation therapy
- Key to diagnosis is physical exam
- Biopsy may help with the diagnosis but more often helps diagnose a cellulitis mimicker

Treatment Ladder

- Oral antibiotics [1]
  - ○ Dicloxacillin 500 mg q6 h
  - ○ Cephalexin 500 mg q6 h
  - ○ Clindamycin 300–450 mg TID
  - ○ Doxycycline 100 mg BID
  - ○ PEARL: Clindamycin and doxycycline may cover MRSA depending on local antibiograms
- Severe cases may require intravenous antibiotics
  - ○ Nafcillin 1–2 g IV q4 h
  - ○ Cefazolin 1 g IV q8 h
  - ○ Vancomycin 30 mg/kg/day IV in two divided doses

Outside the Box Treatment Options [3]

- Adjunctive prednisone (with antibiotics)
  - 30 mg for 2 days, 15 mg for 2 days, 10 mg for 2 days, 5 mg for 2 days
  - Leads to faster resolution
- Adjunctive non-steroidal anti-inflammatory agents (NSAIDs) (with antibiotics)

In the Context Of …

- Immunocompromised patients
  - Empiric broad-spectrum coverage during pathogen analysis
- Human, dog or cat bite [1]
  - Amoxicillin-clavulanate 500 mg q8 h
- Limb threatening diabetic foot ulcer [1]
  - Ampcillin-sulbactam 3 g IV q6 h

Erythrasma

Caused by

- *Corynebacterium minutissimum* (normal skin flora)

Key DDx

- Intertrigo
- Inverse psoriasis
- Contact dermatitis
- Acanthosis nigricans

Work Up Pearls

- Look for risk factors such as DM, obesity, advanced age, humidity, poor hygiene, hyperhidrosis, and/or immunosuppression
  - Treat any underlying condition
- Coral red fluorescence with Wood's lamp due to coproporphyrin III
- KOH (+/−methylene blue) may show chains of bacilli due to concomitant infection

Treatment Ladder [4–6]

- Wash with antibacterial soap to prevent recurrence
- Topical

- o Fusidic acid cream
- o Imidazole (miconazole, clotrimazole)
- o Clindamycin or erythromycin
- o Mupirocin 2% ointment BID × 2–4 weeks
- o Whitfield ointment (salicylic and benzoic acids)
- o 20% aluminum chloride (if hyperhidrosis)
- Systemic
  - o Erythromycin 250 mg q6 h (or 1 g daily) for 14 days
  - o Clarithromycin 1 g once

Genital Warts (Condyloma Acuminatum)

Caused by

- Human papillomavirus (HPV)

Key DDx [7]

- Bowenoid papulosis and erythrodysplasia of Queyrat
  - o Genital lesions consistent with squamous cell carcinoma in situ on histology
  - o Due to high risk HPV sub-type 16
- Buschke-Lowenstein tumor (giant condyloma acuminatum) [8]
  - o Large cauliflower mass in the anogenital area
  - o Locally invasive growth with potential for metastases
  - o Due to low risk HPV sub-types 6 or 11

Work Up Pearls

- Typically, diagnosis is clinical
  - o It should be noted that banal seborrheic keratosis-appearing lesions can mimic condyloma so consider biopsy for new lesions
- Reconsider diagnosis for poorly or non-responsive lesions

Treatment Ladder

- Office-based therapies [6, 9]
  - o Cryotherapy
  - o Bichloracetic acid (BCA) or 80–90% trichloracetic acid (TCA) weekly until clearance
  - o Podophyllin 25% for 6 h repeated weekly
  - o Intralesional interferon-alpha
  - o Surgical excision/Curettage
  - o Electrosurgery/Laser destruction (Dangerous plume)
  - o ALA—PDT (red light) weekly × 3 total treatments

- Home-based therapies [6, 10]
  - Aldara
    - 5% cream M/W/F overnight for max of 16 weeks (wash off after 10–16 h)
    - 3.75% cream nightly for 8 weeks
  - Podofilox gel/solution 0.5% BID on 3 consecutive days per week for 4–6 weeks (i.e. 4 days off per week)

Outside the Box Treatment Options

- Sinecatechins 10–15% ointment TID (max 16 weeks)
  - PEARL: This is an extract of green tea from *Camellia sinensis.*
- Cidofovir gel 1% daily on 5 days per week for up to 18 weeks

In the Context Of …

- Immunosuppression or transplant patients
  - Biopsy any new or non-responsive lesions
  - Consider HPV vaccination

Gram Negative Toe Web Infection [7, 11]

Caused by

- Most commonly *Pseudomonas aeruginosa*

What Not To Miss

- Concomitant tinea infection

Key DDx

- Bullous tinea
- Contact dermatitis to shoe or footwear allergens

Work Up Pearls

- Look for risk factors: tinea, occlusion, hyperhidrosis, antifungal/antibiotic/steroid use, poor hygiene/homelessness ("trench foot") and/or occupations requiring heavy boots
  - Address any underlying co-morbidities
- Bacterial culture

Treatment Ladder

- Topical ciclopirox 0.77% BID
  - PEARL: This covers BOTH gram-negative bacteria and any co-existent tinea
- Ciprofloxacin 500 mg BID for 10 days
- Debridement of hyperkeratotic rim if present

Outside the Box Treatment Options

- Amikacin 5% gel
- Aluminum chloride (for hyperhidrosis) + gentamicin cream
- Povidone-iodine BID
- White vinegar soaks or Domeboro soaks
- Castellani's paint or gentian violet
- Topical gentamicin, polysporin or silvadene for pseudomonas

---

Herpes Simplex (HSV) [6, 12–14]

Caused by

- Herpes simplex virus 1 and 2

What Not To Miss

- Eczema herpeticum
- HSV disseminatum within acne lesions

Key DDx

- Eczema coxsackium
- Herpes zoster
- Bullous impetigo

Work Up Pearls

- Viral culture
- Tzanck smear
- Direct fluorescent antibody assays (DFA)
- PCR
- Serologies

Treatment Ladder

- HSV labialis outbreak (recurrence)
  - Docosanol 5x/day until healed
  - Penciclovir 1% cream q2 h for 4 days
  - Acyclovir 5% ointment q3 h for 7–10 days
  - Acyclovir 5% + hydrocortisone 1% 5 times daily for 5 days
    - Reduces risk of ulceration
  - Acyclovir 400 mg PO TID for 7–10 days
  - Famciclovir 1.5 g PO for 1 dose
  - Valacyclovir 2 g PO BID for 1 day

- Genital Herpes (first episode)
  - Acyclovir 200 mg PO five times daily for 10 days or 400 mg PO TID for 10 days
  - Famciclovir 250 mg TID for 10 days
  - Valacyclovir 1 g PO BID for 10 days

- Genital Herpes (recurrence)
  - Acyclovir 400 mg PO TID for 5 days or 800 mg PO BID for 5 days or 800 mg PO TID for 2 days
  - Famciclovir 1 g PO BID for 1 day or 500 mg PO for 1 dose, then 250 mg PO BID for 2 days or 125 mg PO BID for 5 days
  - Valacyclovir 500 mg PO BID for 3 days or 1 g PO daily for 5 days

- Suppression
  - Acyclovir 400 mg PO BID
  - Famciclovir 250 mg PO BID
  - Valacyclovir 500 mg PO daily for <10 outbreaks per year or 1 g PO daily for >10 outbreaks per year

Outside the Box Treatment Options

- HSV labialis prior to a big event, consider:
  - Intralesional triamcinolone 2.5 mg/mL with injection of 0.1 mL
  - Compeed cold sore patch (available on Amazon.com)

In the Context Of …

- Erythema multiforme (recurrent HSV associated EM)
  - Acyclovir 400 mg PO BID

Herpes Zoster (VZV) [6, 15]

Caused by

- Reactivation of VZV

What Not To Miss

- Zoster in an immunosuppressed patient

Key DDx

- Disseminated VZV
- Herpes simplex virus

Work Up Pearls

- Tzanck smear
  - Rapid and inexpensive
  - PEARL: To do this test: scrape cells from base of lesion, stain with Wright-Giemsa, and look for multinucleated keratinocytes
- Direct fluorescent antibody
  - PEARL: To do this test: scrape cells from base of lesion, smear on glass slide and send to lab for staining
- Biopsy
  - Can aid in inconclusive cases
  - Immunohistochemistry can help confirm diagnosis
- PCR from skin lesion may be helpful
- Consider: HIV testing, lumbar puncture with cerebrospinal fluid analysis and MRI of brain and/or spinal cord if appropriate

Treatment Ladder

- Varicella
  - Acyclovir 20 mg/kg (800 mg max) PO four times daily for 5 days
  - Valacyclovir 20 mg/kg (1 g max) PO TID for 5 days

- Herpes Zoster
  - Acyclovir 800 mg PO 5 times daily for 7–10 days
  - Famciclovir 500 mg PO TID for 7 days
  - Valacyclovir 1 g PO TID for 7 days

Outside the Box Treatment Options

- Consider adding intramuscular triamcinolone for pain
  - Single dose of ~60 mg IM
  - Only consider if the patient does not have any contraindications to corticosteroids

In the Context Of ...

- Immunocompromise [16]
  - Varicella
    - Acyclovir 10 mg/kg IV q8 h for 7–10 days (or up until 2 days after cessation of new vesicles)
  - Herpes Zoster
    - Acyclovir 800 mg 5 times daily for 7–10 days
    - Valacyclovir 1000 mg TID for 7–10 days
      - PEARL: Valtrex can cause thrombotic thrombocytopenia purpura (TTP) or hemolytic uremic syndrome (HUS) in immunosuppressed patients
    - Famciclovir 500 mg TID for 7–10 days
    - Foscarnet 60 mg/kg IV BID to TID
  - Disseminated Zoster in an immunocompromised patient (i.e. HIV/AIDs, solid organ transplant or hematopoietic stem cell transplant
    - IV acyclovir 10 mg/kg q8 h

- Prophylaxis
  - Prevention of VZV with vaccination
  - Post exposure: VZIg 1 vial/10 kg IM, max 5 vials
  - Transplant: acyclovir 400–800 mg q6 h up to 3 months

- Post-herpetic neuralgia [17]
  - Start treatment if patient develops early pain symptoms
  - Gabapentin 100–300 mg up to TID but can use up to 2400 mg/day
  - Pregabalin 150 mg (up to 300–600 mg/day)
  - Nortriptyline 10–25 mg (increase weekly to 75–150 mg/day)
  - Amitriptyline 10–25 mg (up to 100 mg/day)
  - Desipramine 10–25 mg (up to 150 mg/day
  - Lidocaine patch
  - Capsaicin cream
  - Methylcobalamin 1.0 mg daily subcutaneous injection, 6 times per week [18]

Impetigo [19]

Caused by

- Bullous is almost always caused by *Staphylococcus aureus*
- Non-bullous is often *S. aureus* or *Streptococcus pyogenes*

What Not To Miss

- Secondary impetiginization of a primary dermatologic condition
  - Frequently is non-bullous

Key DDx

- Resolving immunobullous disease
- Tinea
- Linear bullous IgA dermatosis

Work Up Pearls

- Bacterial culture
- Clinical lesions are annular with collarette of epidermis
  - Most of the time the bullae are not intact

Treatment Ladder

- No treatment, will self-resolve

- Colonization treatments
  - Bleach baths
  - Chlorhexidine
    - Use as a shower wash in intertriginous areas groin, hands and feet
  - Nasal mupirocin in each nostril BID for 5 days

- Topical
  - Mupirocin
  - Neomycin
  - Bacitracin
  - Polymyxin B
  - Gentamicin
  - Fusidic Acid
  - Topical antibiotic combined with topical corticosteroid

- Systemic [20]
  - Dicloxacillin 250 mg q6 h
  - Amoxicillin/clavulanic acid 875/125 mg BID
  - Cephalexin 250 mg q6 h or 500 mg BID

In the Context Of …

- Focal recurrent lesions
  - Consider fomite, exposures or contaminated equipment

Intertrigo [6, 21]

Caused by

- Most commonly *Candida* species

What Not To Miss

- Cutaneous strep infection in infants

Key DDx

- Inverse psoriasis
- Seborrheic dermatitis
- Subcorneal pustular dermatosis
  - Pustules at the edge
- Hailey-Hailey
  - Erosive
- Extramammary Paget's disease
  - Unilateral affecting axilla or groin

Work Up Pearls

- KOH
- Bacterial culture of pustules or exudate

Treatment Ladder

- Lifestyle
  - Minimize moisture and chafing
  - Powders may increase irritation
  - Wear cotton clothes
- Topical
  - Nystatin BID × 2–4 weeks
  - Miconazole, ketoconazole, clotrimazole cream BID × 2–4 weeks

- ○ Low potency topical steroid/calcineurin inhibitor + topical antifungal (polyene or imidazole)
- ○ Domeboro solution, Castellani paint, or vinegar:water solutions BID × 5–10 min
- ○ 20% aluminum chloride (if hyperhidrosis)
- ○ Consider Vytone (hydrocortisone and iodoquinol-anti-inflammatory and amebocide) if other combinations not covered by insurance
- ○ Consider zeosorb AF OTC

Outside the Box Treatment Ideas

- Interdry sheets under pendulous breasts or pannus
  - ○ Available on Amazon.com

In the Context Of …

- Diabetes
  - ○ If poor response to treatment, search for poorly controlled diabetes

- Immunosupression
  - ○ May need PO fluconazole 100 mg daily for 7 days or PO itraconazole 200 mg daily

Molluscum Contagiosum [6, 22, 23]

Caused by

- Poxvirus

What Not To Miss

- Molluscum disseminatum in eczema
- Other infectious entities that have molluscum-like lesions
  - ○ PEARL: Cryptococcus, penicillium, coccidiomycosis, histoplasmosis can all appear as molluscum-like lesions clinically

Key DDx

- Keratosis pilaris
- Folliculitis
- Flat warts
- Arthropod bites

Work Up Pearls

- Curette one lesion, then perform potassium hydroxide (KOH) preparation to identify Henderson-Patterson bodies

Treatment Ladder

- No treatment—will spontaneously resolve
- Topical
  - Salicylic acid gel 12%, salicylic acid-lactic acid 16.7% combination solution, or salicylic acid plaster
  - Potassium hydroxide
  - 0.7% Cantharidin 0.7% solution or combination 1% cantharidin, 30% salicylic acid and 5% podophyllum resin
  - Hydrogen peroxide
  - Imiquimod 1% five times weekly—max 16 weeks
  - Tretinoin/adapalene

- Office-based treatments:
  - Cryotherapy
  - Curettage
  - Electrodesiccation
  - 40% silver nitrate paste
  - PDL

Outside the Box Treatment Options

- 3% Cidofovir
- 0.5% Podophyllotoxin
- 10% Povidone-iodine with 50% salicylic acid
- 5% Acidified nitrite nightly with 5% salicylic acid under occlusion
- Cimetidine 40 mg/kg/day for 2 months (pediatric dosing) [24]
- Interferon alpha subcutaneous injection
- 10% Sinecatechins ointment BID × 4 weeks
- Lemon myrtle oil
- Intralesional candida antigen

In the Context Of ...

- Adults with groin lesions
  - Counsel on sexually transmitted infections (STI)
  - Offer additional STI testing

- Immunosuppression
  - May see giant molluscum-like lesions

Paronychia [6, 7]

Caused by

- Frequently yeast (*Candida*), particularly for chronic paronychia
- *Staphylococcus* is more common for acute paronychia

What Not To Miss

- Felon

Key DDx

- Irritant or contact dermatitis
  - Nail acrylics/adhesives
  - Cleaning supplies

Work Up Pearls

- Bacterial culture
- Fungal culture

Treatment Ladder [25, 26]

- Lifestyle
  - Avoidance of inciting factors
  - Keep hands as dry as possible and wear gloves for wet work
  - Repeated microtrauma (i.e. frequently trimming cuticles)
- Acute Paronychia
  - Topical antibiotics
  - Incision and drainage
    - PEARL: Antibiotics not necessary if lesion has been surgically drained
  - Soaks (1 part white vinegar: 3 parts H2O)
- Chronic Paronychia
  - Soaks (1 part white vinegar: 3 parts H2O)
  - Potent topical steroids
  - Topical calcineurin inhibitor
  - Consider intralesional or oral steroids if refractory
  - Can combine corticosteroids with antifungals (i.e. Mycolog ©)
    - Solutions are easier to administer
  - If bacterial co-infection, topical or oral antibiotics
    - Consider garamycin ophthalmic solution BID
  - Continue treatment until inflammation resolves (may take months)

In the Context Of ...

- Systemic medications
  - May need to discontinue certain medications (e.g. isotretinoin, EGFRs)
- Immunocompromised patients or concomitant overt cellulitis
  - Consider oral antibiotics directed against likely pathogen

Onychomycosis (Tinea Unguium) [27–30]

Caused by

- Most commonly *Trichophyton rubrum* > *Trichophyton interdigitale*
- Most commonly for distal subungual is *T. rubrum*
- Most commonly for white superficial is *T. mentagrophytes* (adults) and *T. rubrum* (pediatrics and HIV)

What Not To Miss

- Dermatophytoma—often linear lesions
- Keratinocyte cancers—Similarly often appear as linear lesions
  - These can co-exist with dystrophy and/or onychomycosis

Work Up Pearls

- Look for risk factors: age, DM, HIV, peripheral vascular disease, peripheral neuropathy, sports, traumatic nail injuries
  - Address any underlying comorbidities
- Fungal culture
- Nail clipping for PAS
  - PEARL: It is highly recommended that there is a proven positive fungal culture or nail clipping prior to initiating oral therapy per the AAD "Choosing Wisely" guidelines [2]

Treatment Ladder

- PEARL: Combination of oral and topical agents increases cure rate
- Topicals (not very effective but safer than oral)
  - 10% efinaconazole solution (Jublia) once daily for 48 weeks
    - Expensive and only occasionally covered by insurance
  - 5% tavaborole solution (Kerydin) once daily for 48 weeks
  - Ciclopirox lacquer (Penlac) applied daily
    - Not quite as effective as above but less expensive

- o   Naftifine/ciclopirox/imidazole creams/gels
- o   Urea 40% (ointment under occlusion for onychauxis)
- • Oral—Consider baseline LFTs
  - o   Terbinafine 250 mg daily for 6 weeks for fingernails; 12 weeks for toenails (may need to repeat) or pulse regimen: 250 mg 1 week a month every 2 or 3 months
    - ▪ Higher efficacy compared to other oral agents
  - o   Itraconazole 200 mg daily for 6 weeks for fingernails or 12 weeks for toenails
  - o   Pulse dose itraconazole at 200 mg BID 1 week per month for 3–4 months
  - o   Fluconazole 150–450 mg once weekly for 6 months for fingernails or 9 months for toenails
    - ▪ Oral is best treatment for distal subungual affecting lunula and proximal subungual onychomycosis

Outside the Box Treatment Options

- • Surgical removal of nail
  - o   This is a required treatment for dermatophytoma
- • ALA-PDT [31]
  - o   Consider in patients that cannot tolerate oral therapies
  - o   Can also treat more unusual dermatophytes
  - o   Recommend pre-treatment of infected nail with 20% urea to soften the nail plate, microabrasion or complete nail avulsion
  - o   ALA incubation of 1–5 h, followed by photodynamic therapy
  - o   Perform 3–6 treatments every 2 weeks, if using higher fluences during irradiation
- • Nd:YAG [32]
  - o   Moderate results
  - o   Treated every 4 weeks for total of 5 treatments
    - ▪ Settings: 6 mm spot size, 5 J/cm [2] fluence, 0.3 ms pulse duration
- • Diode laser [33]
  - o   Pulsed mode with spot size of 4 mm with power of 8 W, pulse duration of 80 ms and repetition rate of 5.6 Hz
  - o   Total energy delivered around 500–800 J per session
  - o   Patients received treatments every 2 weeks for an average of 4 treatments

In the Context Of …

- • Pediatric patients
  - o   Griseofulvin microsized 15–20 mg/kg/day divided BID (max 1 g/day)
    - ▪ Most common dose is 250 mg daily until nail changes resolve (up to 12 months)

- o Itraconazole
  - If <50 kg: 5 mg/kg once daily for 1 week then no drug for 3 weeks
  - If >50 kg: 200 mg/day (off label)
- o Terbinafine
  - <20 kg: 62.5 mg/day
  - 20–40 kg: 125 mg/day
  - >40 kg: 250 mg/day
  - Treat for 6 weeks for fingers or 12 weeks for toes (off label)

Tinea Capitis [6, 34, 35]

Caused by

- Most commonly *Microsporum* and *Trichophyton*

What Not To Miss

- Kerion
- Mixed infection with bacteria

Key DDx

- Acne keloidalis nuchae
- Alopecia areata
- Seborrheic dermatitis
- Impetigo
- Folliculitis
- Folliculitis decalvans

Work Up Pearls

- Check for posterior cervical and occipital lymphadenopathy
- KOH
- Fungal culture
- Screen contacts

Treatment Ladder

- Adult
  - o Terbinafine 250 mg daily for 4 weeks
    - PEARL: Best for *Trichophyton*
  - o Griseofulvin for 6 weeks
    - Microsized 500 mg daily (can go up to 1000 mg)
    - Ultramicrosized 375 mg daily (can go up to 750 mg)

- Pediatrics
  - ○ Griseofulvin (approved)
    - ■ Microsized 20 mg/kg/day for 6–8 weeks (max 16 weeks)
      - PEARL: Can give up to 25 mg/kg/day if *M. canis*
      - PEARL: To calculate dose: multiply weight in lbs × 10 (22 mg/kg/day)
    - ■ Ultramicrosized 15 mg/kg/day
      - PEARL: Superior for *Microsporum*
  - ○ Itraconazole 5 mg/kg/day capsule or 3 mg/kg/day solution for max 4 weeks
    - ■ Broader spectrum of action
  - ○ Terbinafine
    - ■ <20 kg: 62.5 mg/day
    - ■ 20–40 kg: 125 mg/day
    - ■ >40 kg: 250 mg/day
- Can do adjuvant ketoconazole shampoo or selenium sulfide shampoo

In the Context Of ...

- Kerion [36]
  - ○ Responds best to oral antifungals
  - ○ If bacterial culture positive, add appropriate antibiotic
  - ○ No evidence for oral steroids

Tinea Corporis/Cruris/Pedis

Caused by

- Most commonly *Microsporum* and *Trichophyton*

What Not To Miss

- Majocchi's granuloma

Key DDx

- Intertrigo (in the groin)
- Annular lesion DDx
  - ○ Pityriasis rosea
  - ○ Subcorneal pustular dermatosis
  - ○ Annular psoriasis
  - ○ Pityriasis lichenoides chronica

Work Up Pearls

- KOH

- Fungal culture
- Bacterial culture

Treatment Ladder

- Topical [37, 38]
  - Clotrimazole or miconazole
    - Treat for 2–4 weeks or 1 week beyond clearing
  - 2% Sertaconazole cream daily to BID
  - 1% Terbinafine
  - Ciclopirox
  - *PEARL*: Allylamines are more effective but more expensive
- Oral [6]
  - Griseofulvin
    - Microsized 500 mg/day (can go up to 1000 mg)
    - Ultramicrosized 375 mg/day (can go up to 750 mg)
    - PEARL:
      - Corporis: treat for 2–4 weeks
      - Pedis: treat for 4–8 weeks
      - Unguium: treat for 4–6 months
  - Terbinafine 250 mg daily for 14 days
  - Fluconazole 50 mg daily for 2–4 weeks (up to 6 weeks in pedis)
  - Itraconazole 100 mg daily for 15 days or 200 mg daily for 7 days (longer for pedis or manuum)

Outside the Box Treatment Options

- 20% zinc-undecylenate powder applied BID for 4 weeks [39]
- On the feet, consider keratolytic to help penetration of topical antifungal

In the Context Of ...

- Recalcitrant cases or immunosuppression
  - Use oral therapies

Tinea Versicolor (Pityriasis Versicolor) [6, 40]

Caused by

- Lipophilic yeast: *Malassezia*
  - Normal flora
  - Becomes pathogenic when the yeast phase converts to mycelial phase

Key DDx

- Seborrheic dermatitis
- Pityriasis lichenoides chronica
- Idiopathic guttate hypomelanosis
- Trichrome vitiligo

Work Up Pearls

- Look for risk factors such as heat, humidity, malnutrition, oral contraceptives, hyperhidrosis, genetics, and/or immunodeficiency
- KOH
- Wood's light examination
  o Will fluoresce yellow/green

Treatment Ladder

- Topical
  o Ciclopirox cream/lotion/gel BID for 3–4 weeks
  o Terbinafine cream/lotion/gel BID
  o Clotrimazole
  o Econazole—less effective
  o 2% Ketoconazole cream 1–2 times per day for 2–4 weeks
  o Ketoconazole or selenium sulfide shampoo daily for 3–5 days, then once weekly
- Systemic (Second line)
  o Fluconazole 300 mg weekly for two doses (safest, most evidence) or 400 mg once
  o Itraconazole 200 mg daily for one week with reevaluation 4 weeks
- Prophylaxis
  o Itraconazole 400 mg once monthly for 6 months

Outside the Box Treatment Ideas

- Topical 15% zinc sulfate solution daily for 3 weeks [39]

Pediculosis Capitis [41, 42]

Caused by

- *Pediculosis capitis*—head louse

What Not To Miss

- Purpuric stains on the skin of occipital scalp and neck may be signal of infestation; termed "maculae ceruleae"

Key DDx

- White piedra

Work Up Pearls

- Can visualize organism under the microscope

Treatment Ladder

- Topicals
  - 0.9% Spinosad suspension (first choice)
    - Apply for 10 min, then wash off
    - Repeat in 7 days only if live lice are seen
    - Patients 4 years and older
  - 0.5% Malathion in 78% isopropyl alcohol with 12% terpineol
    - Perform 2 treatments 1 week apart
    - Use contraindicated in neonates and infants
  - 0.5% Malathion lotion
    - Applied for 8–12 h then wash off and repeat in one week
    - Use contraindicated in neonates and infants
  - 1% Permethrin cream (Nix—OTC)
    - Apply for 10 min, then wash off and repeat in one week
    - Resistance is a concern
  - 0.33% Pyrethrin and 4% piperonyl butoxide (RID)
    - Shampoo hair 1st and towel dry, then apply for 10 min and wash off
    - Repeat in one week
    - Patients 2 years and older
  - 5% Benzyl alcohol lotion
    - Apply for 10 min, then rinse off and repeat in one week
    - Patients 6 months and older
  - 0.5% Ivermectin lotion
    - Apply for 10 min and wash off
    - Second treatment is not indicated
    - Patients 6 months and older
  - Eyelashes: occlusive ophthalmic ointment (such as Vaseline) 2 times daily for 10 days
- PEARL: All topical pediculicidal treatments should be rinsed with cool water. Rinsing with warm water could cause vasodilation and increase risk of systemic absorption.

- Oral
  - Ivermectin 400 mcg/kg every 7 days for 2 doses (off label)
- Cleaning
  - Wash clothes, towels, linens used within 2 days at minimum 130 °F dryer at high heat for at least 10 min
  - For combs/brushes, immerse in 130 °F water for at least 10 min
  - If item cannot be laundered or placed in dryer, seal in plastic bag for at least 3 days
  - Vacuum all furniture

Outside the Box Treatment Ideas

- Nit pickers—have the nits manually extracted
- Shave the head (in male patients)

In the Context Of …

- Household contacts
  - All household members and close contacts should be examined for infestation and treated only if live lice discovered
- Pediatric patients
  - Children younger than 2 years old should be treated with mechanical methods

Pediculosis Corporis [6, 43]

Caused by

- *Pediculosis humanus*—body louse

Key DDx

- Other arthropod bites
- Scabies
- Bedbug bites
- Delusions of parasitosis

Work Up Pearls

- Look for risk factors such as homeless patients or patients requiring social services or other assistance, residents of nursing homes, poor living conditions, and/or elder neglect
- Can visualize organism under the microscope or with dermoscopy

Treatment Ladder

- Topical
  - 5% Permethrin cream (Elimite)
    - Wash off after 8–10 h
  - 0.5% Malathion lotion
    - Apply for 8–12 h then wash off and repeat in one week
    - Use contraindicated in neonates and infants
- Oral
  - Ivermectin 200 mcg/kg every 7 days for 3 doses (off label)
- Clothing
  - Destroy infected clothing
  - If not possible, wash clothing, bedding and towels in hot water and machine dry using hot cycle
  - Make sure to use water at least 60 °C for at least 10 min

Outside the Box Treatment Ideas

- Avoid using items for 2 weeks (seal in plastic bag) to ensure mites are killed
- Iron seams of furniture with hot iron

Pediculosis Pubis [6, 44, 45]

Caused by

- *Phthirus pubis*—pubic louse

What Not To Miss

- Check for STDs
- Consider sexual abuse if seen in a minor

Work Up Pearls

- Can visualize organism under the microscope or with dermoscopy
- Macula cerulae—blue macule on the skin surface

Treatment Ladder

- Topical
  - 0.5% Malathion lotion

- Apply for 8–12 h then wash off and repeat in one week
- Use contraindicated in neonates and infants
  ○ 1% Permethrin cream rinse
    - Apply to whole body for 10 min, then rinse and repeat in one week
  ○ 5% Permethrin cream
  ○ Apply to whole body for 10 min, then rinse and repeat in one week

- Oral
  ○ Ivermectin
    - 250 mcg/kg/dose every 7 days for 2 doses
    - 250 mcg/kg/dose every 14 days for 2 doses (off label)

In the Context Of …

- Hair involvement
  ○ Treat axilla and hairy legs

- Eyelash involvement
  ○ Petroleum jelly occlusion
  ○ Mechanical removal

Perleche [46–48]

Caused by

- Often *Candida* or *Staphylococcus aureus*

What Not To Miss

- Angular cheilitis due to vitamin deficiency

Key DDx

- Lip licking dermatitis
- Secondary syphilis "split papules"
- HSV infection

Work Up Pearls

- Culture for candidiasis/bacteria

Treatment Ladder

- Topicals
  - Miconazole/ketoconazole 2% cream/nystatin BID-TID for 2–3 weeks
    - PEARL: Miconazole has anti-candidal and anti-staphylococcal activity
  - Polymyxin B or mupirocin ointment
  - Clotrimazole topically 2–3 times per day for 3 weeks
    - PEARL: Clotrimazole has anti-candidal and anti-Staphylococcal properties
  - Amphotericin B cream, lotion or ointment 3–4 times per day for 2 weeks
  - Short term course of nystatin/triamcinolone (Mycolog)
- Oral
  - Ketoconazole 200 mg daily to BID for 2 weeks
    - PEARL: Ketoconazole has a black box warning for hepatitis
  - Fluconazole 200 mg loading dose followed by 50, 100, 150 or 200 mg for 7–14 days
  - Itraconazole 100–200 mg daily for 2 weeks
    - Good for fluconazole resistant strains
    - Severe disease needs loading dose of 200 mg TID for 3 days

Outside the Box Treatment Options

- Prosthodontic evaluation for mandibular recession
- Soft tissue filler can be used to prevent recurrence if you bolster the commissure

In the Context Of …

- Recalcitrant disease, immunosuppressed patients, or risk of dissemination
  - Work up includes CBC, iron studies, vitamin B, folate, zinc, HbA1C, HIV, and patch testing
  - Use oral treatments
- Chronic perleche, consider suppressive dosing of oral fluconazole
  - Fluconazole 50–100 mg daily
  - Fluconazole 100–200 mg three times weekly
  - Fluconazole 150 mg weekly
- Dentures
  - Remove nightly
  - Clean with 2% chlorhexidine solution
  - Let dry completely before reinsertion

Scabies [49, 50]

Caused by

- *Sarcoptes scabiei*

What Not To Miss

- Norwegian scabies

Key DDx

- Folliculitis
- Excoriations

Work Up Pearls

- With dermoscopy, you can see the triangle or "delta wing jet" sign that corresponds with scabies head parts [51]
- Mineral prep can demonstrate organism
  - Need to scrape more aggressively, higher yield if get pinpoint bleeding

Treatment Ladder

- Topical
  - 5% Permethrin cream overnight
    - Apply after bathing and drying skin from behind the ears down to the toes including creases and web spaces and leave on overnight
    - Wash off the next day with warm soapy water
    - Repeat in one week
  - 1% Lindane—1 oz of lotion or 30 gm of cream
    - Apply for 8–12 h, then wash off
    - PEARL: Side effects include seizures and aplastic anemia
    - Do NOT use after shower or bath, extensive dermatitis, pregnant/breast feeding, kids less than 6 months, or preexisting seizure disorder
  - 6% Precipitated sulfur ointment or 5–10% in petrolatum
    - Apply nightly for 3 nights and wash off last application after 24 h
  - 10% Crotamiton lotion
  - 10–20% Benzoyl benzoate lotion
- Oral
  - Ivermectin 200 mcg/kg
    - Can retreat in 2 weeks
    - Not for use if less than 5 years old or less than 15 kg
    - Best to only use if crusted scabies or repeat exposure

- Clothing
  - Wash all bed linens/clothing/towels with hot water and hot drying cycles
- Treat household contacts
  - Can provide family members with prescriptions for treatment based on physician's comfort
  - 1% Permethrin cream once with repeat application in one week
  - Ivermectin 200 mcg/kg as single dose

In the Context Of ...

- Pregnancy
  - Permethrin is safe (category B)
- Pediatrics
  - Permethrin is safe for kids down to 2 months
    - Apply to scalp, face, palms and soles
    - Avoid the eyes
- Norwegian crusted scabies
  - Best to use ivermectin 200 mcg/kg
  - Combination 5% permethrin with oral ivermectin 200 mcg/kg
    - Permethrin to full body daily for 7 days, then twice weekly until resolved
    - Oral ivermectin given on days 1, 2, 8, 9, 15, 22, 29
- Post-scabetic pruritus
  - Consider topical steroids
    - Can give concurrently with treatment
  - Duration of pruritus can persist for up to 4 weeks post-treatment

---

Syphilis [45, 52, 53]

Caused by

- Bacterium *Treponema pallidum* sp. *pallidum*

What Not To Miss

- Stages of syphilis
  - Early/Incubation (3–90 days)
  - Primary
    - Single painless chancre
  - Secondary
    - Spirochetes disseminate
    - Develops 2–8 weeks after the chancre

- o Latent
  - ▪ Asymptomatic period
  - ▪ Early latent occurs within 2 years of infection
  - ▪ Late latent occurs after 2 years of infection
- o Tertiary
  - ▪ Neurologic, cardiovascular, or gummatous disease
- o Neurosyphilis
  - ▪ Can occur any time after infection
  - ▪ Early affects CSF, meninges and/or vasculature
  - ▪ Late affects brain and/or spinal cord
  - ▪ Most common comorbidity is HIV
  - ▪ Most common ocular manifestation is uveitis

- Concomittant HIV infection
  - o Check for HIV
  - o Beware of the prozone reaction in the context of HIV
    - ▪ HIV positive patients can make an RPR negative, in which case you must order for the FTA antibodies to confirm diagnosis

- Jarisch—Herxheimer reaction
  - o Symptoms include fever, chills, headache, myalgias and exacerbation of skin lesions
  - o Treatment includes NSAIDs +/− systemic steroids

Key DDx

- Chancroid
- Lymphogranuloma venereum
- Herpes simplex virus (HSV)
- Non-STD ulcers like EBV (in pediatric patients) or CMV

Work Up Pearls

- Serology
  - o RPR or VDRL followed by confirmatory testing (TPPA or FTA-ABS)
  - o PEARL: RPR/VDRL titers should decline with treatment but may remain positive
- Dark field microscopy (not commonly used)
- Biopsy
- Don't forget: HIV testing

Treatment Ladder

- Early 1°, 2° or early latent
  - o Mainstay: IM benzathine penicillin G 2.4 million U
  - o Alternate:

- Doxycycline 100 mg BID for 14 days
- Ceftriaxone 1–2 g daily IV or IM for 10–14 days
- Tetracycline 500 mg q6 h for 14 days

- Late latent or 3°
  - Mainstay of treatment is IM benzathine penicillin G 2.4 million U weekly for 3 weeks
  - Alternatives
    - Doxycycline 100 mg BID for 28 days
    - Ceftriaxone 2 g daily IM or IV for 10–14 days

- Neurosyphilis
  - Aqueous penicillin G 3–4 million U IV q4 h or 18–24 million U continuous IV infusion for 10–14 days
  - Pencillin G procaine 2.4 million units IM daily plus probenecid 500 mg q6 h for 10–14 days
  - Alternatives
    - Ceftriaxone 2 g IV daily for 10–14 days

In the Context Of …

- HIV
  - Treatment of choice is IM benzathine penicillin G 2.4 million U
- Pregnancy
  - Treatment of choice is IM benzathine penicillin G 2.4 million U
  - If penicillin allergic, recommend desensitization
- Penicillin Allergy
  - Desensitization for neurologic disease and in pregnancy

Varicella (See Herpes Zoster)

Verruca Vulgaris

Caused by

- Human papillomavirus (HPV)

What Not To Miss

- SCC
  - Consider biopsy of lesions not responding to typical treatments or long-standing atypical appearing warts

Key DDx

- SCC

Work Up Pearls

- Dermoscopy demonstrates verrucous appearance with hemosiderin in the stratum corneum
  - PEARL: Warts lose the normal dermatoglyphics on dermoscopy

Treatment Ladder

- Office-based therapies
  - Liquid nitrogen monthly
  - 0.7% cantharidin or combination 1% cantharidin, 30% salicylic acid, and 5% podophyllin resin
  - Paring
  - Shave removal
- Home-based therapies
  - 5% Imiquimod cream nightly for up to 12 weeks
  - 0.025–0.1% Tretinoin cream nightly
  - 17–40% Salicylic acid applied nightly

Outside the Box Treatment Options

- Topical zinc as 5% or 10% lotion or as 20% paste [39]
- Intralesional 2% zinc sulfate injection [39]
- Oral zinc sulfate 10 mg/kg, max doxing of 600 mg daily [39, 54]
  - Can lower copper levels so consider checking baseline levels

References

1. Bailey E, Kroshinsky D. Cellulitis: diagnosis and management. Dermatol Ther. 2011;24(2):229–39.
2. American Academy of Dermatology A. Choosing wisely. https://www.aad.org/practicecenter/quality/choosing-wisely. Accessed 11 Oct 2018.
3. Cranendonk DR, Lavrijsen APM, Prins JM, Wiersinga WJ. Cellulitis: current insights into pathophysiology and clinical management. Neth J Med. 2017;75(9):366–78.
4. Avci O, Tanyildizi T, Kusku E. A comparison between the effectiveness of erythromycin, single-dose clarithromycin and topical fusidic acid in the treatment of erythrasma. J Dermatolog Treat. 2013;24(1):70–4.
5. Greywal T, Cohen PR. Erythrasma: a report of nine men successfully managed with mupirocin 2% ointment monotherapy. Dermatol Online J. 2017;23(5).
6. Lebwohl MG, Heymann WR, Berth-Jones J, Coulson I. Treatment of skin disease: comprehensive therapeutic strategies. 4th ed. Elsevier; 2013.

7. Bolognia JL, Schaffer JV, Cerroni L. Dermatology. 4th ed. Elsevier; 2018.

8. Kim HG, Kesey JE, Griswold JA. Giant anorectal condyloma acuminatum of Buschke-Lowenstein presents difficult management decisions. J Surg Case Rep. 2018;2018(4):rjy058.

9. Liang J, Lu XN, Tang H, Zhang Z, Fan J, Xu JH. Evaluation of photodynamic therapy using topical aminolevulinic acid hydrochloride in the treatment of condylomata acuminata: a comparative, randomized clinical trial. Photodermatol Photoimmunol Photomed. 2009;25(6):293–7.

10. Werner RN, Westfechtel L, Dressler C, Nast A. Self-administered interventions for anogenital warts in immunocompetent patients: a systematic review and meta-analysis. Sex Transm Infect. 2017;93(3):155–61.

11. Weidner T, Tittelbach J, Illing T, Elsner P. Gram-negative bacterial toe web infection-a systematic review. J Eur Acad Dermatol Venereol. 2018;32(1):39–47.

12. WHO guidelines for the treatment of *Genital Herpes Simplex Virus*. Geneva; 2016.

13. Chen F, Xu H, Liu J, et al. Efficacy and safety of nucleoside antiviral drugs for treatment of recurrent herpes labialis: a systematic review and meta-analysis. J Oral Pathol Med. 2017;46(8):561–8.

14. Hull CM, Harmenberg J, Arlander E, et al. Early treatment of cold sores with topical ME-609 decreases the frequency of ulcerative lesions: a randomized, double-blind, placebo-controlled, patient-initiated clinical trial. J Am Acad Dermatol. 2011;64(4):696. e691–611.

15. Tyring SK. Management of herpes zoster and postherpetic neuralgia. J Am Acad Dermatol. 2007;57(6 Suppl):S136–42.

16. Lewis DJ, Schlichte MJ, Dao H Jr. Atypical disseminated herpes zoster: management guidelines in immunocompromised patients. Cutis. 2017;100(5):321, 324, 330.

17. Johnson RW, Rice AS. Clinical practice. Postherpetic neuralgia. N Engl J Med. 2014;371(16):1526–33.

18. Wang JY, Wu YH, Liu SJ, Lin YS, Lu PH. Vitamin B12 for herpetic neuralgia: a meta-analysis of randomised controlled trials. Complement Ther Med. 2018;41:277–82.

19. Koning S, van der Sande R, Verhagen AP, et al. Interventions for impetigo. Cochrane Database Syst Rev. 2012;1:CD003261.

20. Hartman-Adams H, Banvard C, Juckett G. Impetigo: diagnosis and treatment. Am Fam Physician. 2014;90(4):229–35.

21. Metin A, Dilek N, Bilgili SG. Recurrent candidal intertrigo: challenges and solutions. Clin Cosmet Investig Dermatol. 2018;11:175–85.

22. Forbat E, Al-Niaimi F, Ali FR. Molluscum contagiosum: review and update on management. Pediatr Dermatol. 2017;34(5):504–15.

23. Jahnke MN, Hwang S, Griffith JL, Shwayder T. Cantharidin for treatment of facial molluscum contagiosum: a retrospective review. J Am Acad Dermatol. 2018;78(1):198–200.

24. Dohil M, Prendiville JS. Treatment of molluscum contagiosum with oral cimetidine: clinical experience in 13 patients. Pediatr Dermatol. 1996;13(4):310–2.

25. Rigopoulos D, Gregoriou S, Belyayeva E, Larios G, Kontochristopoulos G, Katsambas A. Efficacy and safety of tacrolimus ointment 0.1% vs. betamethasone 17-valerate 0.1% in the treatment of chronic paronychia: an unblinded randomized study. Br J Dermatol. 2009;160(4):858–60.

26. Tosti A, Piraccini BM, Ghetti E, Colombo MD. Topical steroids versus systemic antifungals in the treatment of chronic paronychia: an open, randomized double-blind and double dummy study. J Am Acad Dermatol. 2002;47(1):73–6.

27. Feldstein S, Totri C, Friedlander SF. Antifungal therapy for onychomycosis in children. Clin Dermatol. 2015;33(3):333–9.

28. Gupta AK, Paquet M. Systemic antifungals to treat onychomycosis in children: a systematic review. Pediatr Dermatol. 2013;30(3):294–302.

29. Gupta AK, Ryder JE, Johnson AM. Cumulative meta-analysis of systemic antifungal agents for the treatment of onychomycosis. Br J Dermatol. 2004;150(3):537–44.

30. Scher RK, Tavakkol A, Sigurgeirsson B, et al. Onychomycosis: diagnosis and definition of cure. J Am Acad Dermatol. 2007;56(6):939–44.
31. Simmons BJ, Griffith RD, Falto-Aizpurua LA, Nouri K. An update on photodynamic therapies in the treatment of onychomycosis. J Eur Acad Dermatol Venereol. 2015;29(7):1275–9.
32. Moon SH, Hur H, Oh YJ, et al. Treatment of onychomycosis with a 1,064-nm long-pulsed Nd:YAG laser. J Cosmet Laser Ther. 2014;16(4):165–70.
33. Weber GC, Firouzi P, Baran AM, et al. Treatment of onychomycosis using a 1064-nm diode laser with or without topical antifungal therapy: a single-center, retrospective analysis in 56 patients. Eur J Med Res. 2018;23(1):53.
34. Gupta AK, Drummond-Main C. Meta-analysis of randomized, controlled trials comparing particular doses of griseofulvin and terbinafine for the treatment of tinea capitis. Pediatr Dermatol. 2013;30(1):1–6.
35. Tey HL, Tan AS, Chan YC. Meta-analysis of randomized, controlled trials comparing griseofulvin and terbinafine in the treatment of tinea capitis. J Am Acad Dermatol. 2011;64(4):663–70.
36. Proudfoot LE, Higgins EM, Morris-Jones R. A retrospective study of the management of pediatric kerion in Trichophyton tonsurans infection. Pediatr Dermatol. 2011;28(6):655–7.
37. Croxtall JD, Plosker GL. Sertaconazole: a review of its use in the management of superficial mycoses in dermatology and gynaecology. Drugs. 2009;69(3):339–59.
38. Rotta I, Otuki MF, Sanches AC, Correr CJ. Efficacy of topical antifungal drugs in different dermatomycoses: a systematic review with meta-analysis. Rev Assoc Med Bras. 2012;58(3):308–18.
39. Gupta M, Mahajan VK, Mehta KS, Chauhan PS. Zinc therapy in dermatology: a review. Dermatol Res Pract. 2014;2014:709152.
40. Faergemann J, Gupta AK, Al Mofadi A, Abanami A, Shareaah AA, Marynissen G. Efficacy of itraconazole in the prophylactic treatment of pityriasis (tinea) versicolor. Arch Dermatol. 2002;138(1):69–73.
41. Chosidow O, Giraudeau B, Cottrell J, et al. Oral ivermectin versus malathion lotion for difficult-to-treat head lice. N Engl J Med. 2010;362(10):896–905.
42. Lebwohl M, Clark L, Levitt J. Therapy for head lice based on life cycle, resistance, and safety considerations. Pediatrics. 2007;119(5):965–74.
43. Foucault C, Ranque S, Badiaga S, Rovery C, Raoult D, Brouqui P. Oral ivermectin in the treatment of body lice. J Infect Dis. 2006;193(3):474–6.
44. Burkhart CG, Burkhart CN. Oral ivermectin for Phthirus pubis. J Am Acad Dermatol. 2004;51(6):1037; author reply 1037–1038.
45. KA W, GA B. Sexually transmitted diseases treatment guidelines, 2015. MMWR Recomm Rep. 2015;64(RR-03):1–137.
46. Park KK, Brodell RT, Helms SE. Angular cheilitis, part 1: local etiologies. Cutis. 2011;87(6):289–95.
47. Park KK, Brodell RT, Helms SE. Angular cheilitis, part 2: nutritional, systemic, and drug-related causes and treatment. Cutis. 2011;88(1):27–32.
48. Sharon V, Fazel N. Oral candidiasis and angular cheilitis. Dermatol Ther. 2010;23(3):230–42.
49. Rosumeck S, Nast A, Dressler C. Ivermectin and permethrin for treating scabies. Cochrane Database Syst Rev. 2018;4:CD012994.
50. Strong M, Johnstone P. Interventions for treating scabies. Cochrane Database Syst Rev. 2007;(3):CD000320.
51. Fox G. Diagnosis of scabies by dermoscopy. BMJ Case Rep. 2009;2009.
52. Clement ME, Okeke NL, Hicks CB. Treatment of syphilis: a systematic review. JAMA. 2014;312(18):1905–17.
53. Hook EWR. Syphilis. Lancet. 2016.
54. Mun JH, Kim SH, Jung DS, et al. Oral zinc sulfate treatment for viral warts: an open-label study. J Dermatol. 2011;38(6):541–5.

Common Cutaneous Side Effects of Anti-cancer Agents

Allison Zarbo and Anna Axelson

Cytotoxic Chemotherapies

- Introduction [1]
  - **Common Terminology Criteria for Adverse Events (CTCAE)**: a grading scale for severity of adverse events with unique clinical descriptions for each adverse event (Version 5 published Nov 27, 2017)
    - Please see version 5 here: https://ctep.cancer.gov/protocolDevelopment/electronic_applications/ctc.htm#ctc_50 to classify for specific entity (e.g., alopecia, bullous eruption, xerosis)
    - Each disorder has a unique set of maximum grade with appropriate description, and not all entities will reach grade 5 (death).
      - Grade 1: mild
      - Grade 2: moderate
      - Grade 3: severe or medically significant but not immediately life threatening
      - Grade 4: life threatening; urgent intervention indicated
      - Grade 5: death related to adverse event
  - **Common alkylating agents**

Common alkylating agents	
Sulfur mustards	Sulfur mustard
Nitrogen mustards	Mustargen (mechlorethamine) Cyclophosphamide Ifosfamide Melphalan Chlorambucil

A. Zarbo
Department of Dermatology, Henry Ford Health System, 3031 West Grand Blvd, Suite 800, Detroit, MI 48202, USA

A. Axelson (✉)
Henry Ford Health System, 3031 West Grand Blvd, Suite 800, Detroit, MI 48202, USA
e-mail: aaxelso1@hfhs.org

© Springer Nature Switzerland AG 2020
H. W. Lim et al. (eds.), *Practical Guide to Dermatology*,
https://doi.org/10.1007/978-3-030-18015-7_14

289

Common alkylating agents	
Aziridines and epoxides	Thiotepa Mitomycin
Alkyl sulfonates	Busulfan
Nitrosureas	Carmustin Streptozocin
Hydrazines and triazine derivatives	Procarbazine Dacarbazine

○ **Common antimetabolites**

Common antimetabolites	
Folate antagonist	Methotrexate Permetrexed
Pyrimidine analog	Capecitabine (prodrug of fluorouracil) Cytarabine Gemcitabine
Purine analog	Cladribine Mercaptopurine Thioguanine Fludarabine
Ribonucleotide reductase inhibitor	Hydroxyurea

○ **Anthracyclines**
  ■ Examples: doxorubicin, daunorubicin, epirubicin, and idarubicin

• **Common Reactions**

  ○ **Hand foot syndrome** [2–4] [5–10] [11–13]
    ■ Clinical presentation: initial tingling sensation in palms/soles, then tender diffuse, symmetric erythema with or without scale on the palms and soles, may progress to blistering and desquamation
    ■ Most often seen with cytarabine, pegylated liposomal doxorubicin, capecitabine, fluorouracil
    • May develop temporary loss of fingerprints with capecitabine
    ■ Different from hand-foot skin reaction seen with multitargeted tyrosine kinase inhibitors (MTKIs)

  ○ **Hair pigmentary changes** [14], [15]
    ■ "Flag sign" with methotrexate: alternating bands of hyperpigmentation of hair on the scalp, eyebrows and eyelashes which corresponds to treatment and no treatment
    ■ Cisplatin, cyclophosphamide, and combination regimens may abruptly change hair color

  ○ **Chemotherapy-induced alopecia** [16] [17][18, 19] [20–23]
    ■ Primarily anagen effluvium with onset 7–10 days, then most prominent 1–2 months after starting chemotherapy

- Cyclophosphamide and busulfan can cause permanent alopecia
- Docetaxol can cause prolonged and/or permanent alopecia
- Scalp cooling may minimize the alopecia, but not completely eliminate it
  - Use 30 min prior to infusion, throughout infusion and 90–120 min after infusion
  - Contraindicated in: Leukemias/lymphomas (systemic treatment required; discuss with primary team if a lymphoma); solid tumors with continuous-infusion chemotherapy > 1 day; cranial irradiation; sensitivity to cold; cold agglutinins; cryoglobulinemia; posttraumatic cold dystrophy; caution with abnormal liver function

○ **Subacute cutaneous lupus erythematosus** [24–26] [27] [28] [29]
  - Classic clinical presentation
  - Most common (MC): Taxanes, fluorouracil and capecitabine, doxorubicin with cyclophosphamide, gemcitabine

○ **Sclerodermoid-like changes** [30] [31] [32]
  - Clinical presentation: trunk and extremities with edema, tightening and indurated skin
  - MC: Bleomycin, gemcitabine, docetaxel

○ **Radiation recall dermatitis** [33, 34] [35] [15] [36] [37–40]
  - Clinical presentation: Previously irradiated skin with new onset acute inflammation with erythema after administration of chemotherapy; May present with vesiculation, desquamation, ulceration
  - MC: Dactinomycin, anthracyclines and anthracycline-like drugs

○ **Hyperpigmentation** [41, 42] [43] [44] [45, 46] [47] [15] [48] [49, 50] [51, 52] [53, 54]

Cutaneous and mucosal hyperpigmentation	
Generalized pattern	**Causative agents**
Diffuse	• Busulfan ("busulfan tan") • Methotrexate • Procarbazine
Diffuse and pressure induced	• Hydroxyurea • Cisplatin
Localized pattern	**Causative agents**
Flexural areas, palmar creases	• Bleomycin • Cyclophosphamide • Busulfan • Doxorubicin
Cutaneous and mucosal hyperpigmentation	• Busulfan • Cyclophosphamide (gingiva) • Tegafur (prodrug of 5- fluorouracil; lower lip, glans penis, also acral) • Doxorubicin (tongue, buccal mucosa) • Cisplatin • Fluorouracil

Cutaneous and mucosal hyperpigmentation	
Generalized pattern	**Causative agents**
Serpentine hyperpigmentation*	• Fluorouracil • Taxanes • CHOP (cyclophosphamide, doxorubicin, vincristine, prednisolone)
Flagellate hyperpigmentation	• Bleomycin (often with preceding generalized pruritus)
Reticular hyperpigmentation	• Pacitaxel • Cytarabine • Fluorouracil • Idarubicin

*Hyperpigmentation overlying vein proximal to injection site of chemotherapy

o **Nails** [55, 56] [57] [58] [48] [15, 59] [60, 61]

Nail changes		
Type	**Description**	**Causative agents**
Melanonychia	Onset 1–2 months after chemotherapy, may be associated with mucosal or cutaneous pigmentation, and may persist for years	•Fluorouracil • Alkylating agents •Taxanes •Antimetabolites •Anthracyclines
Leukonychia	White opaque discoloration	•Taxanes •Doxorubicin •Cyclophosphamide •Vincristine
Red/purple nail discoloration	Secondary to subungual hemorrhage	•Taxanes
Onycholysis	Detachment of the nail from the nail bed; prevent this with cold therapy to hands and feet to prevent the formation of subungual abscesses	•MC: taxanes •Cyclophosphamide •Doxorubicin •Etoposide •Fluorouracil •Hydroxyurea •Capecitabine •Ixabepilone •Bleomycin with vinblastine

▪ Multiple others: Beau's lines, onychomadesis, paronychia with or without pyogenic granulomas, subungual abscesses

o **Photosensitivity** [62] [58] [63] [64] [65, 66] [67–69] [68, 69] [70–73] [74]

Type of photosensitive reaction		
Type	Description	Causative agents
Phototoxic reaction	"Exaggerated sunburn", severe erythema, pain and tenderness of sun-exposed areas arising minutes to hours after exposure to UV light; blistering and PIH possible	•Vandetanib •Vemurafenib •Imatinib •Fluorouracil • Tegafur •Paclitaxel •Hydroxyurea •Dacarbazine •Vinblastine •Epirubicin
Photoallergic reaction	Type IV hypersensitivity with erythema, pruritus, and dermatitis extending beyond sun-exposed areas into the sun-protected areas which occurs 24 hours after UV light exposure	•Flutamide •Tegafur
Photorecall phenomenon	Administration of a chemotherapy triggers a similar sunburn which may have occurred months to years prior	•Methotrexate •Taxanes
Photoenhancement reaction	Chemotherapy administration triggers erythema in sun-exposed areas about 2–5 days after sun exposure	•High-dose methotrexate •Taxanes •Gemcitabine •Pegylated liposomal doxorubicin •Combination therapies •EGFR+ radiation
Photo-onycholysis	Detachment of the nail from the nail bed 2–4 weeks after drug administration	•Mercaptopurine

Targeted Therapies (solid tumors)

Epidermal Growth Factor Receptor (EGFR) Inhibitors [75] [76, 77] [78–81] [82–85] [86] [87] [83, 88] [76, 77, 89–91] [92]

- EGFR inhibitors

  - Monoclonal antibodies: Cetuximab, Panitumumab, Necitumumab
  - Small molecule EGFR inhibitors: Gefitinib, Erlotinib, Lapatinib, Afatinib, Osimertinib

- Papulopustular rashes
  - Clinical presentation: diffuse acneiform eruption with folliculocentric erythematous papules and pustules with or without pruritus on the face, trunk, extremities sparing the palms and soles; no comedonal component
  - Begins 1–2 weeks after EGFRi initiation and improves significantly around 8 weeks of treatment; if persists after 8 weeks of treatment, need to rule out superinfection
    - Dose-dependent

- Severity of rash positively correlated with survival; treatment of rash does not affect survival outcomes
  - MC cutaneous reaction, present in >80% of patients
  - Treatment pearls: petroleum jelly for xerosis, *strict* photoprotection, low-mid potency topical steroid ointments or oils for pruritus, topical antibiotic, systemic antibiotics if needed (doxycycline or minocycline, cautioning on photosensitivity)

- PRIDE syndrome
  - **P**apulopustules and/or **p**aronychia
  - **R**egulatory abnormalities of hair growth
  - **I**tching
  - **D**ryness due to **e**pidermal growth factor receptor inhibitors

Summary of EGFR inhibitor reactions	
Site of reaction	**Type of reaction**
Cutaneous	Papulopustular rashes (see above) Exfoliative eruptions Bullous eruptions Hand-foot skin reaction (see MTKIs) Pruritus Telangiectasias Urticaria Xerosis and desquamation
Mucosa	Aphthous ulcerations or oral, nasal mucosa
Hair	Abnormal or change in scalp, facial hair or eyelash growth
Nails	Paronychia +/− pyogenic granuloma

Multitargeted Small Molecule Tyrosine Kinase Inhibitors
[93] [94, 95] [96] [97, 98] [99] [100] [101–107] [108–110] [111, 112] [113, 114] [32] [115] [116, 117] [115, 116]

- Multitargeted small molecule tyrosine kinase inhibitors
  - Sorafenib, sunitinib, pazopanib, regorafenib, axitinib, cabozantinib

Reactions to sorafenib and sunitinib	
Site of reaction	**Type of reaction**
Cutaneous	Acquired perforating dermatosis Eruptive melanocytic lesions Erythema multiforme and EM-like eruptions Exanthematous rashes Hand-foot skin reaction (see below) Keratoacanthomas, squamous cell carcinoma* Pyoderma gangrenosum** Scalp dysesthesia Seborrheic dermatitis-like reaction SJS Yellow discoloration of skin** Xerosis

Reactions to sorafenib and sunitinib	
Site of reaction	Type of reaction
Mucosa	Mucositis Geographic tongue
Hair	Alopecia - temporary Hair depigmentation - reversible upon drug holiday or discontinuation
Nails	Subungual splinter hemorrhages Periungual erythema

*MC sorafenib
**MC sunitinib

- **Hand-foot skin reaction**: [100] [118, 119] [5, 120] [121] [122–127]
  - MC sorafenib and sunitinib, ~40% of patients; different from hand foot syndrome induced by traditional chemotherapies
  - Clinical presentation: localized areas on the palms, soles, interdigital web spaces, and lateral aspects of the feet with focal hyperkeratotic callus-like lesions on an erythematous base with onset approximately 2–4 weeks after initiation of therapy
  - Associated with paresthesias, tingling, burning, soreness, decreased tolerance with hot objects, and can impair ADLs and QOL
  - Associated with increased tumor response rate and overall survival
  - Manage with cushioned shoes, decrease friction, keratolytics +/- topical retinoids, topical steroids if erythema, topical lidocaine, acitretin, oral/topical gabapentin

BRAF Inhibitors [128] [129] [130–135] [130, 136] [137] [129–132] [130–132, 138] [129] [130, 131, 139] [140, 141] [142–144] [132–135] [145, 146] [129–132] [129–132, 147] [148]

- BRAF inhibitors, and encorafenib
  - Vemurafenib, dabrafenib, and encorafenib

Reactions to BRAF inhibitors	
Site of reaction	Type of reaction
Cutaneous	Eruptive nevi [v] Grover disease [d] Keratoacanthomas* Melanoma—second primary [d] - Unclear if secondary to therapy or higher risk at baseline due to primary melanoma Papulopustular eruption* Photosensitivity [v] Plantar hyperkeratosis [d] Pyogenic granulomas [v] Radiation enhancement [v] SJS/TEN [v] Benign and malignant squamous proliferative disorders * Highest risk in patients >60yo, first 3 months of treatment; occur in sun-protected sites more commonly than sporadic SCCs; risk is decreased when combined with MEK inhibitors Xerosis*

Reactions to BRAF inhibitors	
Site of reaction	Type of reaction
Hair	Alopecia +/– structural hair changes*
Nails	Acute paronychia[v]
	Brittle nails [v]
	Onycholysis [d]

*Vemurafenib and dabrafenib
[v]Vemurafenib
[d]Dabrafenib

MEK Inhibitors [149] [150] [151] [148]

- MEK inhibitors
  - Trametinib and cobimetinib

- Trametinib
  - Cutaneous reactions
    - Acneiform rash
    - Pruritus
    - Xerosis
  - One case report of DVT in patient on trametinib and dabrafenib

- Cobimetinib
  - Cutaneous reactions
    - Acneiform eruption
    - Photosensitivity
  - Nail changes: paronychia and onycholysis

Targeted therapies (hematologic malignancies)

- **Bruton tyrosine kinase (BTK) inhibitors**(ibrutinib, acalabrutinib)[1, 2]
  - MC petechiae, ecchymoses, hematomas, bleeding diathesis
  - Non-palpable petechial eruption
  - Palpable purpuric rash (clinically resembling leukocytoclastic vasculitis)
  - Neutrophilic panniculitis

---

[1]Iberri DJ, Kwong BY, Stevens LA, Coutre SE, Kim J, Sabile JM, Advani RH. Ibrutinib-associated rash: a single-centre experience of clinicopathological features and management. Br J Haematol.
[2]Stewart J, Bayers S, Vandergriff T. Self-limiting Ibrutinib-Induced Neutrophilic Panniculitis. Am J Dermatopathol. 2018 Feb; 40(2):e28–e29.

- **BCR-ABL inhibitors** (imatinib, dasatinib, nilotinib, bosutinib, ponatinib)[3], [4]: cutaneous reactions common, usually low grade
  - Non-specific dermatitis with morbilliform papules on face>trunk>extremities
  - Lichenoid dermatitis
  - Pruritus: common and can be severe
  - Periorbital edema: around 6 weeks after initiation
  - Pigmentary changes: blue-grey hyperpigmentation in darker skin or hypopigmentation

- **Proteasome inhibitors** (bortezomib, carfilzomib, ixazomib)[5]
  - Erythematous nodules and plaques
  - Morbilliform exanthem or maculopapular rash, with small vessel vasculitis on pathology but no associated systemic vasculitis
  - Sweet syndrome

- **PI3Kδ inhibitors** (idelalisib, duvelisib, and copanlisib)[6], [7]
  - Non-specific maculopapular rash in 10–20% but severe in up to 2%
  - Desquamative/exfoliative erythroderma with islands of sparing and keratoderma, "EM-like" epidermal necrosis on pathology
  - May have delayed onset and protracted course

Checkpoint Inhibitors [152] [153] [154] [155] [153, 156] [157, 158] [159] [160]

- **Programmed cell death receptor 1 (PD-1) inhibitors**
  - Nivolumab, pembrolizumab, and cemiplimab
  - PD-1 is on the T cell

[3]Dervis E, Ayer M, Akin Belli A, Barut SG. Cutaneous adverse reactions of imatinib therapy in patients with chronic myeloid leukemia: A six-year follow up. Eur J Dermatol. 2016 Apr 1;26(2):133–7.

[4]Penn EH, Chung HJ, Keller M. Imatinib mesylate-induced lichenoid drug eruption. Cutis. 2017 Mar; 99(3):189–192. Review.

[5]Al-Dawsari, Najla, et al. "Chapter 20: Histone Deacetylase Inhibitors, Proteasome Inhibitors, Demthylating Agents, Arsenicals, Retinoids." Dermatologic Principles and Practice in Oncology: Conditions of the Skin, Hair, and Nails in Cancer Patients, by Mario E. Lacouture, Wiley-Blackwell, 2014, pp. 216–217.

[6]Gabriel JG, Kapila A, Gonzalez-Estrada A. A Severe Case of Cutaneous Adverse Drug Reaction Secondary to a Novice Drug: Idelalisib. J Investig Med High Impact Case Rep. 2017 May 24; 5(2):2324709617711463.

[7]de Weerdt I, Koopmans SM, Kater AP, van Gelder M. Incidence and management of toxicity associated with ibrutinib and idelalisib: a practical approach. Haematologica. 2017 Oct; 102(10):1629–1639. doi: 10.3324/haematol.2017.164103. Epub 2017 Aug 3. Review.

- **Programmed cell death receptor ligand 1 (PD-L1) inhibitors**
  - ○ Atezolizumab, avelumab and durvalumab
  - ○ PD-L1 is on tumor cells
  - ○ PEARL: PD-1 and PD-L1: can get delayed reactions, up to months and years

- **Cytotoxic T-lymphocyte-associated antigen 4 (CTLA-4)**
  - ○ Ipilimumab and tremelimumab (in development)
  - ○ Side effects are due to immunologic enhancement and include dermatologic, rheumatologic, gastrointestinal, hepatic, endocrinologic
    - ■ Treatment includes immunosuppression, dose modification and cessation of therapy

Reactions to checkpoint inhibitors	
Site of reaction	**Type of reaction**
Cutaneous	Bullous disorders including BP Follicular eruption Granulomas to filler and tattoo ink Lichenoid dermatitis Maculopapular eruption Papulopustular eruption Pruritus without dermatitis Psoriasis/psoriasiform dermatitis SJS/TEN Sweet's syndrome Urticarial eruption Vitiligo
Mucosa	Gingivitis Lichenoid mucositis Mucositis (PD-1 inhibitors >> CTLA-4 inhibitors) Sicca syndrome
Hair	Alopecia (c/walopecia areata)

References

1. National Institutes of Health NCI. Common Terminology Criteria for Adverse Events (CTCAE), Version 5.0 Nov, 2017. https://ctep.cancer.gov/protocoldevelopment/electronic_applications/docs/CTCAE_v5_Quick_Reference_8.5x11.pdf.
2. Cohen PR. Acral erythema: a clinical review. Cutis. 1993;51(3):175–9.
3. Burgdorf WH, Gilmore WA, Ganick RG. Peculiar acral erythema secondary to high-dose chemotherapy for acute myelogenous leukemia. Ann Intern Med. 1982;97(1):61–2.
4. Hood AF, Haynes HA. Dermatologic complications. In: Holland JF, editor. Cancer medicine. 4th ed. Baltimore: Williams & Wilkins; 1997.
5. Miller KK, Gorcey L, McLellan BN. Chemotherapy-induced hand-foot syndrome and nail changes: a review of clinical presentation, etiology, pathogenesis, and management. J Am Acad Dermatol. 2014;71(4):787–94.
6. Hoff PM, Valero V, Ibrahim N, Willey J, Hortobagyi GN. Hand-foot syndrome following prolonged infusion of high doses of vinorelbine. Cancer. 1998;82(5):965–9.
7. Eich D, Scharffetter-Kochanek K, Eich HT, Tantcheva-Poor I, Krieg T. Acral erythrodysesthesia syndrome caused by intravenous infusion of docetaxel in breast cancer. Am J Clin Oncol. 2002;25(6):599–602.

8. Ozmen S, Dogru M, Bozkurt C, Kocaoglu AC. Probable cytarabine-induced acral erythema: report of 2 pediatric cases. J Pediatr Hematol Oncol. 2013;35(1):e11–3.
9. Farr KP, Safwat A. Palmar-plantar erythrodysesthesia associated with chemotherapy and its treatment. Case Rep Oncol. 2011;4(1):229–35.
10. Karol SE, Yang W, Smith C, Cheng C, Stewart CF, Baker SD, et al. Palmar-plantar erythro-dysesthesia syndrome following treatment with high-dose methotrexate or high-dose cytara-bine. Cancer. 2017;123(18):3602–8.
11. Wong M, Choo SP, Tan EH. Travel warning with capecitabine. Ann Oncol Off J Eur Soc Med Oncol. 2009;20(7):1281.
12. Chavarri-Guerra Y, Soto-Perez-de-Celis E. Images in clinical medicine. Loss of fingerprints. N Engl J Med. 2015;372(16):e22.
13. Al-Ahwal MS. Chemotherapy and fingerprint loss: beyond cosmetic. Oncologist. 2012;17(2):291–3.
14. Wheeland RG, Burgdorf WH, Humphrey GB. The flag sign of chemotherapy. Cancer. 1983;51(8):1356–8.
15. Susser WS, Whitaker-Worth DL, Grant-Kels JM. Mucocutaneous reactions to chemother-apy. J Am Acad Derm. 1999;40(3):367–98; (quiz 99–400).
16. Hood AF. Cutaneous side effects of cancer chemotherapy. Med Clin N Am. 1986;70(1):187–209.
17. Baker BW, Wilson CL, Davis AL, Spearing RL, Hart DN, Heaton DC, et al. Busulphan/cyclophosphamide conditioning for bone marrow transplantation may lead to failure of hair regrowth. Bone Marrow Transpl. 1991;7(1):43–7.
18. van den Hurk CJ, Breed WP, Nortier JW. Short post-infusion scalp cooling time in the pre-vention of docetaxel-induced alopecia. Support Care Cancer Off J Multinatl Assoc Support Care Cancer. 2012;20(12):3255–60.
19. Komen MM, Breed WP, Smorenburg CH, van der Ploeg T, Goey SH, van der Hoeven JJ, et al. Results of 20- versus 45-min post-infusion scalp cooling time in the prevention of docetaxel-induced alopecia. Support Care Cancer Off J Multinatl Assoc Support Care Can-cer. 2016;24(6):2735–41.
20. Komen MM, Smorenburg CH, van den Hurk CJ, Nortier JW. Factors influencing the effec-tiveness of scalp cooling in the prevention of chemotherapy-induced alopecia. Oncologist. 2013;18(7):885–91.
21. Kluger N, Jacot W, Frouin E, Rigau V, Poujol S, Dereure O, et al. Permanent scalp alopecia related to breast cancer chemotherapy by sequential fluorouracil/epirubicin/cyclophospha-mide (FEC) and docetaxel: a prospective study of 20 patients. Ann Oncol Off J Eur Soc Med Oncol. 2012;23(11):2879–84.
22. Tallon B, Blanchard E, Goldberg LJ. Permanent chemotherapy-induced alopecia: case report and review of the literature. J Am Acad Dermatol. 2010;63(2):333–6.
23. Fonia A, Cota C, Setterfield JF, Goldberg LJ, Fenton DA, Stefanato CM. Permanent alo-pecia in patients with breast cancer after taxane chemotherapy and adjuvant hormo-nal therapy: Clinicopathologic findings in a cohort of 10 patients. J Am Acad Dermatol. 2017;76(5):948–57.
24. Chen M, Crowson AN, Woofter M, Luca MB, Magro CM. Docetaxel (taxotere) induced suba-cute cutaneous lupus erythematosus: report of 4 cases. J Rheumatol. 2004;31(4):818–20.
25. Marchetti MA, Noland MM, Dillon PM, Greer KE. Taxane associated subacute cutaneous lupus erythematosus. Dermatol Online J. 2013;19(8):19259.
26. Adachi A, Horikawa T. Paclitaxel-induced cutaneous lupus erythematosus in patients with serum anti-SSA/Ro antibody. J Dermatol. 2007;34(7):473–6.
27. Weger W, Kranke B, Gerger A, Salmhofer W, Aberer E. Occurrence of subacute cutaneous lupus erythematosus after treatment with fluorouracil and capecitabine. J Am Acad Derma-tol. 2008;59(2 Suppl 1):S4–6.
28. Funke AA, Kulp-Shorten CL, Callen JP. Subacute cutaneous lupus erythematosus exacer-bated or induced by chemotherapy. Arch Dermatol. 2010;146(10):1113–6.

29. Wiznia LE, Subtil A, Choi JN. Subacute cutaneous lupus erythematosus induced by chemotherapy: gemcitabine as a causative agent. JAMA Dermatol. 2013;149(9):1071–5.
30. Passiu G, Cauli A, Atzeni F, Aledda M, Dessole G, Sanna G, et al. Bleomycin-induced scleroderma: report of a case with a chronic course rather than the typical acute/subacute self-limiting form. Clin Rheumatol. 1999;18(5):422–4.
31. Bessis D, Guillot B, Legouffe E, Guilhou JJ. Gemcitabine-associated scleroderma-like changes of the lower extremities. J Am Acad Dermatol. 2004;51(2 Suppl):S73–6.
32. Heidary N, Naik H, Burgin S. Chemotherapeutic agents and the skin: an update. J Am Acad Dermatol. 2008;58(4):545–70.
33. Shenkier T, Gelmon K. Paclitaxel and radiation-recall dermatitis. J Clin Oncol Off J Am Soc Clin Oncol. 1994;12(2):439.
34. Parry BR. Radiation recall induced by tamoxifen. Lancet (London, England). 1992;340(8810):49.
35. Burris HA 3rd, Hurtig J. Radiation recall with anticancer agents. Oncologist. 2010;15(11):1227–37.
36. D'Angio GJ, Farber S, Maddock CL. Potentiation of x-ray effects by actinomycin D. Radiology. 1959;73:175–7.
37. Camidge R, Price A. Characterizing the phenomenon of radiation recall dermatitis. Radiother Oncol J Eur Soc Ther Radiol Oncol. 2001;59(3):237–45.
38. Schwartz BM, Khuntia D, Kennedy AW, Markman M. Gemcitabine-induced radiation recall dermatitis following whole pelvic radiation therapy. Gynecol Oncol. 2003;91(2):421–2.
39. Camidge R, Price A. Radiation recall dermatitis may represent the Koebner phenomenon. J Clin Oncol Off J Am Soc Clin Oncol. 2002;20(19):4130; author reply.
40. Gzell CE, Carroll SL, Suchowerska N, Beith J, Tan K, Scolyer RA. Radiation recall dermatitis after pre-sensitization with pegylated liposomal doxorubicin. Cancer Invest. 2009;27(4):397–401.
41. Korbitz BC, Reiquam CW. Busulfan in chronic granulocytic leukemia, a spectrum of clinical considerations. Clin Med. 1969;76(16).
42. Bandini G, Belardinelli A, Rosti G, Calori E, Motta MR, Rizzi S, et al. Toxicity of high-dose busulphan and cyclophosphamide as conditioning therapy for allogeneic bone marrow transplantation in adults with haematological malignancies. Bone Marrow Transpl. 1994;13(5):577–81.
43. Bronner AK, Hood AF. Cutaneous complications of chemotherapeutic agents. J Am Acad Dermatol. 1983;9(5):645–63.
44. Hendrix JD Jr, Greer KE. Cutaneous hyperpigmentation caused by systemic drugs. Int J Dermatol. 1992;31(7):458–66.
45. Issaivanan M, Mitu PS, Manisha C, Praveen K. Cutaneous manifestations of hydroxyurea therapy in childhood: case report and review. Pediatr Dermatol. 2004;21(2):124–7.
46. Aste N, Fumo G, Contu F, Aste N, Biggio P. Nail pigmentation caused by hydroxyurea: report of 9 cases. J Am Acad Dermatol. 2002;47(1):146–7.
47. Al-Lamki Z, Pearson P, Jaffe N. Localized cisplatin hyperpigmentation induced by pressure. A case report. Cancer. 1996;77(8):1578–81.
48. Payne AS, James WD, Weiss RB. Dermatologic toxicity of chemotherapeutic agents. Semin Oncol. 2006;33(1):86–97.
49. Schulte-Huermann P, Zumdick M, Ruzicka T. Supravenous hyperpigmentation in association with CHOP chemotherapy of a CD30 (Ki-1)-positive anaplastic large-cell lymphoma. Dermatology (Basel, Switzerland). 1995;191(1):65–7.
50. Baselga E, Drolet BA, Casper J, Esterly NB. Chemotherapy-associated supravenous hyperpigmentation. Dermatology (Basel, Switzerland). 1996;192(4):384–5.
51. Todkill D, Taibjee S, Borg A, Gee BC. Flagellate erythema due to bleomycin. Br J Haematol. 2008;142(6):857.
52. Mowad CM, Nguyen TV, Elenitsas R, Leyden JJ. Bleomycin-induced flagellate dermatitis: a clinical and histopathological review. Br J Dermatol. 1994;131(5):700–2.

53. Cohen PR. Paclitaxel-associated reticulate hyperpigmentation: Report and review of chemotherapy-induced reticulate hyperpigmentation. World J Clin Cases. 2016;4(12):390–400.

54. Masson Regnault M, Gadaud N, Boulinguez S, Tournier E, Lamant L, Gladieff L, et al. Chemotherapy-related reticulate hyperpigmentation: a case series and review of the literature. Dermatology (Basel, Switzerland). 2015;231(4):312–8.

55. Robert C, Sibaud V, Mateus C, Verschoore M, Charles C, Lanoy E, et al. Nail toxicities induced by systemic anticancer treatments. Lancet Oncol. 2015;16(4):e181–9.

56. Sibaud V, Fricain JC, Baran R, Robert C. [Pigmentary disorders induced by anti-cancer agents. part I: chemotherapy]. Annales de dermatologie et de venereologie. 2013;140(3):183–96.

57. Sibaud V, Leboeuf NR, Roche H, Belum VR, Gladieff L, Deslandres M, et al. Dermatological adverse events with taxane chemotherapy. Eur J Dermatol EJD. 2016;26(5):427–43.

58. Chapman S, Cohen PR. Transverse leukonychia in patients receiving cancer chemotherapy. South Med J. 1997;90(4):395–8.

59. Alimonti A, Nardoni C, Papaldo P, Ferretti G, Caleno MP, Carlini P, et al. Nail disorders in a woman treated with ixabepilone for metastatic breast cancer. Anticancer Res. 2005;25(5):3531–2.

60. Scotte F, Tourani JM, Banu E, Peyromaure M, Levy E, Marsan S, et al. Multicenter study of a frozen glove to prevent docetaxel-induced onycholysis and cutaneous toxicity of the hand. J Clin Oncol Off J Am Soc Clin Oncol. 2005;23(19):4424–9.

61. Scotte F, Banu E, Medioni J, Levy E, Ebenezer C, Marsan S, et al. Matched case-control phase 2 study to evaluate the use of a frozen sock to prevent docetaxel-induced onycholysis and cutaneous toxicity of the foot. Cancer. 2008;112(7):1625–31.

62. Gonzalez E, Gonzalez S. Drug photosensitivity, idiopathic photodermatoses, and sunscreens. J Am Acad Dermatol. 1996;35(6):871–85; (quiz 86–7).

63. Monteiro AF, Rato M, Martins C. Drug-induced photosensitivity: photoallergic and phototoxic reactions. Clin Dermatol. 2016;34(5):571–81.

64. Leroy D, Dompmartin A, Szczurko C. Flutamide photosensitivity. Photodermatol Photoimmunol Photomed. 1996;12(5):216–8.

65. Usuki A, Funasaka Y, Oka M, Ichihashi M. Tegafur-induced photosensitivity–evaluation of provocation by UVB irradiation. Int J Dermatol. 1997;36(8):604–6.

66. Fujimoto M, Kikuchi K, Imakado S, Furue M. Photosensitive dermatitis induced by flutamide. Br J Dermatol. 1996;135(3):496–7.

67. Goldfeder KL, Levin JM, Katz KA, Clarke LE, Loren AW, James WD. Ultraviolet recall reaction after total body irradiation, etoposide, and methotrexate therapy. J Am Acad Dermatol. 2007;56(3):494–9.

68. Ee HL, Yosipovitch G. Photo recall phenomenon: an adverse reaction to taxanes. Dermatology (Basel, Switzerland). 2003;207(2):196–8.

69. Droitcourt C, Le Ho H, Adamski H, Le Gall F, Dupuy A. Docetaxel-induced photo-recall phenomenon. Photodermatol Photoimmunol Photomed. 2012;28(4):222–3.

70. Williams BJ, Roth DJ, Callen JP. Ultraviolet recall associated with etoposide and cyclophosphamide therapy. Clin Exp Dermatol. 1993;18(5):452–3.

71. Andersen KE, Lindskov R. Recall of UVB-induced erythema in breast cancer patient receiving multiple drug chemotherapy. Photodermatol. 1984;1(3):129–32.

72. Badger J, Kang S, Uzieblo A, Srinivas S. Double diagnosis in cancer patients and cutaneous reaction related to gemcitabine: CASE 3. Photo therapy recall with gemcitabine following ultraviolet B treatment. J Clin Oncol Off J Am Soc Clin Oncol. 2005;23(28):7224–5.

73. Markman M, Kulp B, Peterson G. Grade 3 liposomal-doxorubicin-induced skin toxicity in a patient following complete resolution of moderately severe sunburn. Gynecol Oncol. 2004;94(2):578–80.

74. Gould JW, Mercurio MG, Elmets CA. Cutaneous photosensitivity diseases induced by exogenous agents. J Am Acad Dermatol. 1995;33(4):551–73; (quiz 74-6).

75. Payne AS, Savarese DMF. Cutaneous side effects of molecularly targeted therapy and other biologic agents used for cancer therapy 2018, 24 Apr 2018. https://www.uptodate.com/contents/cutaneous-side-effects-of-molecularly-targeted-therapy-and-other-biologic-agents-used-for-cancer-therapy.

76. Kimyai-Asadi A, Jih MH. Follicular toxic effects of chimeric anti-epidermal growth factor receptor antibody cetuximab used to treat human solid tumors. Arch Dermatol. 2002;138(1):129–31.

77. Van Doorn R, Kirtschig G, Scheffer E, Stoof TJ, Giaccone G. Follicular and epidermal alterations in patients treated with ZD1839 (Iressa), an inhibitor of the epidermal growth factor receptor. Br J Dermatol. 2002;147(3):598–601.

78. Agero AL, Dusza SW, Benvenuto-Andrade C, Busam KJ, Myskowski P, Halpern AC. Dermatologic side effects associated with the epidermal growth factor receptor inhibitors. J Am Acad Dermatol. 2006;55(4):657–70.

79. Cunningham D, Humblet Y, Siena S, Khayat D, Bleiberg H, Santoro A, et al. Cetuximab monotherapy and cetuximab plus irinotecan in irinotecan-refractory metastatic colorectal cancer. N Engl J Med. 2004;351(4):337–45.

80. Perez-Soler R. Rash as a surrogate marker for efficacy of epidermal growth factor receptor inhibitors in lung cancer. Clin Lung Cancer. 2006;8(Suppl 1):S7–14.

81. Perez-Soler R, Saltz L. Cutaneous adverse effects with HER1/EGFR-targeted agents: is there a silver lining? J Clin Oncol Off J Am Soc Clin Oncol. 2005;23(22):5235–46.

82. Jacot W, Bessis D, Jorda E, Ychou M, Fabbro M, Pujol JL, et al. Acneiform eruption induced by epidermal growth factor receptor inhibitors in patients with solid tumours. Br J Dermatol. 2004;151(1):238–41.

83. Busam KJ, Capodieci P, Motzer R, Kiehn T, Phelan D, Halpern AC. Cutaneous side-effects in cancer patients treated with the antiepidermal growth factor receptor antibody C225. Br J Dermatol. 2001;144(6):1169–76.

84. Moy B, Goss PE. Lapatinib-associated toxicity and practical management recommendations. Oncologist. 2007;12(7):756–65.

85. Jatoi A, Green EM, Rowland KM Jr, Sargent DJ, Alberts SR. Clinical predictors of severe cetuximab-induced rash: observations from 933 patients enrolled in north central cancer treatment group study N0147. Oncology. 2009;77(2):120–3.

86. Lin WL, Lin WC, Yang JY, Chang YC, Ho HC, Yang LC, et al. Fatal toxic epidermal necrolysis associated with cetuximab in a patient with colon cancer. J Clin Oncol Off J Am Soc Clin Oncology. 2008;26(16):2779–80.

87. Ensslin CJ, Rosen AC, Wu S, Lacouture ME. Pruritus in patients treated with targeted cancer therapies: systematic review and meta-analysis. J Am Acad Dermatol. 2013;69(5):708–20.

88. Lee MW, Seo CW, Kim SW, Yang HJ, Lee HW, Choi JH, et al. Cutaneous side effects in non-small cell lung cancer patients treated with Iressa (ZD1839), an inhibitor of epidermal growth factor. Acta Derm Venereol. 2004;84(1):23–6.

89. Nowak AK, Byrne MJ. Cisplatin and gemcitabine in malignant mesothelioma. Ann Oncol Off J Eur Soc Med Oncol. 2005;16(10):1711.

90. Dueland S, Sauer T, Lund-Johansen F, Ostenstad B, Tveit KM. Epidermal growth factor receptor inhibition induces trichomegaly. Acta Oncol (Stockholm, Sweden). 2003;42(4):345–6.

91. Pascual JC, Banuls J, Belinchon I, Blanes M, Massuti B. Trichomegaly following treatment with gefitinib (ZD1839). Br J Dermatol. 2004;151(5):1111–2.

92. Dainichi T, Tanaka M, Tsuruta N, Furue M, Noda K. Development of multiple paronychia and periungual granulation in patients treated with gefitinib, an inhibitor of epidermal growth factor receptor. Dermatology (Basel, Switzerland). 2003;207(3):324–5.

93. Severino-Freire M, Sibaud V, Tournier E, Pauwels C, Christol C, Lamant L, et al. Acquired perforating dermatosis associated with sorafenib therapy. J Eur Acad Dermatol Venereol JEADV. 2016;30(2):328–30.

94. Kong HH, Sibaud V, Chanco Turner ML, Fojo T, Hornyak TJ, Chevreau C. Sorafenib-induced eruptive melanocytic lesions. Arch Dermatol. 2008;144(6):820–2.

95. Jimenez-Gallo D, Albarran-Planelles C, Linares-Barrios M, Martinez-Rodriguez A, Baez-Perea JM. Eruptive melanocytic nevi in a patient undergoing treatment with sunitinib. JAMA Dermatol. 2013;149(5):624–6.

96. Ikeda M, Fujita T, Mii S, Tanabe K, Tabata K, Matsumoto K, et al. Erythema multiforme induced by sorafenib for metastatic renal cell carcinoma. Jpn J Clin Oncol. 2012;42(9):820–4.

97. Lewin J, Farley-Loftus R, Pomeranz MK. Erythema multiforme-like drug reaction to sorafenib. J Drugs Dermatol JDD. 2011;10(12):1462–3.

98. Pichard DC, Cardones AR, Chu EY, Dahut WL, Kong HH. Sorafenib-Induced Eruption Mimicking Erythema Multiforme. JAMA Dermatol. 2016;152(2):227–8.

99. Robert C, Mateus C, Spatz A, Wechsler J, Escudier B. Dermatologic symptoms associated with the multikinase inhibitor sorafenib. J Am Acad Dermatol. 2009;60(2):299–305.

100. Lacouture ME, Reilly LM, Gerami P, Guitart J. Hand foot skin reaction in cancer patients treated with the multikinase inhibitors sorafenib and sunitinib. Ann Oncol Off J Eur Soc Med Oncol. 2008;19(11):1955–61.

101. Arnault JP, Wechsler J, Escudier B, Spatz A, Tomasic G, Sibaud V, et al. Keratoacanthomas and squamous cell carcinomas in patients receiving sorafenib. J Clin Oncol Off J Am Soc Clin Oncol. 2009;27(23):e59–61.

102. Dubauskas Z, Kunishige J, Prieto VG, Jonasch E, Hwu P, Tannir NM. Cutaneous squamous cell carcinoma and inflammation of actinic keratoses associated with sorafenib. Clin Genitourin Cancer. 2009;7(1):20–3.

103. Kong HH, Cowen EW, Azad NS, Dahut W, Gutierrez M, Turner ML. Keratoacanthomas associated with sorafenib therapy. J Am Acad Dermatol. 2007;56(1):171–2.

104. Hong DS, Reddy SB, Prieto VG, Wright JJ, Tannir NM, Cohen PR, et al. Multiple squamous cell carcinomas of the skin after therapy with sorafenib combined with tipifarnib. Arch Dermatol. 2008;144(6):779–82.

105. Smith KJ, Haley H, Hamza S, Skelton HG. Eruptive keratoacanthoma-type squamous cell carcinomas in patients taking sorafenib for the treatment of solid tumors. Dermatol Surg Off Publ Am Soc Dermatol Surg. 2009;35(11):1766–70.

106. Kwon EJ, Kish LS, Jaworsky C. The histologic spectrum of epithelial neoplasms induced by sorafenib. J Am Acad Dermatol. 2009;61(3):522–7.

107. Jantzem H, Dupre-Goetghebeur D, Spindler P, Merrer J. Sorafenib-induced multiple eruptive keratoacanthomas. Ann Dermatol Venereol. 2009;136(12):894–7.

108. Nadauld LD, Miller MB, Srinivas S. Pyoderma gangrenosum with the use of sunitinib. J Clin Oncol Off J Am Soc Clin Oncol. 2011;29(10):e266–7.

109. Dean SM, Zirwas M. A Second Case of Sunitinib-associated Pyoderma Gangrenosum. The Journal of clinical and aesthetic dermatology. 2010;3(8):34–5.

110. ten Freyhaus K, Homey B, Bieber T, Wilsmann-Theis D. Pyoderma gangrenosum: another cutaneous side-effect of sunitinib? Br J Dermatol. 2008;159(1):242–3.

111. Rini BI, Escudier B, Tomczak P, Kaprin A, Szczylik C, Hutson TE, et al. Comparative effectiveness of axitinib versus sorafenib in advanced renal cell carcinoma (AXIS): a randomised phase 3 trial. Lancet (London, England). 2011;378(9807):1931–9.

112. Autier J, Escudier B, Wechsler J, Spatz A, Robert C. Prospective study of the cutaneous adverse effects of sorafenib, a novel multikinase inhibitor. Arch Dermatol. 2008;144(7):886–92.

113. Ikeda M, Fujita T, Amoh Y, Mii S, Matsumoto K, Iwamura M. Stevens-Johnson syndrome induced by sorafenib for metastatic renal cell carcinoma. Urol Int. 2013;91(4):482–3.

114. Lee JH, Lee JH, Lee JH, Kim SY, Kim GM. Case of sunitinib-induced Stevens-Johnson syndrome. J Dermatol. 2013;40(9):753–4.

115. Suwattee P, Chow S, Berg BC, Warshaw EM. Sunitinib: a cause of bullous palmoplantar erythrodysesthesia, periungual erythema, and mucositis. Arch Dermatol. 2008;144(1):123–5.

116. Hubiche T, Valenza B, Chevreau C, Fricain JC, Del Giudice P, Sibaud V. Geographic tongue induced by angiogenesis inhibitors. Oncologist. 2013;18(4):e16–7.
117. Gavrilovic IT, Balagula Y, Rosen AC, Ramaswamy V, Dickler MN, Dunkel IJ, et al. Characteristics of oral mucosal events related to bevacizumab treatment. Oncologist. 2012;17(2):274–8.
118. Abdel-Rahman O, Fouad M. Risk of mucocutaneous toxicities in patients with solid tumors treated with sunitinib: a critical review and meta analysis. Expert Rev Anticancer Ther. 2015;15(1):129–41.
119. Zhang L, Zhou Q, Ma L, Wu Z, Wang Y. Meta-analysis of dermatological toxicities associated with sorafenib. Clin Exp Dermatol. 2011;36(4):344–50.
120. McLellan B, Ciardiello F, Lacouture ME, Segaert S, Van Cutsem E. Regorafenib-associated hand-foot skin reaction: practical advice on diagnosis, prevention, and management. Ann Oncol Off J Eur Soc Med Oncol. 2015;26(10):2017–26.
121. McLellan B, Kerr H. Cutaneous toxicities of the multikinase inhibitors sorafenib and sunitinib. Dermatol Ther. 2011;24(4):396–400.
122. Jain L, Sissung TM, Danesi R, Kohn EC, Dahut WL, Kummar S, et al. Hypertension and hand-foot skin reactions related to VEGFR2 genotype and improved clinical outcome following bevacizumab and sorafenib. J Exp Clin Cancer Res CR. 2010;29:95.
123. Kucharz J, Dumnicka P, Kuzniewski M, Kusnierz-Cabala B, Herman RM, Krzemieniecki K. Co-occurring adverse events enable early prediction of progression-free survival in metastatic renal cell carcinoma patients treated with sunitinib: a hypothesis-generating study. Tumori. 2015;101(5):555–9.
124. Nagyivanyi K, Budai B, Biro K, Gyergyay F, Noszek L, Kuronya Z, et al. Synergistic survival: a new phenomenon connected to adverse events of first-line sunitinib treatment in advanced renal cell carcinoma. Clin Genitourin Cancer. 2016;14(4):314–22.
125. Nakano K, Komatsu K, Kubo T, Natsui S, Nukui A, Kurokawa S, et al. Hand-foot skin reaction is associated with the clinical outcome in patients with metastatic renal cell carcinoma treated with sorafenib. Jpn J Clin Oncol. 2013;43(10):1023–9.
126. Otsuka T, Eguchi Y, Kawazoe S, Yanagita K, Ario K, Kitahara K, et al. Skin toxicities and survival in advanced hepatocellular carcinoma patients treated with sorafenib. Hepatol Res Off J Jpn Soc Hepatol. 2012;42(9):879–86.
127. Poprach A, Pavlik T, Melichar B, Puzanov I, Dusek L, Bortlicek Z, et al. Skin toxicity and efficacy of sunitinib and sorafenib in metastatic renal cell carcinoma: a national registry-based study. Ann Oncol Off J Eur Soc Med Oncol. 2012;23(12):3137–43.
128. Cohen PR, Bedikian AY, Kim KB. Appearance of New Vemurafenib-associated Melanocytic Nevi on Normal-appearing Skin: Case Series and a Review of Changing or New Pigmented Lesions in Patients with Metastatic Malignant Melanoma After Initiating Treatment with Vemurafenib. J Clin Aesthet Dermatol. 2013;6(5):27–37.
129. Hauschild A, Grob JJ, Demidov LV, Jouary T, Gutzmer R, Millward M, et al. Dabrafenib in BRAF-mutated metastatic melanoma: a multicentre, open-label, phase 3 randomised controlled trial. Lancet (London, England). 2012;380(9839):358–65.
130. Chapman PB, Hauschild A, Robert C, Haanen JB, Ascierto P, Larkin J, et al. Improved survival with vemurafenib in melanoma with BRAF V600E mutation. N Engl J Med. 2011;364(26):2507–16.
131. Ribas A, Kim KB, Schuchter LM, Gonzalez R, Pavlick AC, Weber JS, et al. BRIM-2: An open-label, multicenter phase II study of vemurafenib in previously treated patients with BRAF V600E mutation-positive metastatic melanoma. J Clin Oncol Off J Am Soc Clin Oncol. 2011;29. Abstract 8509.
132. Sinha R, Larkin J, Gore M, Fearfield L. Cutaneous toxicities associated with vemurafenib therapy in 107 patients with BRAF V600E mutation-positive metastatic melanoma, including recognition and management of rare presentations. Br J Dermatol. 2015;173(4):1024–31.

133. Ascierto PA, Minor D, Ribas A, Lebbe C, O'Hagan A, Arya N, et al. Phase II trial (BREAK-2) of the BRAF inhibitor dabrafenib (GSK2118436) in patients with metastatic melanoma. J Clin Oncol Off J Am Soc Clin Oncol. 2013;31(26):3205–11.

134. Anforth R, Fernandez-Penas P, Long GV. Cutaneous toxicities of RAF inhibitors. Lancet Oncol. 2013;14(1):e11–8.

135. Carlos G, Anforth R, Clements A, Menzies AM, Carlino MS, Chou S, et al. Cutaneous toxic effects of BRAF inhibitors alone and in combination with MEK inhibitors for metastatic melanoma. JAMA Dermatol. 2015;151(10):1103–9.

136. Chapman PB, Hauschild A, Robert C, Larkin J, Haanen JB, Ribas A, et al. Updated overall survival (OS) results for BRIM-3, a phase III randomized, open-label, multicenter trial comparing BRAF inhibitor vemurafenib (vem) with dacarbazine (DTIC) in previously untreated patients with BRAFV600E-mutated melanoma. J Clin Oncol Off J Am Soc Clin Oncol. 2012;30(15 suppl):8502.

137. Zimmer L, Haydu LE, Menzies AM, Scolyer RA, Kefford RF, Thompson JF, et al. Incidence of new primary melanomas after diagnosis of stage III and IV melanoma. J Clin Oncol Off J Am Soc Clin Oncol. 2014;32(8):816–23.

138. Dummer R, Rinderknecht J, Goldinger SM. Ultraviolet A and photosensitivity during vemurafenib therapy. N Engl J Med. 2012;366(5):480–1.

139. Sammut SJ, Tomson N, Corrie P. Pyogenic granuloma as a cutaneous adverse effect of vemurafenib. N Engl J Med. 2014;371(13):1265–7.

140. Boussemart L, Boivin C, Claveau J, Tao YG, Tomasic G, Routier E, et al. Vemurafenib and radiosensitization. JAMA Dermatol. 2013;149(7):855–7.

141. Boussemart L, Routier E, Mateus C, Opletalova K, Sebille G, Kamsu-Kom N, et al. Prospective study of cutaneous side-effects associated with the BRAF inhibitor vemurafenib: a study of 42 patients. Ann Oncol Off J Eur Soc Med Oncol. 2013;24(6):1691–7.

142. Bellon T, Lerma V, Gonzalez-Valle O, Gonzalez Herrada C, de Abajo FJ. Vemurafenib-induced toxic epidermal necrolysis: possible cross-reactivity with other sulfonamide compounds. Br J Dermatol. 2016;174(3):621–4.

143. Jeudy G, Dalac-Rat S, Bonniaud B, Hervieu A, Petrella T, Collet E, et al. Successful switch to dabrafenib after vemurafenib-induced toxic epidermal necrolysis. Br J Dermatol. 2015;172(5):1454–5.

144. Sinha R, Lecamwasam K, Purshouse K, Reed J, Middleton MR, Fearfield L. Toxic epidermal necrolysis in a patient receiving vemurafenib for treatment of metastatic malignant melanoma. Br J Dermatol. 2014;170(4):997–9.

145. Anforth R, Menzies A, Byth K, Carlos G, Chou S, Sharma R, et al. Factors influencing the development of cutaneous squamous cell carcinoma in patients on BRAF inhibitor therapy. J Am Acad Dermatol. 2015;72(5):809–15.e1.

146. Zelboraf (vemurafenib) prescribing information. www.accessdata.fda.gov/drugsatfda_docs/label/2011/202429s000lbl.pdf.

147. Piraccini BM, Patrizi A, Fanti PA, Starace M, Bruni F, Melotti B, et al. RASopathic alopecia: hair changes associated with vemurafenib therapy. J Am Acad Dermatol. 2015;72(4):738–41.

148. Dika E, Patrizi A, Ribero S, Fanti PA, Starace M, Melotti B, et al. Hair and nail adverse events during treatment with targeted therapies for metastatic melanoma. Eur J Dermatol EJD. 2016;26(3):232–9.

149. Kim KB, Kefford R, Pavlick AC, Infante JR, Ribas A, Sosman JA, et al. Phase II study of the MEK1/MEK2 inhibitor Trametinib in patients with metastatic BRAF-mutant cutaneous melanoma previously treated with or without a BRAF inhibitor. J Clin Oncol Off J Am Soc Clin Oncol. 2013;31(4):482–9.

150. Wada N, Uchi H, Furue M. Case of deep vein thrombosis in a patient with advanced malignant melanoma treated with dabrafenib and trametinib. J Dermatol. 2018.

151. Prescribing information for Cotellic (cobimetinib). http://www.accessdata.fda.gov/drugsat-fda_docs/label/2015/206192s000lbl.pdf.
152. Carlos G, Anforth R, Chou S, Clements A, Fernandez-Penas P. A case of bullous pemphigoid in a patient with metastatic melanoma treated with pembrolizumab. Melanoma Res. 2015;25(3):265–8.
153. Naidoo J, Page DB, Li BT, Connell LC, Schindler K, Lacouture ME, et al. Toxicities of the anti-PD-1 and anti-PD-L1 immune checkpoint antibodies. Ann Oncol Off J Eur Soc Med Oncol. 2015;26(12):2375–91.
154. Joseph RW, Cappel M, Goedjen B, Gordon M, Kirsch B, Gilstrap C, et al. Lichenoid dermatitis in three patients with metastatic melanoma treated with anti-PD-1 therapy. Cancer Immunol Res. 2015;3(1):18–22.
155. Postow MA. Managing immune checkpoint-blocking antibody side effects. Am Soc Clin Oncol Educ Book Am Soc Clin Oncol Meet. 2015:76–83.
156. Pintova S, Sidhu H, Friedlander PA, Holcombe RF. Sweet's syndrome in a patient with metastatic melanoma after ipilimumab therapy. Melanoma Res. 2013;23(6):498–501.
157. Robert C, Schachter J, Long GV, Arance A, Grob JJ, Mortier L, et al. Pembrolizumab versus Ipilimumab in Advanced Melanoma. N Engl J Med. 2015;372(26):2521–32.
158. Weber JS, Hodi FS, Wolchok JD, Topalian SL, Schadendorf D, Larkin J, et al. Safety Profile of Nivolumab Monotherapy: A Pooled Analysis of Patients With Advanced Melanoma. J Clin Oncol Off J Am Soc Clin Oncol. 2017;35(7):785–92.
159. Topalian SL, Sznol M, McDermott DF, Kluger HM, Carvajal RD, Sharfman WH, et al. Survival, durable tumor remission, and long-term safety in patients with advanced melanoma receiving nivolumab. J Clin Oncol Off J Am Soc Clin Oncol. 2014;32(10):1020–30.
160. Zarbo A, Belum VR, Sibaud V, Oudard S, Postow MA, Hsieh JJ, et al. Immune-related alopecia (areata and universalis) in cancer patients receiving immune checkpoint inhibitors. Br J Dermatol. 2017;176(6):1649–52.

Correction to: Cosmetics and Lasers

Caitlin Farmer, Matteo Lopiccolo and Alison T. Boucher

Correction to:
Chapter "Cosmetics and Lasers" in:
H. W. Lim et al. (eds.), *Practical Guide to Dermatology*,
https://doi.org/10.1007/978-3-030-18015-7_5

The original version of this chapter was inadvertently published with incorrect authorship in the opening page of Chapter "Cosmetics and Lasers". The first author's name has been changed to "Caitlin Farmer". The erratum chapter has been updated with the change.

The updated version of this chapter can be found at
https://doi.org/10.1007/978-3-030-18015-7_5

© Springer Nature Switzerland AG 2020
H. W. Lim et al. (eds.), *Practical Guide to Dermatology*,
https://doi.org/10.1007/978-3-030-18015-7_15

Index